HISTORY OF MEDICINE IN INDIA

HISTORY OF MEDICINE IN INDIA

The Medical Encounter

Editors
Chittabrata Palit
Achintya Kumar Dutta

Publications

KALPAZ PUBLICATIONS
DELHI - 110052

History of Medicine in India: The Medical Encounter

Rs. 750

ISBN: 81-7835-323-7

Published in **2016** in India by
Kalpaz Publications,
C-30, Satyawati Nagar,
Delhi-110 052
Email: kalpaz@hotmail.com

Laser Type Setting by: Tact Computer Graphics, Delhi
Printed at: Salasar Imaging System, Delhi

Contents

List of Contributors

1.	Chittabrata Palit	:	Professor of History, Jadavpur University, Kolkata
2.	Amiya Kumar Hati	:	Former Director, School of Tropical Medicine, Kolkata
3.	Dhrub Kumar Singh	:	Research Scholar, Centre for Historical Studies, School of Social Sciences, Jawaharlal Nehru University, New Delhi
4.	Amal Das	:	Professor of History, Kalyani University, Kalyani, West Bengal
5.	Simkie Sarkar	:	Research Scholar, Heras Institute, St. Xavier's College, University of Mumbai, Mumbai
6.	Arabinda Samanta	:	Reader in History, The University of Burdwan , Burdwan, West Bengal
7.	Syamal Roy	:	Department of Immunology, Indian Institute of Chemical Biology, Kolkata
8.	Kaushik Roy Choudhury	:	Senior Research Fellow, Indian Institute of Chemical Biology, Kolkata.
9.	Achintya Kumar Dutta	:	Reader in History, The University of Burdwan, Burdwan, West Bengal
10.	Anil Kumar	:	Reader in History, Satyawati College, University of Delhi, Delhi
11.	Deepak Kumar	:	Professor, History of Education, Zakir Husain Centre for Educational Studies, School of Social Sciences, Jawaharlal Nehru University, New Delhi
12.	Brahmananda Gupta	:	Former Professor of Sanskrit, Rabindra Bharati University, Kolkata

and Research Professor of History of Medicine, The Asiatic Society, Kolkata

13. Subrata Pahari : Lecturer in History, Mahishadal Girls' College, Mahishadal, Midnapore, West Bengal

14. Mousumi Bandyopadhyay : Senior Lecturer in History, Sivnath Sastri College, Kolkata

15. Aparajita Dhar : Lecturer in History, The University of Burdwan, Burdwan, West Bengal

16. Sujata Mukherjee : Reader in History, Rabindra Bharati University, Kolkata

17. Vijay Kumar Yadavendu : Post-Doctoral Fellow, Zakir Husain Centre for Educational Studies, School of Social Sciences, Jawaharlal Nehru University, New Delhi

18. Mridula Ramanna : Reader in History, South Indian Educational Society College, University of Mumbai, Mumbai

19. Kabita Ray : Reader in History, Sivnath Sastri College, Kolkata

Preface

This volume has grown out of a national seminar hosted by Corpus Research Institute in Jadavpur University Campus, Kolkata in 2002. There are altogether eighteen essays on various aspects of the history of medicine in India. This is a discipline which is universally acclaimed all over the world as vital for the health care of human civilisation. In India, it is yet to become an academic discipline in the universities. Only medical research institutes had such a wing from before. Fortunately, history of science and medicine is now entering the syllabus of postgraduate studies as a priority area of study as prescribed by the University Grants Commission. As it is a life and death question, the general reading public also have a lively interest in the subject. This book will cater to both levels of readership. It is divided into five sections. The first section deals with epidemics, both policy and practice. At least five epidemics are discussed in detail in this section. The second section deals with western medicine, its emergence and intervention in a traditional society. The third section highlights indigenous medicine which was on the crossroads of revival and survival. This is followed by a crucial section on gender and health especially dealing with the advent of gynaecology and approach to delivery deaths. The last section is on social work which focusses attention on social construction of health and social work in this field, much against the western notion of the lack of public initiative in India. This book is destined to be the first major Indian reply to medical orientalism dominating the area.

Chittabrata Palit

Achintya Kumar Dutta

1

Introduction

—Chittabrata Palit and
Achintya Kumar Dutta

Diseases and medicine have not only gripped the attention of doctors and medical scientists but of social scientists and social workers as well. They have become the subjects of historical scholarship in the east and west in recent past. The history of medicine in British India is gradually emerging as one of the major areas of 'new social history'. A number of scholars, both in India and western countries, have been engaged in research on various aspects of medicine in colonial India for the last couple of decades, and some of them have produced books and articles of very high quality, which throw light on the socio-political significance of the developing concept of public health in British India. The aspects studied in the scholastic discourses are varied — relation between medical knowledge and colonial power, encounter between western medicine and indigenous society, the efficacy and impact of the former on epidemic diseases, mortality, developing concept of sanitation, hygiene and public health, and above all socio-economic and political perspectives of disease and medicine. The study of major pestilence in the past has been enriched by the advances in the field of medicine and disease. It has been recognized that several areas of historical enquiry—from the history of population to the history of material and mental culture—have a common bond in the subject of health and disease. The social history of disease and medicine thus gradually came up as one of the key areas of medical history, which has been treated as a window to see through the nature of development or underdevelopment of a given society at a specified time.[1]

Almost all these aspects have been covered to varying degrees in the essays collected in this volume. But the authors here have studied them with a new thrust and innovative conclusions. The essays contain new approaches and throw some light on the topics hitherto neglected, such as *kala-azar* epidemics, medical works of the scientists other than British, indigenous as well as western approach to delivery deaths, and role of voluntary associations in tackling public health problems. Taken together, these essays point out the adequacy and inadequacy of health measures, nature of British medical intervention and its impact on society. A number of contributors attempt to explore the changing perception of diseases. Others demonstrate the nature of 'colonial' medicine and imperialism in the context of health care facilities and make a critique of health policy in colonial India.

This volume is not a comprehensive account of disease, medicine and empire. The introductory essay is simply a humble attempt to focus on a few major public health issues and problems that come within the purview of these scholastic observations and their significance in the light of historiography of medicine and public health in British India. However, this book covers considerable territory in this emerging area of history of medicine and may be useful to supplement the historiography of medicine in general and colonial India in particular.

I. Tropical or Global

British India had experienced the scourges of epidemic diseases, such as malaria, small-pox, cholera, plague etc. In the imperial literature and also in the history by some western scholars, these lethal diseases have been attributed exclusively to the tropics. Even they have been consigned as Indian epidemics, thriving on her enervating climate, untidiness and obscurantism. But these constructs are empirically untenable. Most of these diseases were of global occurrence and have been worldwide in their distribution. As Thomas McKeown explained it, all these diseases prevailed all over the globe down to the end of the 19th century. Plague plagued Europe since the time of the fall of the Roman Empire. It was common in Elizabethan England and found place in such expression like 'Plague on both the Houses'. Malaria which in Italian means foul air was rampant in Greece, Italy, Spain, and Latin America. Similarly, cholera and small-pox had their regime over United States and the continent. Influenza was endemic in the cold countries. Diseases like syphilis and leprosy are found in many parts of the western countries. Syphilis is of western origin.

It has been pointed out in the *The Wellcome Trust Illustrated History of Tropical Diseases* that it is really difficult to define exactly what is meant by 'tropical disease'.[2] Many of the aforesaid diseases once widespread have been pushed back to the warmer and poorer parts of the world by the success of hygiene and preventive measures in the more developed parts of the world. Is the term indicative of otherisation or inferiorisation? Was it a western way of defining something culturally and politically alien, as well as environmentally distinctive, from Europe and other parts of the temparate zone?

The tropical climate was almost universally considered to be the prime cause of European ill health. India was conceived as a land of dirt, disease, and sudden death. Though not perhaps quite a 'White Man's Grave' like the coast of West Africa, India was regarded as a place where the Englishman was not likely to enjoy a healthy life.[3] Philip Curtin in his work *Death by Migration* describes India as a home of all dreadful diseases and epidemics where the ruling class migrated only to face death.[4] He demonstrates that mortality rates for Europeans were far higher in India than in Britain. This binary contrast between the west and east has also been highlighted before him by Daniel Headrick,[5] and in the writings of colonial medical officers and imperial politicians. The east was dark, while the west was 'enlightened', 'modern', and 'civilized'. Imperialism to them was not only the conquest of territory and people but also a civilizing mission. Conquest of diseases in Asia and Africa was a part of this civilizing process. Indians were held as backward, superstitious, and conservative. The British rule in India meant transformation of Indian society from traditions to moderity.[6] This medical encounter between the east and west was a binary process between diseases and their cure.

However, Curtin also shows that mortality reduces from around the mid-19th century, following improvements in hygiene and medicine. Thus western medicine was projected as a hallmark of the racial pride that underpinned 'new imperialism'. Scholars, however, raised questions on this point. Mark Harrison points out that his study confirms Headrick's point about the vital importance of medicine in maintaining imperial rule.[7] David Arnold is of the opinion that Headrick probably exaggerates the effectiveness of medical intervention. He states that the use of quinine as a prophylactic was by no means as common as in the second half of the 19th century as Hendrick's account would seem to imply.[8]

From the times of the ancient Greeks onwards, health was perceived to be linked widely to an array of topographical and environmental factors—soil, humidity, heat, swamps, etc. This environmental theory of disease presumably based on 'miasma' marked out India as an exotic, and dangerous space. The British blamed India's disease-ridden character on climate, inertia, and superstition. But their homeland was not free from diseases. To be sure, England too, in the 18th century, and into the early industrial era, was a land of cities laden with filth, poverty among the working classes, lives cut short by diseases for which medical science had no cure. Britain was even subject to periodic epidemic devastation of cholera and small-pox.

Until the germ theory of disease was recognised towards the end of the 19th century, the health officials of India generally believed in the miasma theory of diseases.[9] That is disease is caused by some poisonous chemical brought by certain weather conditions. In the light of the germ theory of disease, this hypothesis proved to be incorrect. It was thus recognised that the real cause of the disease was a specific living microorganism. The germs were everywhere, and consequently, the disease. Europe had also experienced diseases like cholera, malaria, small-pox and plague. But disease became a part of a wider condemnation of African and Asian backwardness. British citizens who travelled to India carried incipient germs in them and these flared up in the inter-communicating zone when they met the 'native' population. They thus became the vectors of diseases. The Europeans thus brought venereal diseases, such as syphilis which was noticed as early as the 16th century by Bhava Misra, a noted Vaidya in Benaras, who called it *firangi roga* (disease of the Europeans).[10] The white soldiers were potent disseminators of this disease about which Ballhatehat in his *Race, Sex and Class under the Raj* has so vividly written. David Arnold has rightly remarked that European medical attitudes often remained subjective.[11] Though a number of pestilence had occurred in pre-colonial India,[12] epidemics became frequent with the coming of colonialism.

Epidemics spread in India due to commercial and military penetration and creation of colonial infrastructures—roads, railways, system of labour migration and so on. The unhygienic coolie lines where the labourers were forced to stay by the British capitalists in the plantations, mines, and factories facilitated spread of the epidemic diseases. It is an undesirable fact that the nature of colonial economy and the ecological changes brought about under colonialism had far-reaching consequences on public health. The expansion of irrigation canals and the construction of railway embankments created favourable habitats for malaria-carrying mosquitoes in India. These factors have been mentioned by David Arnold, Ira Klein, and also by many Indian scholars. It is thus clear that colonization was responsible to a great extent for frequent outbreak of epidemics.

II. Western Medicine and Indigenous Medicine

The coming of the British with their science and culture was an epoch-making event in modern Indian history. It introduced the fast developing modern medical system of the west. The result was the encounter between western medicine and indigenous medicine—a cultural encounter between Indian's traditional society and the west. Relationship between western and Indian systems of medicine has been an important issue in medical history. Mark Harrison in 'Medicine and Orientalism: Perspectives on Europe's Encounter with Indian Medical Systems' has described it vividly.[13] He demonstrates both collaboration and contradiction in it as it passed through several stages from 17th century onwards. Though not speaking of hegemonization, he mentions that the European's attitude towards Indian systems of medicine underwent a change after 1820. European medical men borrowed extensively from indigenous medicine. They made extensive use of indigenous medical knowledge, using local medicinal plants and consulting Indian medical texts and practitioners of Indian systems of medicine. But the dominance of western medicine was enshrined in the institutions of colonial state with the abolition of Native Medical Institution in 1835, established to teach both western and indigenous medicine in vernacular language. After 1820, European medical practitioners came to believe that recent advances in medicine had created a gulf between western and Indian systems of medicine. Growing confidence in the achievement of western science and medicine was challenging Orientalism, and European practitioners started to belittle their indigenous counterparts.[14] Thus with the consolidation of British rule and achievements in medicine at home, Europeans' difference from Indians was emphasized, western medicine got official patronage, and Indian medicine was marginalized. Medical paternalism came to an end. The former was marked as 'scientific', based on reason and observation, and superior to Indian systems which followed tradition and intermingled with superstition.

The works of Charles Leslie and David Arnold, provide valuable insights into the whole gamut of relationship between modern and traditional medicine. David Arnold in his *Colonizing the Body* also mentions that the interaction between 'colonial' medicine and indigenous medical systems was limited by a strong sense of superiority of western medical ideas. Indigenous medical system was not incorporated into colonial medicine. Thus there was a process of subordination and marginalization by which western medicine marked its conquest over indigenous medicine. Western medicine assumed a position of clear authority over Indian medicine and Indian bodies. Its attitude was monopolistic not pluralistic.

There seems to be no doubt about the assertion of western historians that western medicine achieved its uniqueness and superior efficacy by the advancement of knowledge in anatomy, physiology, and chemistry. It must be conceded that 'colonial medicine' was a great improvement upon pre-colonial medicine. It became popular in the colonies also. But to belittle Indian medicine as inferior and backward seems to be unhistorical and untenable. The efficacy of Indian drugs could not be denied. Indian method of variolation against small-pox was described by J. Z. Holwell in 1767 as 'rational' and 'well founded', although 'quasi-religious.[15] Even despite the advancement, western medicine had certain limitations. It failed to conquer some of the lethal diseases. For instance, there was lack of knowledge about the causality, transmission, and treatment of *kala-azar* for quite a long time and innumerable victims lost their lives in the 19th and 20th centuries. Western medicine could not save them. Even new breakthroughs in bacteriology and parasitology were not found before the last quarter of the 19th century. There were several areas in which the western and indigenous systems could have collaborated but did not. Revival of Indian medical systems and synthesis between the western and indigenous medicine were preferable to the majority of Indians. But the official policy was to exclude indigenous practitioners entirely from the government ambit.[16] Europe took a radical step away from medical pluralism in India.[17] Medical pluralism might have been more effective in a plural society like India. The concept of superiority of western medicine possessed European doctors' work encompassing not only the understanding and possible conquest of new diseases in the colony, but also an extension of western cultural values to the non-western world.[18] They did not prefer assimilation or synthesis. Absolute supremacy of the one and total subjugation of the other characterized Victorian imperialism for which the colonial medical men worked.[19] This is what has been mentioned by some historians of India as complete hegemonization.[20] Indigenous medicine was ultimately pushed back to the periphery. It felt marginalized and subjugated. The process of hegemonization was perpetuated through the network of medical institutions and hospitals and the Indian Medical Service. Three distinct services, namely covenanted, uncovenanted, and subordinate medical services came to constitute the British medical organization. They are said to have been used for promoting and popularizing western medicine. There was a systematic propaganda against traditional medicine and therefore official patronage was withdrawn from it.

III. Epidemic and Health Policy

Another important issue that comes within the purview of this discourse is the British medical policy and public health service in colonial India. The critics argue that British medical policy in India was impregnated with British self-interest and not guided by the spirit of altruism. Medical historians of the west like David Arnold are of the opinion that it was not only meant for the benefit of the colonial rulers, it also spread beyond that. This is an undeniable fact. But there is much truth in the claim of the critics that the British medical policy originated from and remained subservient to the needs and expediencies of the empire. The rulers primarily concentrated on how to provide the best hygienic, sanitary, and medical facilities to the military and civil population of their own race.[21] It was not devised as a part of welfare policy. The health policy was primarily aimed at catering to the needs of civilians and soldiers.[22] It was mainly extended to urban areas to safeguard the Europeans in the mines, plantation, factories, and administrative centres. Western medicine remained too closely identified with the requirements of the colonial state and so was remote from the needs of the people. It failed to make the transition from state medicine to public health.[23] Despite the much condemned disease-ridden tropics, the British led a healthier and richer life with increased vitality and life expectancy even when compared to the European standards.[24] India was not the 'White-man's grave'; rather she became the graveyard of Indians under British rule. Thus colonial medicine appeared to be 'uncanny imperialism par excellence'.[25] The majority of the Europeans in India had managed to escape the lethal diseases. The civic amenities were confined to business centres and administrative enclaves. With excellent sanitary measures in and around the cantonments and civil lines, they warded off cholera to a great extent, and with the help of quinine, they managed malaria quite well.[26] The real victims were the indigenous people who fell in droves at the outbreak of every epidemic. The rural areas having the bulk of the population were to a large extent neglected and left to their fate.

British medical intervention to tackle the outbreaks of epidemic diseases is considered as one of the significant aspects of western medicine in India. That these diseases were a cause of concern for the colonial rulers is an undeniable fact. But the question has been raised whether this concern was for the Indian people as a whole or for the army, European civilians, plantations, trade, and industry. It is evident from the historical fact that the government started taking measures against these diseases when they posed serious threat to plantations, trade, and industry. For instance, the government immediately organized anti-*kala-azar* measures when *kala-azar* rapidly progressed in the 1880s towards the prosperous upper Assam valley, the main centre of tea industry. The government was least concerned about the impact of the malaria epidemic on the native civil population. It was only when the epidemic fever threatened the health of the military personnel that the government intervened and took some ameliorating steps.[27] The colonial administrators increasingly realized that if the surrounding areas of military barracks, civil lines and even the secluded abodes of Europeans remained diseased and uncared for, it would be difficult to fully protect themselves.[28] Bengal's Sanitary Commissioner observed in 1865, 'even if we look no further than the protection of the health of the European soldiers, it will be evidently insufficient if we endeavour to improve the condition of our cantonments alone, and ignore the existence of the masses of the native population by which our troops are surrounded'.[29] Thus military needs largely dictated British concern for native health.

However, the government adopted certain medical measures, both preventive and curative, when epidemics broke out. It is true that these anti-epidemic measures had a bearing upon the incidence of the diseases and mortality due to them. But the question does arise as to the inadequacy and efficacy of these measures as well as public health service in colonial India. Most of the research work on history of public health in India refers to the fact that the governmental measures to combat epidemic diseases were not adequate. Anti-malaria measures in Bengal were found to be unsatisfactory.[30] C. E. Bentley in *Malaria and Agriculture in Bengal* (1925) reported that only a very small proportion of malaria-affected people of Bengal received treatment sufficient to afford them relief. The vast majority of the sufferers from malaria received either no medical attention whatsoever or entirely depended on the treatment of village practitioners.[31] Even the government could not check the marketing of spurious quinine. Since the European population was concentrated in the town of Calcutta, attempts were made to insulate the British population in the town from the ravages of epidemic malaria.[32] There were very few qualified doctors to run dispensaries. The native doctors under a Sub-Assistant Surgeon looked after them.[33] V. R. Muraleedharan in his study on Madras has also referred to the lukewarm response of the government against malaria. He points out that malaria was more severe in the countryside where little anti-malaria operations were taken up compared to urban areas.[34] What had actually followed was an increasing reliance on palliative measures.

Similarly, the methods adopted by the government to tackle the *kala-azar* epidemic in Bengal too were limited. The number of centres for *kala-azar* treatment were very small compared to the population.[35] Many places affected with small-pox were left unprotected. Segregation on sanitary principles in case of cholera proved to be inadequate. The

British officials in India were frenzied over the plague epidemic. The government was guided primarily by the British business lobby in Bombay to protect their commercial interest, mainly cotton trade. Under the Epidemic Diseases Act (1897), draconian measures of quarantine were undertaken. On mere suspension of infection, people were forcibly removed to hospitals. There was ruthless segregation of the mind from the body in the treatment of plague cases. Their houses were dug up and insecticides sprayed into them. The anti-plague measures were so stringent and coercive that they resembled more military than medical and were directed more against the natives than the plague bacillus.[36]

Anil Kumar in his *Medicine and the Raj* has given an objective and rational interpretation about the weakness of anti-plague measures of the government in India. He has rightly asserted that plague revealed western medicine's crisis of confidence. It had no answer to its causation, cure, and prevention. The government failed to understand as to how to deal with the plague epidemic effectively without jeopardizing British commercial interests and eventually relied on administrative rather than medical policy. The British bureaucracy and the army took over the reins of medical works.[37] The tensions of the empire dictated the British colonialists to unleash a reign of terror, most inhuman and callous. which resulted in chaos and conflict. People's opposition to government measures and anti-plague riots broke out in Bombay. Some western historians are of the opinion that though there was severity in the government measures, its intention was not foul. I.J. Catanach points out the role of the political leaders in fanning people's hysteria making it a political issue.[38] This seems to be an attempt to undermine the problem involved. These upheavals were reactions to the severity of strict controls and police regulations imposed by apparently insensitive and uncaring authorities.[39] A sober opinion, however, comes from Arnold who tries to explain the conflict as a mass opposition to the government's interventionist policy without rapport from the people.[40] It underscores the embedded ruthlessness and selfishness of colonial rule which could not be alleviated even by a benign health policy during plague epidemic. The anti-plague measures proved to be counterproductive and demonstrated an utter failure of British medical policy.

In view of government's plague policy, Mark Harrison argues that the government had a well-intentioned and sincere commitment to the welfare of the people which is evident from incurring huge public expenditure by the government since 1896 on medical administration and medical research. The appointment of the Plague Commission by the government and the initiative to implement its recommendations by setting up laboratories for further research on this disease provided sound 'foundation for the growth of medical science in India'. He does not agree with Radhika Ramasubban's argument that the British Indian government only did some 'piecemeal' and 'adhoc' development of medical research and refutes her claim that government chose to 'escape into medical research' as a means of avoiding any further commitment to public health reform.[41] Moreover, he emphasizes the fact that there were many well-meaning doctors and administrators who differed with the official policies and served the cause of the people in their individual capacities.[42] Anil Kumar criticizes Harrison's argument on the ground that the laboratories set up by the government in this context were mainly erected 'as little factories for the production of vaccine and sera'. These were not meant for research on disease. The scientific community of India looked to the metropolis where works on the tropical diseases had been undertaken in right earnest. Therefore, he argues that Harrison's claim that anti-plague drives facilitated medical research work greatly in India does not seem to carry much weight. Secondly, despite the differences in opinions, those doctors and administrators could hardly ever influence the health policies. Policy-making was a one-way affair.[43] There is much truth in Harrison's assertion that the laboratories established in early 20th century contributed to the promotion of scientific researches and activities in India to some extent. But the ruthlessness of the plague policy had actually overshadowed the benefits of government investment in medical laboratories.

The critics claim that British India's health care system was not so effective to control epidemic diseases and removing health hazards of the people. The discriminating attitude of the government to the native people in connection with medical relief has also been condemned. The government's lukewarm attitude to safeguarding the lives of rural people may be illustrated by the following incident.

Baboo Dinanath Bandopadhyay and other inhabitants of Gorulgacha, a village in Serampur subdivision of Hooghly district, submitted a petition in 1877 to Sri Ashley Eden, then Lt. Governor of Bengal, praying for the opening of a charitable dispensary in their village. Mr. Haggard, Subdivisional Officer of Serampur, responded to their petition in the following words:

> If you are willing to guarantee a monthly subscription of Rs. 40 I can hold out to you hopes of a dispensary being established but not otherwise. You will have to provide a suitable house for the purposes of a dispensary and proper furniture, Almerah and Cabinet for the safe custody of the medicines. A legal guarantee will also have to be drawn up in order to secure the payment of all subscription.[44]

The British Indian government has been criticized for its poor infrastructure for rural health care. Though the government set up hospitals, dispensaries, and research institutes to tackle the health problems, existing public health organization was not satisfactory. A proper executive health service of all ranks was not devised for rural India. The British who formed health boards and built up sewage, piped water, and medical facilities in England during the 19th century to control epidemic diseases, did not take similar steps in India.[45] Measures for sanitary improvement were very limited. Bulk of the revenue was derived from land but nothing in the way of sanitary attention was done, and the machinery was not well devised for striking swiftly and surely at epidemics.[46] The rural areas are said to have received little benefits of western medicine. Mark Harrison also points out that the low priority given to the health of India's rural population was undeniable.[47] Government's policy to save rural people of India particularly during malaria epidemics had been vehemently criticized by the press. *The Patriot* pointed out that 'many millions had been spent to make barracks healthy for a few thousand soldiers' while 'a thousandth part of that sum would not have been required for the restoration of the salubrity of the fever-stricken villages'.[48]

Sanitary management was the primary and essential step for combating infective diseases. Ronald Ross advocated it for combating malaria, but he was very much disappointed with the government's attitude to control it.[49] Improved sanitation was suggested as remedy for *kala-azar* by Leonard Rogers. Improvement in sanitation in rural areas and liberal use of lime wash might possibly have been effective in making condition unfavourable for sandfly, the *kala-azar* vector. But the question of village sanitation remained almost unheeded in Assam, the hotbed of *kala-azar*. In fact, improvement in this field was very meagre. Government funds for sanitation were inadequate. On the contrary, Indians were blamed for their apathy and resistance sanitary programmes and other health measures. The conservative and superstitious beliefs of indigenous people might possibly have stood in the way of sanitary reforms to some extent. But this cannot be a defensive argument for inadequate sanitary improvement. The government also failed to overcome these constraints. Considering the situation in the 19th century, sanitation should have been forced upon the people of India, as was done by the home government in the mother country.[50] In fact, the shoestring budget for public health of the colonial government did not cater the medical facilities to the 'native' population. The Commissioner of Nadia pleaded in 1863 for necessary sanitary measures to check the ravages of malaria in

Bengal. But the government's response was tardy. It sanctioned very small amount for it.[51] The financial grant for anti-*kala-azar* work in Bengal was 'very adequate'.[52] The facilities for examination and treatment of *kala-azar* cases were inadequate or non-existent in the rural areas in Bengal. Mridula Ramanna also mentions that a constraint on sanitary progress in Bombay in the 19th century was governmental reluctance to make financial commitments.[53] The sanitary measures of public health, including the drainage of subsoil, the destruction of mosquitoes, and mass quinization as advocated by Ronald Ross for eradication of malaria in Bengal, were rejected by the colonial government for the enormous expenditure involved, though it would have been a fragment of the drain of wealth from India. These sanitary measures were the determinants of public health in the developed countries and helped eradicate malaria from many countries in the world. But they were not properly taken up at the place where knowledge about the life cycle of malaria parasite was discovered.

In fact, the main criticism of the policy is that public health service in colonial India was run on a very small budget and mainly catered to the needs of the Europeans. Only the metropolitan cities and the district headquarters were covered by this policy. The rural areas were served by ramshackle sub-divisional dispensaries manned by compounders having an inadequate supply of vital medicines. There was no dearth of people's cooperation in the field of public health. People's voluntary work was not lacking in the domain of public health in Bengal and other provinces.[54] In Assam the people cooperated with the health officials in maintaining regulations under the Epidemic Diseases Act for checking the progress of *kala-azar*.[55] The villagers reported *kala-azar* and requested for medical assistance and attended anti-*kala-azar* campaign conducted by the Health Department. But the health policy of the government had a very limited coverage. For instance, there was one doctor for 42,000 population in rural Bengal in the 1920s, while there was hardly one doctor per 6,300 population in India compared to 1 per 1000 population in United Kingdom in the 1940s.[56] The number of public health officials were small and they were not ready to leave the comfort of their District Headquarters and sallied forth with their black bags and hypodermics into remote villages.[57] Roger Jeffery is of the opinion that despite so many attributes of imperial health policy in India, the impact of many measures was restricted to a small sector of the population, first, to the European civil and military servants and their families, later to Indians with access to urban facilities. Therefore, even if 19th century medical services had been beneficial, the mass of the Indian population could not have benefited. Preventive campaigns were never fully pushed through; vaccinations and plague control, demonstrated the failure of British health policy to come to terms with local society.[58]

It is claimed by most recent studies on public health in India that the health progress was slow during British rule. Radhika Ramasubban has pointed out that the health policy in British India was a 'colonial mode of health care' characterized by segregation and neglect of the indigenous population.[59] Ramasubban holds that only metropolitans missed the benefits of sanitary reforms which swept through most of Europe in the 19th and early 20th century. Roger Jeffery, however, dismisses this view. He argues that the army and European civil population did not need so many hospitals and dispensaries. Secondly, European sanitary reforms were largely urban; many rural areas in Europe were without centralized water-supply or drainage or refuse disposal for many years. Jeffery points out that the poverty of the Indian population was the most important problem in connection with public health. Though it seems to be partly true, there is no gainsaying the fact that health care services for the Indians and sanitary improvement works for rural areas received low priority. That government's commitment to the health of the Indian people was weak had been illustrated on many occasions, even in periods of epidemics. The government's reluctance to promote drainage in fever-stricken areas of Bengal is one such glaring example.[60]

A proper Public Health Ministry came to function only after 1920 with the passing of the Local Self-Government Act. The responsibility to tackle the epidemics and funding of rural health was now put on the shoulder of the District Boards and Union Boards. But they failed to cope with the situation because of scanty reasons and scarcity of health personnel. The district dispensaries set up in rural areas were ill-equipped to tackle the health problems. Many municipalities and local boards were unable to raise sufficient revenue for vital sanitary reforms. More government aid and better supervision on the local bodies were necessary. David Arnold also implies the need for greater government participation in public health, and is critical of the transfer of sanitation to financially ill-equipped and inexperienced municipalities.[61] A more concerted effort by government to assist the local bodies would undoubtedly have done much to improve the situation.[62] Although mortality due to epidemic diseases was reduced in the 20th century by the remedial measures, there was no remarkable progress in their prevention and eradication programme. What was followed in regard to anti-epidemic policy and public health development were small-scale measures. Truly speaking, compared to the progress registered in public health in western countries, India was lagging behind in public health services abysmally. During the five pre-war years 1934–39, the condition of public health in India was highly shameful. Death rate for general population in 1941 was 21.8 per thousand and child mortality was 138 per thousand births.[63] Hundred million people suffered from malaria, of which 20 lakh died every year. Even in 1947, after independence of the country, it was estimated that about 75 million people suffered from malaria every year.[64] Moreover, five lakh people died of tuberculosis, while 2.5 million suffered from this disease annually.[65] In 1944, in North Bihar alone, two lakh people died of cholera and malaria.[66] *Kala-azar* was still widely prevalent in north-eastern India.[67] Malaria, cholera, and tuberculosis were the three most dreadful diseases causing havoc among the rural population of India and the government had not taken adequate steps to eradicate them. Of 47,400 doctors available in India, in 1944, only 13,000 were reported to be on the staff of medical institutions maintained by government and other agencies.[68] The remaining were in private practice concentrated mostly in urban areas. Hence, the rural population were the worst sufferers. Consequently, the people had to depend on the *Kavirajs* and *Hakims* who were easily available in the interior to provide treatment in their own ways. But it should not be explained as native opposition to western medicine. It is true that there were contradictions in Indians' attitude and responses to western medicine. But at the same time, it is also true that they were not culturally opposed to it. That western medicine was gaining popularity among Indian people is indicated by the increasing number of patients attending hospitals and dispensaries. In the case of malaria epidemic in Bengal, it was found that rural people walked many miles to stand in the queues for a phial of quinine.[69] In different instances, *kala-azar* patients in Assam arrived at the hospital unexpectedly for treatment on their own initiative, at their own expenses after selling up their property to provide themselves with funds.[70] What was required was a more concerted effort by the government with the positive intention of providing health care facilities for the native people in the formulation of public health policy.

It thus appears from what has already been said that health policy of the British Indian government had certain weaknesses and rural people of India became prey to them. The health policy was indeed a one way game. There was little scope of being involved with the indigenous people in its making. Even the officers of the IMS, who made valuable contributions to the development of medical science in India, could hardly influence British health policy. The development of health standard and diffusion of health care services meant little, for almost everyone in

India did not receive any priority in the health policy. In view of deteriorating condition of public health in India, R.P. Dutt had rightly pointed out in 1940 that provision for the most elementary needs of public health, hygiene, and sanitation was very low in respect of the working masses in the towns or in the villages. This point has also been referred to in other works.[71] Even many of the western historians have been critical of the weak commitment of the government to the health of the Indian people.

What seems to be interesting to note in this context is that the British Indian Government also realized the weaknesses of the health care service and gave due attention to it towards the end of the Second World War, though a belated one. Among the social services, Lord Wavell placed communications, public health, and education in order of priority. Consequently, the Government of British India appointed Health Survey and Development Committee with Sir Joseph Bhore as its chairman in 1943 for reviewing existing health conditions and health organizations in British India and making recommendations thereon for the future development of health services. The appointment of the committee is an important phenomenon in the history of public health in India. For it is on the recommendations of this committee that modern health care system of India was build up. But the survey report of the Committee gives a gloomy picture of public health in India[72] and thus confirms the defects and weaknesses of public health policy of the government. The members of this committee inspected hospitals, medical colleges, public health organizations, and a number of rural areas. They point out the following lacunae in the health administration and other related matters. (1) The relations of the central government to the provinces in the field of health were not clearly defined and in the matters of epidemics, nutrition, medical educational standard, research etc. the influence of the centre seemed weak. (2) The central government had not availed expert medical and scientific advice in a measure proportionate to the urgent health needs. (3) Financially the government was not ready to do things on a generous scale for health. (4) Overall health situation was weaker in India than even in the Philippines and Panama. (5) Preventable diseases had in a varying degree been prevented by that time in other parts of the world. But in India many of those diseases were still prevalent. The then expenditure per head on medical relief and public health for India was between 3 and 4 annas per annum. Of this only one-third goes to preventive medicine. It was very small compared to the UK, where Rs. 54/- per head per year was spent on medical relief alone. The failure to develop the public health services and to staff and finance them adequately was therefore a very obvious criticism. (6) The ravages of the infectious diseases and malnutrition were so widespread that the relief provided by hospitals, dispensaries, and individual doctors could only make a very small impression upon the general mass of disease and suffering. Dispensary provision was for the most part of the year low standard. The local authorities in Bengal failed to deal adequately with the outbreak of epidemics. Over and above, the Health Department was not well-organized.[73]

However, the recommendations of the Bhore Committee provided the framework for modern health care system. It is an undeniable fact that western medicine had efficacy to successfully combat the epidemics. Developing concept of public health and hygiene, medical institutions and hospitals, IMS and subordinate medical service and so on provided an organized medical system and an iron framework of public health administration in independent India. It gave certain benefits to Indian people. Compared to the development in western medicine, medical science in India did not advance much during the middle ages.[74] Indian medical system was rather disorganized and parochial. Medical researches based on the method of experiment and observation carried out by experts on different diseases also provided knowledge about preventive and curative aspect of medicine. Thus knowledge of theory and practice of medicine developed. Therefore, western medicine, though often condemned, was summoned up and welcomed by the Indians.

The high mortality caused by epidemic diseases became a matter of concern to the government and it provided the initiative for carrying out scientific investigations by the experts from IMS and AMD (Army Medical Department) to control them. Thus Cunningham, Lewis, Giles, Rogers, and Ross were assigned to work on cholera, malaria, beri-beri, and *kala-azar*. The government also sought the services of international experts in the bacteriology like Robert Koch and W.M. Haffkine. But it could not successfully challenge the lethal diseases. In many cases the colonial government was completely helpless. For instance, the government was incapable of adopting any curative measure for *kala-azar* cases when this disease broke out in the form of epidemic in late 19th century in Assam and continued to take a heavy toll on human lives well into the 20th century, for, there was no clinical medicine for its cure. The available indigenous or western drugs could not save the victims in Assam.[75] The role of modern medicine was still limited. But the government did not sit idle keeping its hands folded. The anti-*kala-azar* measures like segregation and evacuation as well as medical relief, though unsuccessful, continued. With the introduction and successful use of effective drugs in Assam from 1919 onwards, the public health measure constituted of rapid mass treatment of *kala-azar* cases for a couple of decades.[76] The sustained and extensive treatment had a great effect in saving lives.[77] By the mid 1920s, more than 400 hospitals and dispensaries with their out-centres were working in Assam for the treatment of this disease.[78] Thus the government showed a very positive gesture for the treatment of *kala-azar* cases and consequently the mortality reduced to a great extent. The co-operation of the local people and active participation of health officials in anti-*kala-azar* measures had undoubtedly subscribed to the success of medical measures here. The government appointed a special commission in 1924 to study this disease in Assam (known as *Kala-azar* Commission) with S.R. Christophers as its director. But here again government health policy failed to prevent and stamp out this disease.

In fact, the colonial administration did not pursue a coherent policy for the improvement of public health in India. Lack of political will and overpowering commercial interests prevented the rulers from organizing western medicine to effectively deal with the challenges of the epidemics. Nevertheless, western medicine evoked interest among the local populace.

IV. About the Book

In this collection of essays, the opening essay by Chittabrata Palit is a general critique of public health policy in colonial India. Medical Orientalism in under scrutiny and a contrast has been made between western and eastern medicine and approaches to public health. This sets the tune for the section on epidemics. This is followed by a general survey of all the epidemics causing holocaust in public health in colonial India by Amiya Hati.

Then comes case-studies of a few epidemics which swept over India in the colonial period. Dhrub Kumar Singh writes a penetrating essay on the changing perceptions of cholera. Amal Das probes Calcutta plague with enphasis on colonial intervention into indigenous society. Simkie Sarkar takes up leprosy in 19th century Bombay with reference to policy and people. Arabinda Samanta brings out the demographic dimensions of malaria in rural Bengal which hit different sections of people differently. Kaushik Roy Chowdhury and Syamal Roy explore the causes of *kala-azar* epidemics in India while Achintya Kumar Dutta gives the enthralling account of Upendranath Brahmachai's pursuit of this dreaded disease and his discovery of urea stibamine.

In the section on western medicine, there are two fascinating articles, one by Anil Kumar on the contours of western medical institutions in India between 1822–1911 and the other by Deepak Kumar who delves into the details of the medical works of the eccentric Russian mistrusted medical scientist W.H. Haffkine. In the next section on indigenous medicine, Brahmananda Gupta traces the evolution of Ayurveda from pre-colonial times while Subrata Pahari traverses the chequered career of traditional medicine in colonial India.

The discourse on gender and health is opened by Mousumi Bandyopadhyay who evaluates indigenous approach to delivery deaths which assumed epidemic proportions in colonial Bengal while Aparajita Dhar makes a critique of western approach to the same subject. Sujata Mukherjee's essay softens this critique with reference to patronage and philanthropy of western medicine in British India.

The last section on social work begins with Vijay Kumar Yadavendu's insightful essay on changing paradigms of social construction of health which deals with responses of the receiving side of public health. The next essay is by Mridula Ramanna who sketches the remarkable career of a pioneer of public health in Ahmedabad and a doyen of self help in the setting of a denial policy. Last but not the least is the essay by Kabita Ray in the same vein. She highlights voluntary associations which arose in 20th century Bengal to grapple with public health problems where the government was found wanting.

References

1. Biswamoy Pati and Mark Harrison (eds.), *Health Medicine and Empire Perspectives on Colonial India*, OUP, New Delhi, 2001, p.1.
2. F. E. G. Cox, *The Wellcome Trust Illustrated History of Tropical Diseases*, The Wellcome Trust, London, 1996, Introduction.
3. Thomas R Metcalf, *Ideologies of the Raj*, Foundation Books, New Delhi, 1998(PB), p. 171.
4. Philip D. Curtin, *Death by Migration Europe's Encounter with the Tropical World in the 19th Century*, CUP, 1989.
5. Daniel Headrick, *The Tools of Empire: Technology and European Imperialism in the 19th Century*, Oxford, 1981.
6. Allen J. Greenberger, *The British Image of India: A Study in the Literature of Imperialism 1880-1960*, London, 1969, pp. 43-44.
7. Mark Harrison, *Public Health in British India: Anglo-Indian Preventive Medicine 1859-1914*, Foundation Books, New Delhi, 1994, p. 2 (hereafter *Public Health*); Biswamay Pati and Mark Harrison, *op. cit.*, p. 12.

8. David Arnold (ed.), *Imperial Medicine & Indigenous Societies*, Manchester University Press, New York, 1988, p. 10 (hereafter *Imperial Medicine*).
9. Ralph Shlomowitz and Lance Brennan, 'Mortality and Migrant Labour in Assam, 1865–1921', *Indian Economic and Social History Review*, 27, 1, Jan-March 1990, New Delhi, pp. 85-110.
10. Deepak Kumar (ed.), *Disease and Medicine*, Tulika, New Delhi, 2001, p. XVII.
11. David Arnold (ed.), *Imperial Medicine*, p.7.
12. Extract from *Record of Past Epidemics in India*, no date, passim.
13. Biswamay Pati and Mark Harrison, *op. cit.*, pp. 37-87.
14. *Ibid.*, pp. 62-65.
15. Deepak Kumar, *op. cit.*, p. XVII.
16. Roger Jeffery, *The Politics of Health in India*, London, 1988, p. 99.
17. David Arnold, *Imperial Medicine*, p. 12; for early British attitude to Indian Medical systems, see also David Arnold, *Science, Technology and Medicine in Colonial India*, CUP, 2000, pp. 66-67.
18. Deepak Kumar, *op. cit.*, p. XVIII.
19. Anil Kumar, *Medicine and the Raj British Medical Policy in India 1835–1911*, New Delhi, 1998, p. 10.
20. Deepak Kumar, *op. cit.*, Introduction.
21. Anil Kumar, *op. cit.*, pp. 88, 216.
22. Mridula Ramanna, *Western Medicine and Public Health in Colonial Bombay 1845–1895*, Orient Longman, New Delhi, 2002, p. 234.
23. David Arnold, *Colonizing the Body State Medicine and Epidemic Disease in Nineteenth Century India*, OUP, Delhi, 1993, p. 3 (hereafter *Colonizing the Body*).
24. Anil Kumar, *op. cit.*, p. 216.
25. *Ibid.*, p. 218.
26. *Ibid.*, p. 216.
27. Arabinda Samanta, *Malarial Fever in Colonial Bengal 1820–1939: Social History of an Epidemic*, Kolkata, 2002, p. 120.
28. Anil Kumar, *op. cit.*, p. 88; Arabinda Samanta, *op. cit.*, p. 149.
29. David Arnold, *Imperial Medicine*, p. 14.
30. C. E. Bentley, *Malaria and Agriculture in Bengal*, Calcutta, 1925, Ch. VI & VII; Kabita Ray, *History of Public Health Colonial Bengal 1921–1947*, Calcutta, 1998, pp. 109-129.
31. C. E. Bentley, *op. cit.*, p. 103.
32. Arabinda Samanta, *op. cit.*, p. 120.
33. *Ibid.*, p. 131.
34. V. R. Muraleedharan, 'Malady in Madras: The Colonial Government's Response to Malaria in the early Twentieth Century', in Deepak Kumar (ed.), *Science and Empire: Essays in Indian Context 1700–1947*, Delhi, 1999, p. 103.

35. Kabita Ray, *op. cit.*, pp. 71-72.
36. Anil Kumar, *op. cit.*, p. 197.
37. For details, see Anil Kumar, *op. cit.*, pp. 190-203.
38. I. J. Catanach, 'Plague and the Indian Village 1896–1914' in Peter Robb (ed.), *Rural India, Land, Power and Society under British Rule*, London 1983; 'Plague and Tensions of Empire 1896–1918' in R. McLeod and Milton Lewis (eds.), *Disease, Medicine and Empire: Perspectives of Western Medicine and the Experience of European Expansion*, London, 1988; 'Poona Politicians and the Plague' in J. Marselos (ed.), *Struggling and Ruling: The Indian National Congress 1885–1985*, New Delhi, 1987.
39. Terence Ranger and Paul Slack (eds.), *Epidemics and Ideas.: Essays on the Historical Perception of Pestilence*, CUP, 1992, p.12.
40. David Arnold, *Colonizing the Body*, Ch. 5.
41. For details see Mark Harrison, *Public Health*, pp. 152-157; Anil Kumar, *op. cit.*, p. 203.
42. Anil Kumar, *op. cit.*, p. 203.
43. *Ibid.*, pp. 203-204.
44. Dinonath Benerjea, *The Success of My Efforts From 1873 to 1877*, Victoria Press, Cuttack, 1877, pp. 8-9. The photocopy of this document was borrowed from Somnath Roy, Retd. Professor of History of the University of Burdwan, who visited Harvard University in 1996 and collected this document from Harvard University Library.
45. Ghanshyam Shah, *Public Health and Urban Development: The Plague in Surat*, Sage Publication, Delhi, 1997, p. 28.
46. Andrew Balfour and H. H. Scott, *Health Problem of the Empire Past, Present and Future*, London, 1924, p. 136.
47. Mark Harrison, *Public Health*, p. 190.
48. Cited in Mark Harrison, *Public Health*, p. 190.
49. Ronald Ross, *Memoirs*, p. 363 and *Studies on Malaria*, London, 1928, pp. 137-139.
50. Ghanshyam Shah, *op. cit.*, p. 28.
51. Arabinda Samanta, *op. cit.*, pp. 121-122.
52. Kabita Ray, *op. cit.*, p. 72.
53. Mridula Ramanna, *op. cit.*, p. 236.
54. For details, see Kabita Ray, *op. cit.*, Ch. III.
55. *Annual Sanitary Report, Assam for the year 1921*, p. 10.
56. Girindra Kumar Mitra, *Malaria O Kala-azar Pratikar Samasyar Parikalpana* (in Bengali), Calcutta, 1924, p. 6; Madhu Nagla, *Sociology of Medical Profession*, Gaipur, 1997, p. 60.
57. MSS/Eur C 188 (OIOC), British Library, The Memoirs of Sir Arthur Dash, Pt. 3: Diary (1927–1935), p. 4.
58. Roger Jeffery, *op. cit.*, p. 100.

59. Cited in Mark Harrison, *Public Health*, p. 227; Roger Jeffery, *op. cit.*, p. 100.
60. Mark Harrison, *Public Health*, p. 234.
61. Cited in Mark Harrison, *Public Health*, p. 233.
62. *Ibid*, p. 234.
63. S. B. Singh, *Second World War as Catalyst for Social Changes in India*, Delhi, 1998, p. 125.
64. P. K. Dutta, *A Study of NMEP: A System Approach*, New Delhi, 1993, p. 3.
65. S. B. Singh, *op. cit.*, pp. 125-126.
66. *Ibid.*
67. For details, see Achintya Kumar Dutta, 'The Profile of Kala-azar: A Historical Review', in Abhijit Dutta *et. al.,* (ed.), *Explorations in History*, Calcutta, 2003, pp. 149-171.
68. *Health Survey and Development Committee Report*, vol. I, p. 13 cited in S. B. Singh, *op. cit.*, Ch. 8.
69. J. M. G. Bell, ICS, Tour Diary 1941–47, Mss in the Centre of South Asian Studies, Cambridge; J. T. Donovan, ICS, Tour Diaries, 1927–31, Mss in *Ibid.*,
70. *Report of the Pasteur Institute, Shillong, Third Annual Report for the Year ending December, 1919*, p. 7.
71. Mark Harrison, *Public Health*, p. 233.
72. Wellcome Institute Archives, GC/186/6, Papers on Health Survey Committee, India by Dr. Janet Vaughan, Memorandum pt. I, pp. 4-18.
73. *Ibid.*
74. Satpal Sangwan, *Science, Technology and Colonisation: An Indian Experience 1757–1857*, Delhi, 1991, p. 4.
75. For details, see Achintya Kumar Dutta, 'The Pursuit of Kala-azar and Upendranath Brahmanchari', in *History*, 2000, vol. III, no. 1, The University of Burdwan, Burdwan, pp. 48-60.
76. *Annual Report of the Working of the Civil Hospitals and Dispensaries in the Provinces of Assam for the year 1938*, p. 3.
77. British Library, MSS / EUR C435, In the Days of the Raj, and after: Doctor, Soldier, Scientist, Sikari by Col. H E Shortt, IMS, p. 70; *Indian Medical Research Memoirs No. 25: Reports of the Kala-azar Commission, India Report No II* (1926–30), Calcutta, 1932, p. 48.
78. *Health Bulletin No. 9: Treatment Campaign Against Kala-azar, Assam* by D. Murrison, Calcutta 1927, p. 1.

Epidemics, Policy and Practice

2

Epidemics and Empire: A Critique of Public Health Policy in Colonial India

—Chittabrata Palit

Preamble

A study of the subject has become imperative in view of the growing neocolonial literature depicting India as a dark subcontinent as much as Africa has been branded as the white man's grave. Both are imagined as quagmires of lethal epidemics and decimating diseases. Some of the stereotypes used by British officials in a period of medical imperialism from around 1835 are being recycled from the past by western historians like David Arnold, Ira Klein, Charles Leslie, Paul Brass, Ian Catanach etc. Roy McLeod, Michael Worboys, Paul Greenough and J.C. Hume are some exceptions.

I. Tropical/Temperate

In African Studies today, the dichotomy between tropical and temperate diseases has come to be increasingly challenged. It has been argued that the colonial hangover to regard a group of lethal diseases as 'tropical' is distinctly racist. These diseases like plague, malaria, small-pox, cholera, influenza, and syphilis are still being held as native to the dark continent or subcontinent. They are assigned to either climatic or genetic causes. Even some typically temperate diseases like tuberculosis and AIDS are being dumped on these countries. It has been contested that some of the so-called tropical diseases have disappeared from the west in the 20th century entirely due to heavy investment in sanitary reform and nutrition. The binary contrast in diseases, in the final analysis, boils down to that between poverty and wealth. The latter can be traced to two hundred years of colonial rule in the third world which caused so much drain of wealth from the colonies to the metropolis (Feierman 1974, Mcleod 1988). It can be maintained that most of these diseases originated in Europe. Plague had been the most dreaded epidemic since the days of ancient Rome. St. Benedict died of it in mid-6th century. Britain was pulverized by plague in the 17th century. It did not abate until the 19th century in some form or other. It has been in Shakespeare as 'plague on both the houses' to describe Elizabethan parliament. It has found its way into the nursery rhyme, 'Ringa Ringa Roses' and as a regular verb of menace in English vocabulary. Malaria (mal=foul, aria=air in Italian) was also of European origin and was rampant in Latin countries from 17th to 19th centuries and beyond. Spain took it to her colonies in Latin America. England suffered from small-pox in the late 19th century and the disease was transmitted to settler colonies of Australia and New Zealand as well as the subject colonies of India. Cholera was chronic in France, England, and the USA from the mid-19th century. It was carried to the Philippines. Russia also had an epidemic of cholera. Syphilis, a dog-borne European disease was carried by seaman into Afro-Asia. (Ross 1910, Scott 1939, Snow 1936, Rosenberg 1962, Sullivan 1988, McLeod 1988, Hirst 1953, McNeil 1976). Of the two stories leading to the discovery of the medicinal bark of a wild tree in Peru, one is associated with the illness of the Duchess of Cinchon, wife of the Spanish Governor of Peru who got cured of her fever by taking a concoction of the herb, which came to be known as cinchona after her name. The other story is that the Spanish Jesuits brought it to Europe as a prophylactic to such remittent and intermittent fever (ague, yellow fever, dengue, and malaria) and an English apothecary made a trade of it in 17th century England. Oliver Cromwell would rather die of malaria than take the 'Popish' remedy. Scott lends credence to the first story. It is confirmed by E. Laurie. Italian scientists Grassi and Bignani in 1097 discovered the anopholes female mosquito as the vector of malaria and Italy had no tropical colonies as yet. Alphonse Laveran discovered the plasmodium that invades the bloodstream in 1880. Quinine was in use in French Algiers since 1835.

By then the germ theory of Louis Pasteur had overtaken 'miasma' as the root of these diseases. Yet the tropics were blamed for these epidemics. The heat of the tropical sun and humidity of swampy lands were still held responsible for the diseases. The mosquitoes, lice, rats were condemned as vectors but the root of the virus was not traced. But similar climate prevailed in Latin countries of Europe and parts of USA and England. There was no swampy land nor even a blade of grass in Kalat, Waziristan, the frontier of modern Pakistan, yet blackwater fever was rampant there in the early 20th century. As to lice, rats, and cockroaches, the P & O lines carried loads of them along with passengers from Europe to Asia and Australia. Yet when plague came to Bombay in 1896, only Hong Kong connection was blamed. But there was plague epidemic in Karachi and Punjab, Calcutta, and Rangoon in the 1910–20 period. It was a shippy disease and one has to turn to Europe for its source. Britannia ruled the epidemics as well. The hosts of the diseases were ignored, only vectors and the tropics were condemned. It is true that the tropical climate was too hostile to whitemen and flared up the germs in their bodies and overpowered their natural resistance in the inter-communicating zone while the local population remained for a while immune in the initial period. But the lethal contact caused a holocaust among the original people of Africa, Asia, Australia, Latin and North America who were left out of the pale of the so-called conquest of epidemics. It was of the whites, by the whites and for the whites. The rhetoric of conquest of disease is a concomitant of territorial expansion. In fact, the first conquered and consolidated more terriotories than gunboats, breechloaders, and canonnades. It was medical imperialism par excellence. The Indian Medical Service was a wing of the British Indian Army and catered only to cantonments and actual fields of action. Gradually, it extended to urban areas—civil lines of white population and vested white interests in mines, plantations, and factories. The rural areas having the bulk of the native population were left to their fate and demonology. The sanitary measures of public health as advocated by Ronald Ross for eradication of malaria in Bengal alone was ridiculed by the official circle as chimerical for the enormous expenditure involved. Ross meekly wanted to apply it only to white installations and living quarters. Even that was turned down though it would be a fragment of the drain of wealth from India. As McKeown shows, those very measures were the long-term determinants of public health in the developed countries, including USA. It also helped eradicate malaria and yellow fever in Panama, Cuba, Suez, Malaysia, and West Africa.

Even if one admits that upto the middle of the 19th century, many such epidemics were global in nature, both tropical and temperate, it is this colossal investment in public health in both sanitary reform and research for prophylactics which made the world of difference between the so-called tropical and temperate zones, an investment generated by colonial extraction but denied to the colonies. They got the disease but not the remedy. It was indeed a case of colonizing the body. Cholera is a case in point. Cholera was rampant in France, England, Russia, and USA in the second half of the 19th century, and not just in India on the banks of Ganga. Whereas sanitary reform, especially, water treatment for this water-borne disease eradicated it in the west, nothing similar was carried out in India. Only Punjab derived some such measure after considerable foot-dragging by the bureaucracy. (Scott 1939, Laurie 1938, Headrick 1981, Ross 1910, Megroz 1931, Arthur Dash Memoirs 1910–1947, Curtin 1964 & 1989, McKeown 1976, Worboys 1988, Snow 1936, Rosenberg 1962, Sullivan 1988, Hume 1984).

II. Military/Civil

It has already been stated in the preceding section that western medicine entered India as military medicine. It was to cater to the cantonments and forward lines to win battles of expansion. The main enemies were not the native princes alone but the diseases and epidemics which decimated the British Army. The Indian Medical Service, a wing of the British Army set up in the early 19th century fought this part of the more lethal battle and it can be said that medical imperialism actually consolidated the empire. The IMS fought blackwater fever in Waziristan. It prevented plague in the port cities of Bombay, Karachi, Calcutta, and Rangoon and kept the flow of trade and commerce unabated. In the plains, it grappled with malaria, cholera, small-pox. None of them were tropical diseases per se. Most of them were European in origin and some global in character given the state of public health management in the mid-19th century. They had nothing to do with tropical miasma. Yet western histories are replete with stories of victory over tropical diseases and triumph of empiricism. They project the tropics as the contemptible other, chockful of malignant diseases. The so-called victory was not the victory over the disease as a whole as should have been the criterion of medical science. The whites contaminated the native population with their lethal contact and left them economically impoverished in the grip of malnutrition and epidemics without extending equal treatment to the occupied.

The victory was in a narrow sense over the inherited diseases of the whites in a hostile climate. The dark continent and the subcontinent remained the white man's grave for a long time till they became the graveyard of the native population. This was achieved through a dual policy of drain of wealth and health of the subject-nations. The dialogue between epidemics and empire has been hopelessly one-sided. It has been only the success story of the hegemonist. Though Headrick calls western medicine one of the tools of empire, he does not bring out the full implication of medical imperialism. He is also taken up with the success of metropolitan medicine and has no space for its fall out on the periphery. Yet Mcleod in his superb introduction to *Disease, Medicine and Empire* queries this smugness. In a stunning book, Kenneth

Ballhatchet exposes this hypocrisy. In dealing with a delicate subject like the immoral traffic between the army and the prostitutes, he narrates how lustful white soldiers had to be provided with prostitutes in the red bazaars around the cantonments and the Veneral Diseases (VDs) were blamed on the loose women alone. Contagious Diseases and Cantonments Acts were passed in the 1860s to register prostitutes, carry out their health inspection, and put them in lock hospitals forcibly for treatment to safeguard army. The vector of VD had to be the hapless professional without a thought that the white soldier could also be its carrier, as he was of syphilis, a European disease. Yet within the purview of army requirement, the lock hospitals provided the minimal treatment to the abused women. Even this was gradually withdrawn after 1872 raising the incidence of the VD phenomenally again. Lal bazaars apart, the orderly bazaars skirting the barracks as in Barrackpore were vulnerable to European contact and contagion without any scope of treatment.

The civil native population were left out of the scope of public health service. A section of the IMS personnel was periodically transferred to man the civil hospitals in the presidency towns and district headquarters. They mostly attended white population in urban areas and the precincts of plantations, mines, and factories. The military duty of the IMS was of such priority that even within the white cadre, there was strong grievance against it. Ronald Ross in the middle of intense research on mosquitoes and malaria at Hyderabad, was subjected to hectic transfer to N.W. Frontier, Rajputana, Burma, Madras, and Calcutta affecting his work. It also affected other members like Laurie who was engaged in his research in *kala-azar* and black water fever in Waziristan but transferred to Calcutta. The masses of the civil population who lived in the rural areas remained virtually beyond the purview of western medicine. (Ross 1910, Headrick 1981, Ballhatchet 1980, Scott 1939, Laurie 1938).

III. Urban/Rural

The urban set-up of the IMS for the civil population was itself peripheral to the military establishments. A few metropolitan hospitals in the district headquarters were meant for the urban elites and there too, the white ruling class was privileged. Besides, the civil surgeon (white) and the Indian sub-assistant surgeons in the district headquarters who did a lot of private practice were mostly unavailable for rural masses. The government virtually disowned them. There was no public health department nor any budgetary provision for sanitary reforms even in periods of malaria and cholera epidemics. Only in the 1920s, when the Local Self-Government Act was passed and District Boards and Union

Boards took over the responsibility and bulk funding of rural health, the district dispensaries in rural areas were set up. But they were ramshackle huts with few medicines and barefoot doctors trained in the medical schools. More often the local vaids and hakims were pressed into service.

The indigenous systems of medicine were discouraged and discontinued, which were both cheap and readily available at the doorstep without allopathic replacements. The vaids and hakims were castigated as quacks depending on folklore and no exact science though they were the ultimate resort of the villagers. The epidemics of malaria, cholera, small-pox, and plague were brought to the countryside by government policy of immigration, railway transportation, and embankments. White-owned plantations, mines and factories herded colonies of coolies (labour) in the cooly lines of dingy barracks spreading the contagion. Many of the diseases were spread from the ship to the field in this way (Ramasubban). In the district gazetteers and settlement reports, it is clearly pointed out that some of the districts like Jessore, Hooghly, and Bankura in Bengal which were known as healthy were becoming death traps over the 19th century.

The rural masses did resort to their gods and goddesses like Sitala and Olabibi for moral and mental reinforcement against the mighty epidemics but they were not culturally averse to allopathic medicine and treatment. From the district magistrates' tour diaries, it is evident that villagers travelled many miles and stood patiently in queue for a phial quinine or inoculation. But these were in chronic short supply. The government clearly had no infrastructure for rural healthcare. While epidemics were transported to the interior, there was no remedy. Traditional medicine had been languishing without patronage and its practitioners had not been incorporated in the health care programme. The villagers were allegedly religious obscurantists and this cultural opposition stood in the way of the introduction of western medicine. Rumour-mongering against official doctors and medicine by villagers made it difficult for the government to penetrate villages. This official escapism has been harped on by Ian Catanach, Arnold, and Klein. The truth of the matter has been spelt out by Frantz Fanon and Steven Feierman in the African context. It was the question of trust between the occupier and the occupied which had been destroyed by centuries of exploitation and foul play. Going to see a doctor was thought as hazardous as going to the police. (Tour diaries of Bell 1941–1947, Donovan 1927–1931, Bengal civilians, R. Nicholas 1981, D. Arnold 1988 & 1990, Ira Klein 1986 & 1988, I.J. Catanach 1983, Frantz Fanon 1978, Steven Feierman 1974).

IV. Segregation/Community Healing

Segregation was the watchword of imperial medicine. It was primarily a racist outlook which treated the indegenous population with contempt for having filthy and unhygienic habits and being vectors of all kinds of infectious diseases. Cantonments and civil lines inhabited by the whites were generally separated from the native dwellings. The duality of white towns having civic amenities and black towns having none of it was typical of British India. Yet most of the epidemics spread from the ports and cities inhabited by white sailors, soldiers, merchants vegabonds. It has been shown in a previous section that the white town still needed their lal bazaars and orderly bazaars for service, sexual and manual. In the event of diseases following such intercourse, the indigenous people were blamed and segregated. Lock hospitals were not only for the prostitutes but all city hospitals became virtually lock hospitals during epidemics like the plague which gripped Bombay from 1896 and Calcutta in 1912.

As plague threatened not only civilian and military life but also international trade in cotton, oilseeds, and grain due to panic among the European governments, the British officials in India were frenzied over the epidemic. There was blatant and brutal intrusion into the private houses of the native population on mere suspicion of disease. Their hearths and homes were virtually demolished, floors dug up and insecticides sprayed, walls cracked up and limewashed and any inmate suspected of the disease was pulled up and carried in vans to the infectious diseases hospitals for quarantine. They were cut off from their relatives and many died on their way to the hospital. Their dead bodies were not even handed over to the relatives for cremation. It was nothing but ruthless segregation without treatment. It was clear that the authorities only wanted to safeguard themselves and did not care to save the lives of the unfortunate victims. There was no compassion, care or empathy essential for healing.

This was a culture shock of a different kind borne out of enormous credibility gap and not religious and cultural obscurantism. Traditional medicine and medical care depended on community healing and family care. The patient was treated in body and mind in his personalized circumstances. The spread of rumour against government intentions was not due to any fundamental cultural opposition. It was due to lack of credibility and treatment backed by brutal intervention and segregation. The Plague Commissioner Rand was murdered in Bombay because of his excesses. Benign intervention and segregation in cases of infectious disease would not be challenged. It was the dehumanized treatment of the patient which was resented by the local people. Hence the rumour of waterpoisoning and outright poisoning of the patient during the plague epidemic in Bombay. Panic and rumour were not necessarily rustic propensities. The authorities also suffered from the same and took drastic action. In Bengal the rural people came from a long distance for cholera vaccination when mutual trust was built up between the government and the governed. (Arnold 1993, Klein 1988, Catanach 1988, Chandavarkar 1992, Nicholas 1981, Donovan and Dash memories 1931, 1947, Frantz Fanon 1978, Feierman 1974).

Apart from racism, western medicine by itself was concerned with the etiology of the disease limited to the vital parts repaired. The whole concept is based on segregation of the patient from the community and body from the mind. The total perception of the patient as a human being, a member of a family and community and having an interactive mind is missing in it. But these considerations are important in effecting a cure. It is being increasingly recognized in the west that almost all diseases are psychosomatic, needing community or at least family care. (John Ehrenreich 1978, Dubos 1968, Selye 1976, J. Cell 1986).

V. Traditional/Western Medicine

Before the medical intervention of the British, both Ayurvedic and Unani systems of medicine were prevalent in India. Though traditional medicine was not so much institutionalized, it was fairly professionalized and there existed schools of *vaids* and *hakims* founded by stalwarts like Gangadhara Roy in Bengal and Hakim Ajmal Khan in Delhi during the mid-19th century and later. The standard Arabic and Sanskrit texts were read and acted upon in these schools and the British authorities encouraged them in government institutions like the Benares Sanskrit College, Calcutta Sanskrit College, and Native Medical Institution in Calcutta till 1835. But then there was the end of paternalism and government patronage was diverted to western medicine and medical colleges set up in metropolitan cities. With the consolidation of British rule and achievements of western medicine at home, traditional medicine was dismissed as folklore and western medicine was the only stream taught at the Medical College and practised in government hospitals and dispensaries. Meanwhile, traditional medical texts were translated and ransacked and the pharmacopoeia was appropriated in the British pharmacopoeia and many traditional herbal medicines were converted into western drugs by chemical analysis and standardization. The indigenous *vaids* and *hakims* were still recruited as barefoot doctors to man medical care in the countryside after some training in medicine.

Traditional medicine was undoubtedly effective for elemental chronic diseases born out of imbalance of wind, biles and cough, and even in many other viral diseases of the tropics which were much less in appearance than the later epidemics imported from the west. It was not given a fair trial by suitable encouragement and allowed to exist by sufferance in the rural areas where western medicine never reached. The treatment was personalized and cheap and there was a good rapport between the vaid and the patient. Later the Indian practitioners founded their own institutions and formulated an integrated course having the best of both traditions. Drugs were also produced accordingly. Still there was no official recognition and all public health expenditure was lavished on western medicine alone. Against this derecognition there was considerable politicization of the issue and regional and national ayurvedic congresses were formed to press its case on merit. But the withering touch of colonial rule did not allow it to grow even in the vast rural sector which was denied medical care altogether. The solution lay not in the absorption of traditional into the hegemonic regime of western medicine to be euphemistically called 'cosmopolitan' medicine, but the development of an alternative medical system standardized by the logistics of western laboratorics as it is being done in free India today. Obviously, microbial diseases, especially those coming from the west could not be tackled by traditional medicine but still it had efficacy in many other diseases for which there was no western remedy. (Leslie 1976, Brass 1974, Bala 1991, Palit 1996).

VI. Eastern Sounding Board for Western Medicine

It has already been observed that the empire was half won in medical laboratories and empirical work in the empire itself. It was a life and death question for the imperial army against the invisible enemies, the microbes in full play under the tropical sun. The tropics have been variously described as the white man's grave or the process of east-west encounter as migration to death. If diseases and epidemics could be surmounted, the army would be in full strength and military battles could be won. It was medicine for empire or medical imperialism at large. Medical research was directed to the conquest of 'tropical' diseases among the army (mainly white) and next the white ruling class. Thus, Ronald Ross was engaged in research in mosquito-borne malaria at Hyderabad and Robert Koch in tuberculosis and cholera at Calcutta. Macnamara and Rogers followed up research in cholera at Calcutta, Haffkine worked on plague at Bombay and Laurie on *kala-azar* in Waziristan. Take the example of Ronald Ross. Ross, an IMS officer began his research at Hyderabad and ended it at Calcutta at the end of the 19th century. He went on mosquito-keeping, feeding them on malarious patients and healthy poor people who volunteered to be the guinea-pigs on pittance alternately. When he was transferred to Calcutta he found it difficult to get such volunteers. So he carried on the experiment with cageful of parrots until he located the bacteria in the vector mosquito (female anopheles variety). The theory that was propounded by Manson, Laveran, Grassi, and Ross himself was thus experimentally proved and he received the Nobel Prize for this discovery. Its therapy was already known in Europe and its other colonies in Africa, Asia, and Latin America. It was the graduated dose of quinine, an extract of cinchona naturally grown in Latin America and successfully transplanted in Indonesia and India by the Dutch and the British authorities. It was finally synthetically produced from the same alkaloids during the Second World War. Ross's discovery led to the other measure: sanitary reform on war-footing by clearing of jungles and swampy areas and killing of mosquitoes by sprays of insecticide and petrol in ponds, canals, and embankments forming pools of rainwater. The Liverpool School of Tropical Medicine that he founded and directed, carried out commissioned medical expeditions to Malaysia, West and South Africa, Suez, Panama, and Cuba where scheduled sanitary reform was undertaken at a huge expense, more than compensated for by gain in life in the plantations. The entire west benefited from Ross's research, most of all, Britain but when he suggested that such reforms be carried out in at least Bengal, the authorities ignored it on grounds of expense. Even his suggestion for urban areas, plantations, and mines was turned down despite so much drain of wealth and health from India as a whole and Bengal in particular. Only the quinine industry thrived, first the natural produce and then the synthetic product while malaria raged in village India. (Megroz 1931, McKeown 1976, Worboyc 1988).

VII. Public Health/Private Practice

We have already seen that colonial experience was put to good use in other parts of the empire of Britain and other western countries. Britain was cured of most of the fatal diseases due to heavy government investment in public health programmes of sanitation and nutrition. But when it came to implementing it in India, the government dragged its feet on grounds of expense. Sanitary reform was relegated to a secondary position and germ theory and prophylactics made overriding considerations in official policies aided and abetted by the London School of Tropical Medicine headed by Manson. Hume shows convincingly in the case of Punjab how a successful plan of public health with the help of a brigade of *vaids* and *hakims* achieved wonders and the effort to prevent water pollution, in the wake of similar reform in London after its connection with cholera epidemic was convincingly proved by John Snow, saved the region from cholera epidemics. But this was gradually obfuscated and abandoned in favour of the doctor and his clinic. In Bombay, it was the same before the plague epidemic. There was a dualistic development of the city having concrete jungles skirted by slums. The civic amenities were confined to the business district and the administrative enclaves. Public health was not the concern of the government. It was left to the private practice of the government. It was left to the private practice of the fee-fleecing doctors and cartels of chemists and drugguists. If this was not satellization, what else was? Yet Ira Klein argues to the contrary. She blames the rising commercial middle class for the haphazard growth of the city and makes public health a private responsibility of the citizens. The government only leapt into brutal intervention during the plague epidemic when it affected international grade in cotton and grain. Private practice only fattened the purse of the European doctors and Indian practitioners of western medicine in urban areas. Privatization of public health in a poor country of rural masses was denial of equal treatment. McKeown has demonstrated from vital statistics in Britain, that nutrition and hygiene more than therapy and prophylactics, had been responsible for the decline of mortality there. Yet this essential aspect of public health was never given a fair trial in India. Instead, traditional medicine was dismissed as folklore and indigeneous *vaids* and *hakims* ridiculed as quacks, thus sapping the only possible alternative medical care by sheer neglect. A proper Public Health Ministry came to function only after 1920 with the passing of Local Self-Government Act when people in the interior had to pay various cesses for their health care and after 1937, the portfolio passed into Indian hands. (Hume 1984, Snow 1936, Klein 1987 & 1988, Palit 1996).

VIII. Western Drugs: Eastern Medicine

The cheap, locally procurable indigenous medicine was already languishing due to lack of patronage. It was being increasingly replaced by western drugs from the 1880s when they could be mass-produced and tableted at a cheap rate. The vast area of medically unprotected hinterland was left to the imperial drug industry to flood with pills, capsules and syrups. It was a bonanza for the private practitioners and chemists of western medicine. It was medical imperialism of another kind. In the monopoly market, many experimental drugs were pushed to test their prophylactic power at the cost of humanity. Such a human laboratory was nowhere to be obtained. The refined drugs were retained by the west and the rejected ones known for their toxicity and other side-effects were dumped by multinational companies till independence. It continues even now through neocolonial devices of patenting and monopoly. (Bala 1991, Samaddar 1987).

References

1. David Arnold, *Colonizing the Body: State Medicine and Epidemic*, Berkeley, 1993; (ed.), *Imperial Medicine and Indigenous Societies*, Manchester, 1988.
2. Ira Klein, 'Death in India', *Journal of Asian Studies*, 32.4 (1973); 'Malaria and Mortality in Bengal', *Indian Economic and Social History Review* 9.2 (1972); 'Urban Development and Death: Bombay City, 1870–1914', *Modern Asian Studies* 20(4) 1986; 'Plague, Policy and Popular Unrest in British India', *Modern Asian Studies* 22(4) 1988.
3. Charles Leslie (ed.), *Asian Medical Systems: A Comparative Study*, Berkeley & Los Angeles, 1976. Articles by A.R. Beals, B. Gupta and himself.
4. Paul Brass on Ayurvedic Education and Politics in L. &. S. Rudolph (eds.), *Education and Politics in India*, Chicago, 1974.
5. I.J. Catanach, 'Plague and the Indian Village, 1896–1914' in P. Robb (ed.), *Rural India: Land, Power and Society under British Rule,* London, 1983, 'Plague and Tensions of Empire, 1896–1918' in D. Arnold (ed.), *Imperial Medicine and Indigenous Societies*; 'Poona Politicians and the Plague' in J. Massalos (ed.), *Struggling and Ruling: The Indian National Congress 1885–1985*, New Delhi, 1987.
6. Roy McLeod & Milton Lewis (eds.), *Disease, Medicine and Empire: Perspectives on Western Medicines and the Experience of European Expansion*, London and New York, 1988.
7. M. Worboys, 'Manson, Ross and Colonial Medical Policy: Tropical Medicine in London and Liverpool, 1899–1914' In *Ibid.*
8. P.R. Greenough, 'Violation and Vaccination in South Asia, c 1700–1865', *Social Science and Medicine* 14: 345-47.
9. J. C. Hume, 'Colonialism and Sanitary Medicine: The Development of Preventive Health Policy in the Punjab, 1860-1900', *Modern Asian Studies* 20(4) 1984.
10. S. Feierman, 'The Struggle for Control: The Social Roots of Health and Healing in Modern Africa', *African Studies Review* 28 (2/3), 1974.
11. Ronald Ross, *Memoires*, London, 1910.
12. R. L. Megroz, *Ronald Ross: Discoverer and Creator*, London, 1931.
13. H.H. Scott, *A History of Tropical Medicine,* 2 vols, London, 1939.
14. John Snow, *Snow on Cholera*, Reprint, New York, 1936.
15. C.E. Rosenberg, *The Cholera Years: The United States in 1832, 1849 and 1866*, Chicago, 1962.
16. R.E. McCrew, 'Russia and the Cholera, 1823–32' in Roy Mcleod, *op. cit.*

17. R. Sullivan, 'Cholera and Colonialism in the Philippines, 1899–1903' in Roy Mcleod, *op. cit.*
18. L. F. Hirst, *The Conquest of Plague: A Study of the Evolution of Epidemiology*, Oxford, 1953.
19. R. Pollitzer, *Plague*, Geneva, 1954.
20. W. H. McNeill, *Plagues and Peoples*, Garden City, New York, 1976.
21. D. H. Headrick, *The Tools of Empire: Technology and European Imperialism in the Nineteenth Century*. New York 1981, ch. 8.
22. W. Laurie, *Blackwater Fever in Waziristan*, 2 vols., 1938 (Mss. in the Centre of South Asian Studies, Cambridge, U.K.).
23. A.J. Dash, ICS, *A Bengal Diary*, vols. 1–9, 1910–47, cf: chapters 2, 4, 6, 1947.
24. Philip Curtin, *The Image of Africa: British Ideas and Actions 1780–1850*, 2 vols., Madison, 1964, Part III; *Death by Migration: Europe's Encounter with the Tropical World in the 19th Century*, Cambridge, 1989.
25. Thomas McKeown, *The Modern Rise of Population*, London, 1976.
26. K.A. Ballhatchet, *Race, Sex and Class under the Raj*, New York, 1980.
27. Radhika Ramasubban, 'Imperial Health in British India' in McLeod (ed.) *Imperial Medicine*.
28. J.M.G. Bell, ICS, *Tour Diary, 1941–47* (Mss in the Centre of South Asian Studies, Cambridge).
29. J.T. Donovan, ICS, *Tour Diaries 1927–31* (Mss in the Centre of South Asia Studies, Cambridge).
30. R. Nicholas, 'The Goddess Sitala and Epidemic Small Pox in Bengal', *Journal of Asian Studies* 61(1) Nov., 1981.
31. Frantz Fanon, 'Medicine and Colonialism' in J. Ehrenreich (ed.), *Cultural Crisis in Modern Medicine*, New York 1978.
32. R. Chandavarkar, 'Plague Panic and Epidemic Politics in India 1896–1914' in T. Ranger & P. Slack (eds.), *Epidemics and Ideas: Essays on the Historical Perception of Pestilence*, Cambridge, 1992.
33. Rene Dubos, *Man, Medicine and Environment*, New York, 1968.
34. Hans Selye, *The Stress of Life*; New York 1976, revised edition.
35. J.W. Cell, 'Anglo-Indian Medical Theory and the Origins of Segregation in west Africa', *America Historical Review* 91(2) 1986.
36. Poonam Bala, *Imperialism and Medicine in Bengal*, New Delhi, 1991.
37. C. Palit, 'From the Raj to the Panchayati Raj: Local Self-Government in Bengal 1920–55' in C. Palit (ed.), *Political Economy and Protest in Colonial India,* Calcutta, 1997. 'Ayurveda in Colonial Bengal' in the *Souvenir of the International Seminar on Traditional Medicine* sponsored by the Indian Pharmacological Society, Calcutta, 1993.
38. R. Samaddar, 'Health Administration in India since 1947—A Critique', *Socialise Perspective*, vol. 13, November, 1987.

3

Epidemics, Empire and Public Health

—Amiya Kumar Hati

An empire is a larger group of states ruled over by a single monarch or ruling authority. The English word empire comes from a Latin word imperium.

An epidemic (Greek epidemia) means a wide occurrence of an infectious disease in a community at a particular time. This paper will essentially deal with the British empire in India and epidemic that did occur under its grip, extending about 200 years.

There is no denying the fact that British rule was a rule of oppression. The country suffered in every respect, such as economy, agriculture, science, culture, education, human rights, and last but not the least, health. The attitude of the number one empire of that period, where the sun did never set, was to grab the resources of this rich country by hook or by crook. They were merely foreign invaders. Though the rule was essentially the same, a change came when the handover from 'Company' to 'Crown' occurred in 1858. India was only one of the colonies of the British empire. Our destiny was not in our hands. How could a dependent nation progress? The literacy rate was very meagre. Health, specially public health was given the least priority. In such a situation, epidemics were bound to occur and there was no dearth of epidemics.

This account will not be merely a stale statement of epidemics, citing diseases and years. There are many other aspects related to epidemics, such as background, role and responsibilities of the ruling authority in aiding or abetting epidemics, condition of the people, their attitude, miseries and sufferings, venture of Indian scientists, etc. The epidemics had serious impact on economy, agriculture, science, culture, education, human rights, and the public health of this unfortunate country.

There was another noteworthy feature. Several discoveries in the field of medicine took place in this land, some of which were epoch-making. All these pictures taken together can really make a vibrant history of that age for which very little attempt was made by our own people.

Epidemics of malaria, *kala-azar*, plague, cholera, tuberculosis, amoebic dysentery, hook-worm, dengue, small-pox, and epidemic dropsy in British occupied India and their consequences will now be discussed.

Malaria

The word malaria comes from Italian *mala aria*, meaning bad air. It is a misnomer, as the disease does not spread through bad air. The protozoan parasite is transmitted through the bite of infected female anopheline mosquitoes. Nobody has however dared to change the name. Malaria, however, has many other synonyms such as tertian fever, Roman fever, marshy remittent fever, Bengal fever, Roman fever[1] *kampazar, palazar, pilezar*[2] etc.

Long ago in India, this disease was known as '*King of Diseases*'. In the Veda (1500–800 BC) and *Brahmana* (800–100 B.C.) malaria was described as 'death fever'. About 600 BC Charaka and Shushruta, the two renowned Ayurvedic physicians had described three types of malaria fever.[3] Even in the Veda, it has been told that mosquitoes can carry malaria and there are five types of such mosquitoes.[4]

British India was a depot of malaria, except Kashmir. Malaria reigned uninterruptedly in N. W. Frontiers, Delhi, Rajputana, U. P., Terrai area, C. P., Bombay, Goa, Hyderabad, Madras, South Bihar, Orissa, Bengal, Assam, Andaman and Nicobar islands. Only in the Punjab during 1890–1908, in several malaria epidemics 250,000–310,000 people died. In India, about 10 million people used to suffer from malaria annually with one million deaths.[5] Total loss of income due to malaria was estimated to be 400 million dollars per year.[6]

In the Indian subcontinent, out of 19,433 persons surveyed through blood examination, during 1900–1929, the percentage of *Plasmodium vivax, P. falciparum* and *P. malariae* (the three human malaria parasites) was 47.1, 45.9, and 6.9 respectively.[7]

The distribution of three malaria parasites in 1906 and 1930[8] in Bengal and Kolkata is given in Table 1.

Table 1: Distribution of three malaria parasites in Bengal and Kolkata

Year	*Plasmodium Falciparum*		*Plasmodium Vivax*		*Plasmodium malaria*	
	Bengal	*Kolkata*	*Bengal*	*Kolkata*	*Bengal*	*Kolkata*
1906	53.1	58.7	29.7	36.9	17.2	-
1930	46.3	56.0	41.4	37.0	12.5	-

Malaria was endemic in Kolkata and in the 30s, cases reached a peak in 1936, taking an epidemic magnitude (Table 2).[9]

Table 2: Malaria in Kolkata 1930–1937

Year	*1930*	*1931*	*1932*	*1933*	*1934*	*1935*	*1936*	*1937 upto June*
People affected	9,429	10,056	12,195	13,243	14,919	12,427	23,547	11,422

Not much effort was given to contain malaria. During 1899, Calcutta Corporation used to spend Rs. 30/- only per month for mosquito control operation and this was a subject of discussion in a famous science journal *Lancet*, where the discovery of Ronald Ross was first published. During those days kerosine oil was spread over water surface to control mosquitoes.[10]

A malaria conference was held in Simla (where malaria was non-existing) in 1909 and the Malaria Survey of India was formed in Kasauli. Malaria Bureau was instituted and in 1911, Malaria Institute of India was established in Delhi.[11]

Actually Kolkata was under the grip of malaria since its birth in 1690, when Job Charnock landed in Kolkata with 1200 Englishmen, of whom 400 died of malaria within 6 months from August 1690 to January 1691.[12] In 1756, Sirajuddulla recaptured Kolkata from the hands of British merchants, and at that time, many British soldiers captured in the warships suffered severely from malaria.[13]

Malaria incorporates several stories, most of which are contemporary, but are historically interesting:

1. There is an interesting romantic story about how the cinchona bark which yielded quinine came to Europe. The wife of the Spanish ambassador (Countess of Chinchon, mind the spelling) was attacked with malaria. She was cured by taking 'fever bark' in 1638. The kind-hearted Countess brought with her this bark (and also the plant) to Spain for distribution to poor cultivators, who used to suffer from malaria. This fever bark was named Cinchona (the original spelling of chinchona was changed).[14] Swedish Scientist, Carolus Linnaeus named the plant *Cinchona febrifuge*, remembering the name of the Countess of Chinchon in 1742. It is said Linnaeus himself used this bark for the treatment of his wife.[15] There are several discrepancies regarding this popular story. Recently a scientist claimed that the story is totally fictitious.[16] According to this researcher, Charles Ledger, a Britisher had stolen better quality of

cinchona seeds from Bolivia, risking his life. He expected wealth and honour for this from his country, but the British Government did not show any interest. He then sold the seeds to the Dutch Government and received less than 100 pounds as reward. The Dutch grew chinchona plants in Java (Indonesia). The plant was definitely superior to other cinchona plants, so far as yield of quinine was concerned. This type of cinchona plant is scientifically known as *Cinchona ledgeriana*. Ledger however remained poor for ever. He used to receive 100 pounds per year as pension which was very meagre. He was almost penniless when he died in 1905 in Sydney, Australia.

This story does not end here. During World War II Japanese troops captured Indonesia. Americans employed three airships to carry cinchona seeds to South America. Two aeroplanes were destroyed by the enemies. The last one survived and reached safely to the destination and cinchona plantation was started in the vast areas of Latin America.

Malaria was prevalent in different parts of the earth during World War II (1939–1945). In 1934, the Germans invented chloroquine in the name of resochin, a very patent synthetic drug of malaria. The Germans developed another compound named santochin, that was not so effective in malaria. But the Germans gave more importance to santochin than chloroquine. In fact, chloroquine was the magic medicine. The French scientists confirmed it and utilized this medicine alongwith another synthetic drug, mepacrine, developed by the British scientists. These drugs played an important role in treating malaria of soldiers of the allied forces. Of many factors, this is also an important factor for their victory, which acted as the fifth columnist against Hitler.

2. The life and achievements of Ronald Ross (1857–1932), born in Almora in the year when the first independence struggle against the British rule was launched, were no less dramatic. Ross was described as an 'unlikely hero' in the field of discovery of malaria. He wanted by turn, to be a painter, composer, a mathematician, a poet, and a novelist. The one thing he certainly did not want to be was a doctor. That was the wish of his father which he had to fulfil, almost reluctantly. But there were certain qualities in his character more essential to his eventual victory, the discovery of 'Ross's cycle',[17] clearly showing that 'malaria is conveyed from a person

or bird to healthy one by the proper species of mosquitoes and is inoculated by the bite.'

Ross was sent to India in 1885 with the specific assignment to investigate whether mosquitoes transmit malaria or not. He had neither any practical experience about malaria, nor had he any knowledge about mosquitoes. He was even a disbeliever of the theory of Laveran. Moreover, for this very critical problem his time was extremely short. Actually Patrick Manson, a versatile British physician and scientist was his mentor, as well as friend, philosopher, and guide. He was Ross's remote control. In Secunderabad in 1897, he discovered pigmented cells (oocysts, a stage of the life cycle of malaria parasites) from blood in the stomach of a mosquito, imbibed from a falciparum patient 10 days ago. This was a major breakthrough. Ross himself, however, was attacked with malaria prior to his Secunderabad discovery.

Ross was then transferred to Kolkata. He was posted at the P.G. Hospital (now SSKM Hospital). At that time there were not many malaria cases here. Ross turned to bird-malaria. There was also a myth that Ross turned to bird-malaria because a plague scare deprived him of human subjects. It was partially true.

However, his success was remarkable. He discovered the life cycle of bird-malaria parasite, *Plasmodium relictum* (at that time it was known as *Proteosoma*) in the grey mosquito, *Culex guinguefasciatus*. This is known as Ross's cycle. No doubt, this was an epoch-making discovery, which took place in Kolkata in 1898. So Ronald Ross discovered how bird-malaria was transmitted. Italian scientists Grassi, Bignani, and Bastianelli in November, 1898 showed exclusively that *Anophelies* mosquitoes transmit malaria from man to man.

3. Historical events amounting to contradiction and quarrel in the field of Nobel Prize centering around malaria were no less interesting. A proposal came to share the Nobel Prize between Ross and the Italian scientists. Manson and Koch opposed it vehemently. The British lobby was naturally very much powerful at that time. Ross alone won the Nobel Prize in 1902.

But think of Laveran, who was the pioneer in malaria research. He discovered the malaria parasite in 1880, eight years before the discovery of Ross. At last the Nobel Committee felt the prick of conscience. The fault was understood and Laveran was awarded with the Nobel Prize in 1907.

Meanwhile, the relation between Manson and Ross was shattered. Was it due to envy as Patrick Manson was not in the track of the Nobel Prize?[18]

4. R. Knowles and B. M. Dasgupta, in 1932 in the School of Tropical Medicine, Kolkata discovered *Plasmodium knowlesi* from the monkey *Macaca irus*. It was a significant discovery as it facilitated experimental drug research in malaria.
5. There was no participation of any Indian scientist in early malaria research which was a sad aspect. The Britishers perhaps did not want this. They were not so liberal, even in the field of science, so far as participation of natives was concerned.
6. But in the contemporary literature, in the writings of Vidyasagar,[19] Swami Vivekananda,[20] Bankimchandra,[21] Rabindranath,[22] and Saratchandra[23] we get rich references to malaria. Vivekananda and Vidyasagar probably suffered from malaria.
7. How far British rule was concerned with the increase in the magnitude of the malaria problem? Sarda canal was constructed during 1920–1929 which was responsible for the rise of malaria. Unplanned construction of railways was also a great factor in disturbing the environment.[24] But who would make the empire understand these petty affairs? Greed and profit were their ultimate motive, not the upliftment of the natives in the colony. It is to be noted that malaria was rapidly disappearing from England since 1864, after existing there for twelve centuries.[25]
8. In the total darkness was there light anywhere? This was lit by Rabindranath who was concerned with certain fundamental questions. Elimination of malaria? When will it be possible? When will people participate, when will they form co-operatives, when will they come forward? Very rightly he said that although there is malaria in the country, it is not a big problem. The bigger problem is that there is inertia in the minds of people of our country.[26]

Kala-azar or Black Fever (visceral leishmaniasis)

India is the oldest *kala-azar* endemic area in the world. Devastating epidemics once swept through most of Bengal, Bihar, and Assam during British rule. *Kala-azar* was also prevalent in Madras, and in some parts of Orissa and the United Provinces. Though the disease is said to have existed in India for quite a long time, its actual history in this country prior to 1875 is by no means clear. There are reasons to believe that *kala-azar* had existed in Bengal before this date. A kind of fever was stated by Twining as early as 1835[27] which resembled *kala-azar*, and had been found in several districts including Mymensingh (now in Bangladesh) in sporadic form. The disease described by French in 1872[28] in the district of Burdwan, which prevailed from 1862 to 1872 by the name of Burdwan fever, was in all probability *kala-azar*. A similar type of *jwar vikar*, a sort of illness with fever in Jessore district (now in Bangladesh) during the same time was supposed to be *kala-azar* that took a toll of 75,000 lives.

In those days *kala-azar* was endemic in almost every district of undivided Bengal and dispensary returns for 1922 showed 15,556 cases, which according to Napier gave very inadequate idea of the number of cases that were there in the province. In the out patient department of School of Tropical Medicine, Kolkata, *kala-azar* patients were treated regularly every year (see Table 3). The patients used to come from all over Bengal and the number of each district usually varied in inverse ratio to the distance of the particular district from Kolkata. Before the introduction of special treatment with *urea stibamine*, discovered by Brahamachari, the mortality rate was very high.

Kala-azar probably first appeared in Bihar. In 1822, in Purnea district, a disease called '*kala-dukh*' existed which according to Ross[30] could be *kala-azar*. Epidemics of *kala-azar* occurred in Bihar between 1890 and 1900 and again from 1917–1929.[31] An intensified situation was observed in Bihar from 1933–1937 when 55,044, 58,547, 57,400, 68,252, and 91,942 cases from hospitals and dispensaries were recorded in 1933, 1934, 1935, 1936, and 1937 respectively.

Table 3. *Kala-azar* patients treated in School of Tropical Medicine (1921–1948)

Year	*Case of Kala-azar*	*Year*	*Case of Kala-azar*
1921	217	1934	N. A.
1922	631	1935	164
1923	1117	1936	215
1924	1118	1937	213
1925	1108	1938	195
1926	696	1939	170
1927	682	1940	N. A.
1928	670	1941	N. A.
1929	450	1942	132
1930	236	1943	267
1931	234	1944	182
1932	228	1945	558
1933	190	1946	817

The disease first made its appearance in Assam about the year 1875. Full scale epidemic broke out between 1890 and 1900, thereafter a severe epidemic again ravaged the eastern part of the country from 1917 to 1929. In 1897, about 14,500 people died of this fever in Nowgong. A study[32] indicated that *kala-azar* resulted in a decline of population in Assam, primarity affecting children and young adults. Thus *kala-azar* literally sapped the vitality of the people. Vast land had to be left uncultivated and became almost valueless in those areas, where *kala-azar* prevailed. Many tea gardens were practically ruined. Bengal lost a great versatile litterateur, Sukumar Roy, who died of *kala-azar* in Kolkata at the age of thirty-six only.[33]

In 1900, W. B. Leishman discovered certain bodies in the spleen of a British soldier who had been invalidated home from Kolkata with Dum Dum fever (a synonym of *kala-azar*). He published this observation much later in May 1903. C. Donovan in the same year in July found the same bodies in a material from the spleen puncture in Madras. This is the amastigote form of the parasite found in man, which has been named Leishman Donovan bodies or LD bodies. In 1904, Rogers was successful to culture the parasite in the laboratory.

The *Kala-azar* Commission was appointed by the Government of India in 1924. Why did the crown constitute such a commission? Was it for research? Perhaps, but poor people were on many occasions utilized as experimental guinea-pigs. They were compelled to take some injections known to be toxic and some barbaric control measures were adopted according to their whims. Two instances are worth citing. In 1920, a person was appointed to treat *kala-azar* patients with tartar emetic, through injections. The treatment was made compulsory. In subsequent four years, 7,188, 15,888, 19,659 and 37,300 patients received treatment. There were many severe reactions and even deaths. But for experimental purposes, the compulsory treatment was carried out. For control purposes in tea gardens, patients were removed forcibly 300–1200 yards from infected areas and their houses, beddings, and clothings were all burnt.

Investigations related to transmission, carried out by Indian *Kala-azar* Commission were not conclusive.[34] In 1930, the committee brought its investigation to an end. Conclusive proof was obtained in 1942. This has been reviewed in detail in a paper.[35] The main events are summarized here. Knowles *et al.* (1942)[36] demonstrated promastigotes (a flagellate stage of the parasite) in female laboratory-bred sandflies, *Phlebotomus argentipes,* fed on *kala-azar* patients.

Shortt and his co-workers (1925)[37] recorded a massive infection of the pharynx and buccal cavity of the sandfly on the 8th day after feeding (during which time sandflies would attempt feeding for the second time to transmit the infection), and subsequently in 1931,[38] reported successful transmission by the bite of the sandflies in animal. The vectorship of *P. argentipes* was not proven, until Swaminath *et al.* (1942)[39] succeeded in transmitting the disease in Assam to 5 volunteers but only after the infected sandflies had previously been fed on raisins, which probably stimulated ascent of promastigotes to the tip of the beak (probocis) of the fly, wherefrom they could readily enter the wound.

So far as diagnosis was concerned, U.N. Brahmachari demonstrated a very simple procedure in 1917. This is known as globulin precipitation test. As much globulin is present in this disease condition, he invented this test in a novel way. Some serum of the patient was added to twice its quantity of distilled water. A precipitation occurred which signified the presence of the disease.[40] Napier in 1929 put forward aldehyde test or formal gel test, where he demostrated that when a few drops of 40 per cent formaline is added to a serum of the patient it solidifies like the white of an egg.[41]

In the history of treatment of *kala-azar*, U. N. Brahmachari made a major breakthrough by inventing a very potent medicine, *urea stibamine* in 1922,[42] which was unique.[43] This drug completely replaced the toxic drugs stated above, i.e. tartar emetic or sodium antimony tartrate. Brahmachari conducted his research in a small room at the Campbell Hospital, Kolkata (now NRS Medical College), provided with minimum facilities. The drug saved millions of lives and helped to contain epidemics. The adverse reactions were practically nil, the tolerance was excellent, the course was short and for the patient resistant to other toxic drug was effective. In Scott's excellent book[44] entitled *A History of Tropical Medicine*, except for a brief mention of Neostan or stibamine glucose (Burroughs Wellcome) and urea stibamine being of greater value in *kala-azar,* having a relatively low toxicity, and being well tolerated by men in comparatively large doses, nothing was mentioned about Bramachari and his discoveries. This basically reflects the colonial bias towards Indian medical practitioners.

Brahmachari for the first time described a skin condition in some cured *kala-azar* patients which he designated as Post Kala-azar Dermal Leishmaniasis (PKDL).

Plague

Plague is caused by a bacterium, *Yersinia pests* discovered independently by Yersin and Kitasato in Hongkong in July, 1894. Plague was mentioned by Homer in Greece in 1200 BC. It once created havoc and in the 14th century, 'black death' killed ¼th of the world population, including Europe. Since the 1840s, epidemic plague disappeared from Europe.

What about India?

A report on vital statistics of Kolkata, 100 years ago published in *The Statesman*[45] pointed out total number of death registered in the city during the week ending 12 September, 1902. There were 16 deaths from plague, 15 from cholera and 19 from tetanus.

Plague was a great scourge in our country. As in the case of cholera, so with plague, its chief home in the British empire was India. In 1815, plague was present in the mountaneous districts of Hindustan.[46] But the epidemic of 1896 was probably the worst. Plague appeared in Mumbai and Kolkata in 1895.[47]

Between 1889 and 1948 more than 1 crore and 23 lakhs of people died of plague (Table 4). Specific mortality rate was 183.3/100,000 population during 1898–1908. In 1930 alone, 23,825 deaths took place. From 1898 to 1918, average yearly death was 500,000, while it was 100,000 for 1921–1930 and 50,000 for 1931–1935.

Table 4. Deaths due to Plague in India

1889–1908	6032693
1909–1918	4221529
1919–1928	1762718
1929–1938	422880
1939–1948	368596

So many deaths were occuring, but it was quoted in 1930s that the importance of plague was less than cholera and small-pox! The states mostly affected were the Punjab, UP, Bihar, Madhya Pradesh, Andhra Pradesh, Madras, Karnataka, Bengal, Maharashtra, and Gujarat.

The Indian Plague Commission in Bombay made a notable contribution in 1905–1906, related to transmission of the disease. On definite experimental evidence, it was established that a rat flea (*Xenopsylla cheopis*) was the transmitter of plague from rat to rat (and from rat to man), thus confirming the report of Gautier and Rayband's work in Marseilles. Before that Oyata (1897) and Simond (1898) in Bombay injected infected flea extract in mice and produced plague.

No doubt, plague was a disease of horror. But certain measures adopted by the government were more horrible than that horror. In some places all the suspected cases, including beggars were compelled to be segregated in camps. In some areas tax was imposed on inhabitants for relief of the plague-stricken, in some localities infected houses were quarantined and isolated for several weeks, and in some occasions huts and belongings were burnt. During some journeys (ships, railways) the passengers were examined shamelessly and inhumanly. It has been reflected in the works of Rabindranath[48] and Saratchandra.[49] Such harassment and oppression by the colonial authorities have not been completely revealed, which requires a detail retrospective study by the competent authority.

In 1902, in the Punjab one deplorable event took place. Anti-plague inoculation was given to the public. No standardization was maintained. As a result, 18 persons died of tetanus by taking contaminated injections.

Laboratory-cultured plague bacilli were implicated in a homicidal case in 1933 in Kolkata, where a person of the School of Tropical Medicine was involved in a case (Bhattacharya-Pundey case, 1933), reported by the Director of the Haffkine Institute, Bombay and under the title the Pakur Murder, by captain D.P. Lambert, IMS.

When plague invaded Kolkata, a great panic gripped the city. Vivekananda told his followers in 1898 that he would rather sacrifice himself if required to fight against plague in Kolkata, where he was born. At that time he was in the USA, wherefrom he sent a letter to his mother Dhira, telling her of his deep concern related to the plague. He was very much perturbed to know that 500 people had died of plague in the city in one week. Rabindranath returned from Selaidaha in spite of his ill health to stand by the side of the common people at that dark and critical period. A plague committee was constitued in the city and Sister Nivedita as its secretary wholeheartedly engaged herself to serve the plague victims. As those illustrious personalities stood by the side of the people, the people of Kolkata got back their courage to fight against the dreaded disease.

Cholera

It is also known as '*murri*'. It is stated that Asiatic cholera spontaneously developed in India or in other words, India was its home or endemic centre. Six pandemics of cholera occurred between 1817 and 1923. The first epidemic started in Kishnagar on the Hooghly river in 1817. There was little doubt however that in 1816 cholera was already becoming endemic in Bihar. The route of spread of first pandemic was Ceylone (Sri Lanka) 1819, Mauritius–East Africa 1820, Philippines–China–Japan 1822, Arabia 1821, Persia–Seria–Russia 1823. The 2nd, 3rd, 4th, 5th and 6th pandemic always originating from India occurred during 1826–1837, 1842–1862, 1867–1875, 1881–1896 and 1899–1923 respectively.

Europe once suffered much from cholera. During 1840–1849, one million people died of cholera in Russia. In England and Wales, a number of 53,293, 20,097, and 14,378 persons succumbed to the disease in 1849, 1854, and 1866 respectively. Since then cholera virtually disappeared from England.

When we turn to India, we see that cholera was taking another leading part in the procession of death. A record states that during a pilgrimage in Bengal in 1783, 20,000 people died of cholera. The population of British India in 1921 was 318,942,000. In 1821 and 1824 half a million and 300,000 cases were recorded. During the last part of the 19th century, annually 2-8 lakhs of people died of cholera.[50] During 1923–1934, the number of deaths due to cholera amounted to 2,490,401, average 207,533 per annum.

Derozio and David Hare died of cholera in Kolkata in 1831 and 1842 respectively.[51] Robert Koch (1843–1910) isolated the comma bacilli (*Vibrio cholerae*) from cholera patients in Egypt in 1823 [though it had been observed earlier by Pacini (1854) and others], and he confirmed the discovery in Kolkata when he found it in the dejecta of all cholera cases which he examined in 1884.[52] He visited Kolkata as a member of the German Cholera Commission.[53]

In the treatment of cholera, IV saline was first used in Shanghai in 1875.[54] But at that time, normal saline was used and the death rate was above 63 per cent. E.J.U. Meara used it in India in 1908. He recommended it for adult natives, but did not consider it suitable for Europeans and children. He however gave no reason for distinguishing them. He used 0.625 per cent saline. It produced many deaths. Who was there to protest? People were used as laboratory animals at the whims of several so-called researchers. Leonard Rogers in Medical College, Kolkata first used hypertonic saline in 1908. The death rate was reduced to half (32.6 per cent). The treatment was further modified during 1915–1917, the death rate with this treatment was about 19 per cent.

Cholera deaths in Kolkata from 1841 to 1873 is given in Table 5.

Table 5: Cholera deaths in Kolkata (1841–1875)

Year	*People Died*	*Year*	*People died*
1841	5127	1857	3838
1842	6545	1858	5195
1843	3739	1859	4676
1044	5811	1860	6553
1845	6420	1861–1864	N. A.
1846	6427	1865	5076
1847	3041	1866	6825
1848	2502	1867	2268
1849	3867	1868	4178
1850	3348	1869	3592
1851	4374	1870	1560
1852	4189	1871	790
1853	5632	1872	1068
1854	3082	1873	1140
1855	3744	1874	1216
1856	4540	1875	1668

Sambhunath De, working in Medical College, Kolkata, proved the existence of cholera exotoxin. This was a very significant research, opening a new path of investigation, which attracted the attention of many foreign researchers.

In 1896, Kolle's heat killed bacterial vaccine was produced. Roy in 1919 reported a decrease of an epidemic with the vaccination in Hazaribag. But vaccine supplied was too meagre to cater to the need of the country. Moreover, practically no sincere attempt was made to improve water sanitation, specially in the villages.

It is also worthwhile to mention here that malaria, plague, and cholera virtually disappeared in England from 1864, 1841, and 1866 respectively.[55] But its colony/colonies continued to suffer bitterly from these menaces. This is surely due to the double standards adopted, for so many epidemics the empire cannot deny its responsibilities.

Amoebiasis

Amoebiasis and its grave complication liver abscess was very much prevalent at that time. India was one of the worst regions affected by amoebiasis. Next to malaria came bowel complaints and the danger to health and life was more than in the case of malaria.[56]

Most of the Indians did probably suffer from amoebiasis in those days. In a report, coming from Madras in 1844, out of 59 such cases 40 died.[57]

F.A. Losch, in Russia in 1857 descibed the pathogenic nature of the causative organism, *Entamoeba histolytica.*[58] *E. histolytica* is of two types, one is pathogenic, *E. histolytica* (Schaudinn 1903) and the other *E. dispar* (Brumpt 1925) which is not pathogenic. Rogers studied pathogenicity of liver abscess. This was the subject of his Lettsomian Lecture in 1922. Actually, in 1902, Rogers announced amoebae to be founded in the liver abscess and he advised use of emetine in that disease, which he standardized in the treatment of amoebic dysentery between 1912 and 1914.

Dengue

Dengue comes from the Spanish word '*denguero*' meaning an affected or dandified person from the delicate gait assumed or compelled owing to the pain caused by movement. In English it is known as break-bone or break-back fever.

Dengue was first recognized in Cairo in 1779. Epidemics of dengue occurred in India in 1824–1925, 1836, and 1871. Kolkata was worst hit in 1824–1825 and 1836 epidemics.[58] Rabindranath had to shift from Joransako, Kolkata to Peneti or Panihati and yes, it was a judicious scientific shift as vector mosquitoes were not present in suburbs.

Incidentally, Rabindranath had never suffered from malaria or dengue. He was a man who had developed a fine scientific acumen. It was known to him that only female mosquitoes bite. Leman grass oil is a good repellent. He had referred to day mosquitoes which could transmit dengue.

In 1907, Leonard Rogers described seven day fever of Kolkata, which according to Campbell was actually a variety of dengue.[59] It is to be noted that dengue is incapacitating, but it cannot kill a person. Dengue haemorrhagic fever (DHF) was not known in British India. In 1907, Ashburn and Craig said that the organism is a filtre passer, i.e. a virus. Finally in 1916, J. B. Cleland, B. Brddley and W. Mcdonald in Australia showed experimentally '*Aedes aegypti mosquito*' as the vector.[60]

Small-pox

This ancient disease was once prevalent in most parts of the world, believed to have originated in India or China. It ceased to be endemic in the UK in 1935, but in India played a devasting role killing millions (Table 6). Unfortunate superstitious people invented Sitala Mata, the goddess of the disease with a hope to protect them through her grace, which went in vain. Deaths, sufferings, miseries, agonies, and panic were unfathomable. It is to be pointed out that vaccination reached India in 1802, just 4 years after Jenner's original report, but it was not properly or systematically introduced before 1927. Even then the supply was grossly inadequate. There was no serious agenda, program or attempt to eliminate the disease. Indians continued to suffer.

Table 6. Yearly deaths due to small-pox in India (1920–1948)

Year	*People Died of small pox*	*Year*	*People Died of small pox*
1920	98,476	1934	82,327
1921	39,454	1935	89,441
1922	34,397	1936	103,451
1923	41,238	1937	54,810
1924	52,879	1938	39,444
1925	82,134	1939	48,103
1926	111,727	1940	7,287
1927	116,439	1941	59,307
1928	93,298	1942	27,137
1929	71,043	1943	52,374
1930	71,893	1944	216,538
1931	36,782	1945	136,953
1932	42,441	1946	N. A.
1933	102,135	1947	N. A.

Source: Dixon, c.w. 1962. *Small pox*, J & A Churchill Ltd., London, p. 512.

Tuberculosis

TB was also a great killer. Specific medicine was not discovered before 1948. Our progressive poet Sukanta Bhattacharya died of TB at Jadavpur TB Hospital.

Hook Worm

Angelo Dubini in Italy discovered the worm *Ancylostoma duodenale* in 1838. The infected persons did suffer from anaemia. This type of anaemia was known as miner's anaemia. The miners were compelled to live in insanitary condition. Most of them were illiterate. Infected persons were sometimes excluded from employment. Invariably, latrine accommodation was not installed. Their health condition was really wretched. Almost all workers had to bear this infection. This was widespread in rural community responsible for anaemia in 75 per cent of the rural population.

Epidemic dropsy

In 1881, Colonel Kenneth Mcleod, described a new disease in *Indian Medical Gazette* occurring in epidemic form in Kolkata and Howrah, where there was dropsical swelling starting in the feet and extending up even to the face. Pleural and pericardial effusion were not uncommon, but ascites was rarely found. He christened the disease epidemic dropsy. Some 16–17 years later Sir Pardey Lukis observed the same thing.[61] This disease occurred in epidemic form in 1901 (Kolkata), 1902 (Bombay), 1905 (Boro Hills), 1907 (Kolkata), 1914 (Kolkata with 433 deaths), 1919 (Kolkata with 96 deaths), 1920 and 1922 (Allahabad), 1924 (Rangoon, Kolkata), 1926–1927 (Kolkata with 1569 deaths). Mustard oil was suspected while tracing the distribution of the disease. Actually *Argimon mexicana* seeds contaminated mustard oil was held as the culprit, which was discovered by the scientists of the School of Tropical Medicine, Kolkata in 1939. A very easy method to detect the adulteration (Hydrochloric acid test) was also developed at the Tropical School.[62]

Conclusion

Devastating epidemics in the empire took millions of lives. The empire practically adopted no step to contain or eliminate epidemics, displaying a double standard, where health was promoted in its own country and demoted in the colonies. Many oppressive measures were enforced and many death-dealing experiments were carried out, Indians were debarred from the scientific field. The nation became crippled with no real progress. Indian struggle for freedom was definitely hampered.

Will History Repeat Itself?

In this era of globalization, health care as a commodity is under the grasp of powerful multinationals, a much stronger empire than even the colonial one. A commercial colonialism is spreading and at the same time we hear the hurried soft steps of epidemics old and new which may shatter all our lives and dreams.

Acknowledgements

I wish to record my sincere thanks to Sri Kamal Kumar Mukim, Goutam Laboratories, 9A, Kali Krishna Tagore St., Kolkata–700 007, Dr. Hiranmoy Mukherjee, Head of the Department of Entomology, School of Tropical Medicine, Kolkata and Mrs. Bharati Datta, my wife, for various helps.

References

1. H. H. Scott, 1939. *A History of Tropical Medicine*, Edward Arnold Co., London, 1939, p. 1165.
2. A. K. Hati, 1980þ, *Malaria: Protection and Cure*, Published by the organizing committee, Hundred years of Malaria Research, Kolkata, p. 4. (in Bengali).
3. B. L. Raina, *Introduction to Malaria Problem in India*, New Book Co., Bombay,1951.
4. P. E. Russel, *Man's Mastery of Malaria,* Oxford University Press, London, 1955.
5. J. A. Sinton, 'What Malaria Costs India Nationally, Socially and Economically', *Records of the Malaria Survey of India*,1935–36, 5, pp. 413–481.
6. A. K. Hati, *Medical Entomology*, (2nd edn), Allied Book Agency, Kolkata, 2002, p. 201.
7. R. Knowles, R. Senior White, and B. M. Das Gupta, 'Studies in Parasitology of Malaria', *Indian Medical Research Memoir No. 18*, 1930.
8. A. K. Hati, and N. C. Mukherjee, *Distribution of Plasmodium falciparum* in West Bengal, 74,1980, pp. 420–421
9. P. Sen, *'Anopheles sundaicus* (Ludlowi) and malaria in Calcutta (Kolkata)', *J Mal Inst. Ind*, 1, 1938, pp. 83–98.
10. H. N. Cook, *Report of the Health Officer of Calcutta for the year 1899.* Corporation Press, Kolkata, 1900.
11. G. Harrison, *Mosquito, Malaria and Man*, John Murray, London, 1978, p. 314.
12. A. K. Hati, 'To Free Calcutta from Mosquito', *Dainik Basumati*, 10 April, 1983, (in Bengali); L. S. S. O'Malley, *Bengal District Gazetteer, 24 Parganas District*, Kolkata, 1914.

13. G. Covell, *Malaria in Calcutta, Rec Mal Sur Ind.*, 3, 1932, pp. 1-82.
14. A. S. Lyons, and R. S. Petrucelli II, *Medicine, An Illustrated History,* 1978, p. 616.
15. H Goerke, *Linnaeus*, Scribner, N. Y. 1973.
16. G. Gramiceia, *The Life of Charles Ledger (1818–1905)*, London, 1988, p. 222.
17. A. K. Hati, 'One Hundred Years of Discovery of Ross's Cycle' (Ed) *JIMA*, 96,1998, pp. 233–237.
18. A. K. Hati, *Malaria*, West Bengal State Book Board (in Bengali).
19. Vidyasagar, *Complete Works* (in Bengali).
20. Swami Vivekananda, *Complete Works*, vols. 5 and 6 (in Bengali).
21. Bankimchandra, *Complete Works* (in Bengali).
22. R. N. Tagore, *Malaria Protection in Co-operatives*, *Complete Works* (in Bengali), Centenary Edition, vol. 13; pp. 549–562.
23. A. K. Hati, 'Malaria in Saratchandra's Writings', *Sarat Commemoration Volume*, Sarat Memorial Library, Panitras, Howrah (in Bengali); Bharati, Dutta, 'Disease and Patient in Saratchandra's Bulletin,' *Calcutta Public Health Fair III*, pp. 53–56 (in Bengali).
24. R.N. Tagore, *op. cit.*, pp. 552-558.
25. H. H. Scott, *op. cit.*, p. 1165.
26. A. K. Hati, *op. cit.*, see reference 23.
27. L. E. Napier, 'An Epidemiological Consideration of the Transmission of Kala-azar in India'. *Indian Med Record Memoirs 1924–1925*, 1924–25, 219.
28. P. C. Sengupta, 'Kala-azar in Bengal its Incidence and Trends'. *Ind Med Gaz.* 79, 1944, p. 547.
29. U. N. Brahmachari, *Treatise on Kala-azar*. John Ball and Rannielson Ltd., London, 1928.
30. R. Ross, *Report of Nature of Kala-azar*, Calcutta, 1899.
31. M. Dutta, & T. K. Ghosh, 'Review of Current Status of Leishmaniasis Epidemiology', *Proceedings of the Indo-UK workshop on Leishmaniasis*, ICMR, 1983, 1997.
32. Mc Combie, T. C. Young, *Kala-azar in Assam*. H. K. Lewis, London, 1924.
33. A. K. Hati, '300 Years of Calcutta and Public Health', *West Bengal, Public Health issue*, No. 27, 1993, pp. 34-52.
34. 'Report of Kala-azar Commission, India, Report No.1 (1924–25)', *Ind. Med. Res. Memoirs*, No. 4, 1925.
35. A. K. Hati, 'A Review on **Phlebotomus** (Enphlebotomus) **argentipes** Annardale & Brunetti, the vector for Kala-azar (visceral leishmaniasis) in India', *Indian Rev life Sci*, II. 1991, pp. 53-75.
36. R. Knowles, L. E. Napier, and R. A. Smith, 'On a Herpetomonas Found in the Gut of the Sandfly Fed on Kala-azar Patient', *Ind. Med. Gaz.*, 59, 1924, pp. 593–597.

37. H. E. Shortt, P. J. Barraud, and A. C. Craighead, 'Note on a Massive Infection of the Pharynx of **Phlebotomus argentipes** with **Herpetomonas donavani**' 1925.
38. H. A. Shortt, R. O. A. Smith, and C. S. Swaminath 'Transmission of Kala-azar through **Phlebotomus argentipes** by the Oral Route', *Ind. J Med. Res.* 19, 1931, pp. 351–352.
39. C. S. Swaminath, H. E. Shortt, and L. A. P. Anderson, 'Transmission of Indian kala-azar to man by bite of **Phlebotomus argentipes** Ann & Brun'. *Ind. J Med. Res.* **30**, 1942, pp. 473–477.
40. H. H. Scott *op. cit.*, p. 1165.
41. *Ibid.*
42. U. N. Brahmachari, 'Chemotherapy of antimonial compound in kala-azar infection. Part - I. The toxicity of antimony tartrate'. *Ind. J Med. Res.*, 10, 1922, pp. 492–522.
43. A. K. Hati, H. Mukherjee, and B. D. Banerjee, 'Urea stibamine' (mini review), *J of Basic and Applied Biomedicine*, **3**, 1995, pp. 61–65.
44. H. H. Scott, *op. cit.*, p. 1165.
45. *The Statesman*, 13.09.02, '100 years ago today'.
46. H. H. Scott *op.cit.*, p. 1165.
47. A. K. Hati, *Medical Entomology* (2nd Ed.), Kolkata, 2001, p. 201.
48. Bharati, Dutta, 'Outline of Diseases Calcutta in Bengali Literature', *Souvenir, Calcutta Public Health Fair*, 1994, pp. 38–45 (in Bengali).
49. *Medicolegal Review*, 1937, p. 297.
50. R. Pollitzer, *Cholera*, WHO Geneva, 1959, p. 1019.
51. Bharati, Dutta, 'Disease and Death of Some Eminent Person of Calcutta', *Souvenir, Public Health Fair*, April-June 2001, pp. 8-11. (in Bengali).
52. H. H. Scott, *op. cit.*, p. 1165.
53. A. K. Hati, '100 Years of Treatment, Bengali Tradition and Promice,' *West Bengal*, 27, 1994, pp. 88–98 (in Bengali).
54. H. H. Scott, *op. cit.*, p. 1165.
55. *Ibid.*
56. *Ibid.*
57. *Ibid.*
58. A. K. Hati, *Medical Parasitology*, Kolkata, 2002, pp. 188, 190.
59. H. H. Scott, *op. cit.*, p. 1165.
59. *Ibid.*
60. *Ibid.*
61. *Ibid.*
62. A. K. Hati, *op. cit.*, see reference 53.

4

Cholera: Changing Perceptions of Its Casualty in the Last Two Centuries—A Cursory Appraisal

—*Dhrub Kumar Singh*

The intention in this essay is to very briefly chart out some of the benchmark shifts in the etiological and epidemiological understanding of cholera. How the politics of empire permeated the conceptualization of this 'representative' but 'inscrutable malady' will also be cursorily alluded to. The fact that the conceptualization differed in the colony and the metropole underscores the linkages between colonialism and cholera. An appeal for a more consistent public health perspective is made by critiquing the residual ambivalences still persistent in the definition of the disease. Let us start with the definitial dilemma of the present.

The Diarrhoeal Dilemma

'Cholera is an acute diarrhoeal disease, that can in a matter of hours result in profound, rapidly progressive dehydration and death'.[1] This contemporary understanding of cholera is urbane, individualistic, and Eurocentric in approach wherein the public health perspective gets blurred. In the above definition, cholera gets almost entirely subsumed under the generic name of 'diarrhoeal disease'. Moreover, under this rubric, it loses its distinctiveness and specificity as an epidemic disease. In many recent textbooks on Internal medicine, cholera is classified under the rubric of 'diarrhoeal diseases'. The term cholera, according to Harrison's textbook on Internal medicine, is occasionally 'applied to severely dehydrating secretory diarrhoeal illness whether due to *vibrio cholerae* or not, and indeed whether infectious in etiology or not'.[2] Clearly, the boundary between infectious and non-infectious diarrhoeal diseases stands dissolved.

Among the infectious diseases, there could be a large number of causative organisms and each has its own importance from the public health perspective. A classic example of this is cholera, 'a devastating diarrhoeal disease', responsible for seven pandemics and much suffering over the past two centuries.[3] This epidemiological[4] understanding, which entails in itself the distinction between infectious and non-infectious, is very important regarding diarrhoeal diseases. Otherwise no epidemiological logic remains whatsoever in making cholera a notifiable disease.

But, how exactly is one to define cholera within a social context, given the ambivalence in determining its nature? After receiving a case of diarrhoea, the onus lies upon the doctor to understand and ascertain whether it is infectious or not while probing the causes and, therefore, the definition of cholera should reflect this aspect of the disease. A very general definition of diarrhoea without alluding to the infectious and non-infectious aspects can serve as the basis of medical management of an individual clinical case. However, an individual diarrhoeal case, if infectious in origin and choleraic in nature and symptoms, in due course, can trigger off an epidemic depending upon a host of other social, economic, and environmental factors. Therefore, any definition of cholera should be such that it incorporates in itself a public health perspective. This is important for doctors in developing countries like India where seventy per cent of the population still lives in rural areas. Medical infrasturcture available in the rural hinterland may not have the wherewithal to handle an epidemic situation on its own. And by the time the disease is understood as cholera and the alarm sounded, the damage would have already been done. But, while dealing with diarrhoeal diseases, if the doctor remains alert about its infectious aspect and its epidemic potential, he will have the time and energy to notify and alert the nodal agencies so that the necessary machinery can be geared up to combat the situation.

However, if the boundaries of infectious and non-infectious are blurred with regard to 'diarrhoeal diseases' in their definition itself— and hence by extension from the pedagogic enterprise—the fact that a diarrhoeal disease could be a choleraic case will hardly dawn upon the doctor and its public health importance will not strike his mind. The term 'diarrhoeal diseases' is a very loose nosological[5] or epidemiological entity. Rather, it merely signifies a group of diseases in which the predominant symptom is diarrhoea. But the form and ways in which cholera behaves and could behave in a community, marks the importance of considering it as a separate epidemiological entity among the various diarrhoeal diseases.

Besides being a biological event, cholera, and in that respect any other disease with epidemic[6] potential, is also a social and cultural crisis and therefore the affected community behaves or responds according to its socio-cultural milieu. This aspect demands a close understanding of the society which in turn can inform policy formulation. Instead of being an imposition, any ameliorative strategy should be a socially mediated measure bearing in mind the socio-cultural location of the concerned community or society.

Diseases can be defined either on the basis of their characteristic clinical picture or according to their causative agents. But it may happen that the most frequently observed clinical appearance of a disease might not necessarily prove to be the characteristic of that malady. Also, it may be the case that the same etiological agent may provoke a broad spectrum of clinical manifestations in different individuals. Cholera also sometimes presents itself with varied intensity and form, ranging from simple diarrhoeal to symptomless carrier status. Mild varieties or less severe clinical types of cholera may bear every earmark of an illness caused by pathogens other than *vibrio cholerae*.[7]

While defining cholera the above aspects should be kept in mind so as to make the definition a guide to practice as well. Finally, cholera can be defined as 'a bacterial infection of man caused by *vibrio cholerae* (of classical or *El. Tor* bio-types) which characteristically causes severe diarrhoea, and death (in those severely affected), from water and electrolyte depletion. Spread is directly from person to person by the faecal oral route or indirectly by infected food or water. It can spread to any part of the world, and may become endemic where standards of environmental sanitation and personal hygiene are low. Man is the only reservoir of infection'.[8] According to Kamal, 'endemicity[9] is characterized by the presence of an illness or infection in a community in which socio-economic conditions are such that they do not offer effective barriers against its spread'.[10] This applies more to cholera than to other infectious diseases.

Cholera in History

From this task of defining cholera let us take a brief peep into its history. It has almost become habitual to write that all the cholera pandemics of the nineteenth century originated in deltaic Bengal. 'Each major epidemic spread of cholera since 1817 appears to have originated in the epidemic home of the disease in India, where the infection has been entrenched since long before 1817, probably since ***immemorial times*** (emphasis added).'[11]

Macnamara's *History of Asiatic Cholera* (1876) has been mischievous in this regard. In his account, cholera epidemics have been construed as synonymous to the 'Asiatic form' and Europe has been absolved deceitfully[12] from the stigma of this malady 'even though a malady clinically identical with true cholera, and often designated by this name, has been described by Hippocrates and many subsequent writers, some of whom used other names for the ailment, example, that of Weisse Ruhr'.[13] Macnamara and many subsequent commentators emphasized that since the disease, as described, never showed a truly epidemic spread and was only sporadic, it was something different from the true or *Asiatic Cholera.* Even Sydenham's description of cholera during the period 1679–1682 in London has been discounted on this basis.

In the colony, the 'Oriental' framing of the disease was reinforced by alluding to the timeless existence of *Ola Bee Bee*—the goddess of cholera[14]—and, in many accounts, even mythical delineations and allusions have been further mythicized by establishing role exchanges between *Sitala* the goddess of small-pox, and *Ola Bee Bee* the goddess of cholera.[15] The real classical cholera was designated as *Cholera Asiatica,* or epidemic, malignant, Indian or pestilential cholera, clearly differentiating it from *Cholera Nostras, Cholera Morbus, British, English, European, Biliary or Summer Cholera.*[16]

One of the most impartial and medically valid arguments with regard to the nomenclature of cholera was incidentally given by a rebel colonial doctor—Dr. Mahendra Lal Sarkar in the late nineteenth century. Sarkar's analysis, unlike that of his European counterparts, instead of being geographically and culturally coloured, was impassioned. He, being well read in the literature existing in his age on the natural history of cholera, made symptoms the yardstick both, as presented in the pre nineteenth century European medical literature and in the Indian Ayurvedic literature, in order to compare with the cholera symptoms of the nineteenth century. Sarkar dismissed '*Visuchika*' as described in Ayurvedic texts as having no major symptomatic resemblance with the then prevailing cholera, but found that Greek cholera (i.e. cholera which prevailed sporadically in Europe before 1817) had some overlap and resemblance with nineteenth century cholera. His critical survey of the symptomatology of cholera in Europe before 1817, and the cholera of India in and after 1817, convinced him that 'the two diseases ***though allied***, were ***distinct*** (emphasis added)'.[17]

In the former, i.e. in Greek cholera, European cholera or *Cholera Morbus*, the 'rice water stool and vomiting are the exception, coming on very rarely at the end in only the gravest cases'.[18] Similarly, 'suppression of urine is a rare symptom in *Cholera Morbus'*,[19] which appears only as a very late symptom and only in the gravest cases. All these symptoms, i.e. rice-water stool and vomiting and suppression of urine are constant symptoms of true cholera or Indian or *Asiatic Cholera or Cholera Indica*. According to Sarkar, these symptoms are 'present ***as a rule*** (emphasis added) coming on at once or after the first evacuation or two, even in very mildest of cases'.[20] Moreover, 'in the former the evacuations are passed with pain and effort; in the latter they are passed with greatest ease, and as if with no knowledge of the patient, being simply poured out'.[21]

So, Sarkar stresses upon the 'sudden and painless discharge of rice-water liquid from the stomach and bowels, devoid of all trace of bile, as the pathognomonic and therefore truly diagnostic of the modern disease'.[22] Sarkar, on the basis of these diagnostic symptoms of cholera in the nineteenth century, argues against the geographical and cultural connotative epithets attached as adjectives to the disease by European medical men of his age. Instead, he appeals for and employs symptomatological and epidemiological characters to describe the disease. The fatality and epidemicity versus sporadicity contrasts are employed by him to distinguish between the disease as it occurred in Europe and India in the nineteenth century. In this light he avers that 'malignant cholera', 'cholera maligna', or simply cholera or even '*Cholera Morbus*', as used by Sydenham, are appropriate terms for medical descriptions.

Through a parallel reading of the two delineations by contemporary historians of cholera, Macpherson (1872) and Macnamara (1876),[23] one clearly understands how the disease was attributed to India. The entire history of cholera in Britain prior to 1817 was consciously erased from public memory by employing a Eurocentric delineation. Jingoism of national glory did not permit the dissemination of that diseased history. An imperial race could not afford to have such a past. The venerable history of cholera in her own land before 1817 made her national glory vulnerable! The pretentious mother faced by the death and hardships of her own ailing and labouring children forgot her own shady past and blamed the stepchild for the mischief.[24] As alluded to earlier, in contrast to the European medical men's expatiation, we see a heretic,[25] native medical man of the late nineteenth century taking a judicious medical standpoint devoid of any cultural prejudice and not succumbing to the cultural rhetoric of the dominant medical literature of the age. Heretics sometimes show more critical faculty than conformists.

Nevertheless, in the entire colonial period, as the British connection grew intimate, cholera (and the cultural prejudice entailed in its conceptualization) figured prominently in each other's destiny. If colonialism was to foster civilization in the savage lands, then cholera supposedly emanating from a distant colony was undermining that civilizational endeavour. Cholera reciprocated the benevolence entailed in the colonial /civilizational endeavours by sapping the vital energies— the very imperial spirit by its destructive embrace. Perhaps it was a sweet revenge inflicted upon the smiling metropole by the choleraic colony. Cholera blurred the balance sheet of civilization and savagery in more than one way.

The Metropole Infected

During the 1820s, it was hoped 'that the actual presence of the disease in Britain (would) ***never afford*** (emphasis added) more immediate means of judgement'.[26] But cholera belied this hope and the metropole all along the nineteenth century was haunted by its presence. The pious hope of the metropole 'that the imminent of the faculty there (would) be more successful in the researches into its nature, cause and cure'[27] than their bretheren in the choleraic colony, was undermined by the disease. 'East India Company administrators estimated that over one-and-a quarter million died annually of the disease between 1817 and 1831; some eithteen million in total.'[28] As the disease swept through Europe in the years 1830 to 1832, it killed 'one citizen in twenty in Russia, one in thirty in Poland and Austria, and many in every European country before "burning itself out"'.[29] Emanating from a town of Bengal, cholera finally established connections with the town of Sunderland in England which claimed the 'dubious honour of recording the first case of *"Asiatic Cholera"* of the 1831–32 epidemic, when sixty year old William Sproat Senior developed symptoms on October 19, 1831'[30] and died on 26th October 1831.[31] Treatment with ***opium*** and ***brandy*** by two attending surgeons could not save him. The cholera history of the British Isles had begun. William Sproat Senior had left 'cholera' as his legacy, which gripped his granddaughter and her father William Sproat Junior on the next day.[32] 'The epidemic had begun and it spread rapidly throughout the U K, peaking in mid 1832 and eventually burning itself out later in the same year. An estimated 21,882 people died, and the mode of their demise was horrible.'[33]

Cholera deaths dropped out after 1832 but not before instigating riots at Liverpool in May and June in 1832. Fear of the mysterious and horrific disease and frustration caused due to the failure of the medical profession to 'cure' fuelled discontent, which the fear of 'burking' accentuted, and created riotous situations.[34] From 1838 we see the number of deaths due to cholera dwindling. It again rose in 1842 from three digits to 1,620 deaths and in 1849, it claimed 53,293 lives in England.[35]

Before the 1840s, there prevailed a general atmosphere of confusion and medical men often adopted shifting standpoints regarding cholera causality. It was covered under the mist of miasma. The breaking of the third pandemic wave that reached the shores of Britain coincided with the declaration by the newly formed Board of Health that the disease was non-contagious. The simple question that 'why cholera should be severe at one time and at one place and relatively milder at others',[36] and how were the occurrence of isolated cases of cholera to be accounted, made its communicability a riddle.

Amidst the 'mist of miasma', a vague notion of 'a pestilential virus' as the proximate cause of the disease existed among some of the contagionists, but they were unable to solve the riddle convincingly. Generally, the disease was attributed to atmospheric disturbances because the vague 'seed' or 'poison' was thought to take this highway to spread far and wide. Therefore, the understanding of meteorological phenomenon in conjunction with the epidemic's natural history, it was thought, would provide the capacity to predict the outbreak of the disease in certain weather.

John Snow, Cholera, and his 'Lateral Vision'

It was in the 1850s that the existence of a specific '*materia morbis*' a living, multiplying, distinct species was thought to cause and excite the cause of cholera. The seat of multiplication was understood to be the intestinal canal though without convincing reasons. Snow and Budd, interestingly, attempted to understand the causality by focusing on the communicability. For Snow, the ***lateral vision***, i.e., concentrating upon the communicability, was to yield more information about the nature of cholera than the straight vision of directly accounting for the causality. They established that the disease was spread by the use of water which had been contaminated by the faeces from cases of cholera. The 'mist of miasma' could be penetrated by the 'lateral vision' of John Snow. Actually, as one of the founding fathers of anaesthesia, Snow was an expert on respiration and this expertise allowed his lateral vision to discern some very useful clues and plausible insights. These newfound insights accorded consistency to his casual explanation and he was able to dismiss many of the earlier held theories of causalities pertaining to cholera.

The primary symptoms of cholera, i.e. copious rice-water diarrhoea and vomiting convinced him that the disease had nothing to do with the respiratory system, and so, the latter could not be the site of the disease. If the disease was due to '***miasma***' he reasoned, the lungs would have got affected first. As this was not the case, Snow ***rejected*** the prevalent telluric origin and explanation of the disease. The symptoms of cholera led him to the conclusion that cholera was primarily a disease of the alimentary canal. Extending his argument further, he proposed that ***if***[37] there exist a '*materia morbis*' or a cholera poison then it must be swallowed, in order to reach the alimentary canal, and 'the increase of the morbid material, or cholera poison, must take place in the interior of the stomach and bowels'.[38] Snow could thus elicit the 'attention of the microbe hunters to the intestines and their discharges'.[39]

With the above facts in mind, he tried to focus on the ***'communicability'*** aspect of cholera. Though cholera often killed the poor, it also killed the rich. The disease, many a times, revealed its constraint 'to confine itself chiefly to the crowded dwellings of the poor' and to reach the many well off localities to get new victims. This puzzling but egalitarian behaviour of cholera led Snow to conclude that there should be some 'opening' for cholera to 'extend itself more widely and to reach the well-to-do classes of the community'.[40] To account for this 'opening', Snow alluded to the possibility of the 'the mixture of cholera evacuations with the water used for drinking and culinary purposes, either by permeating the ground, and getting into wells, or by running along channels and sewers into rivers from which entire towns (were) sometimes supplied with water'.[41]

During the epidemic outbreak of the disease in London in 1854, Snow set out to test his grand hypothesis. With untiring zeal he conducted his epidemiological investigation going door to door in chosen districts in and around London where cholera had taken its toll. He gathered data about the water supplies, and also accounted the overlap of the water supply to these different localities. In his statistical analysis he calculated and tabulated deaths per thousand in various districts and also accounted for the overlapping supplies to these districts by various water companies. By following the comparison and contrast method, Snow 'sought statistical evidence for or against his particular theory of cholera'.[42]

Needless to say, Snow not only faced the cold behaviour of the medical establishment but also had to surmount many practical impediments. Meanwhile, the outbreak of cholera to the north of the Thames in Soho, 'within roughly 250 yards of the spot where Cambridge Street meets Broad Street and where mortality rate was ***exceptionally*** (emphasis added) high', provided Snow an opportunity to conduct a much more focused epidemiological investigation. Within the limited area in Soho around Broad Street, 500 fatal attacks of cholera occurred. This even surpassed and rekindled the horrific memories of the plague years of bygone centuries, as a good number of those attacked by cholera died within hours.[43] Snow in his investigation naturally 'fixed his attention on the Broad Street pump as the source and centre of the calamity'.[44]

Dr. Snow as the stranger-investigator asked the Parish authorities to remove the pump handle. Amidst the horror of such a death dance, the strange prescription of this doctor was obeyed. As the legend goes, the 'pump handle was removed and the epidemic halted'. This episode shifted the attention towards this strange doctor, who now stood convinced about his water-borne theory of cholera causality and communicability.

Snow soon busied himself in drawing a new type of 'cholera map' of the Broad Street outbreak, which, in a very unique way, not only reduced all human suffering and misery of this small area in 'little black bars on a sheet of paper', but also conveyed to the world a comprehensive understanding of an otherwise 'inscrutable malady'.

Snow's comprehension of the problem and his analytical rigour in attempting to solve it was remarkable. From the symptoms of the disease Snow moved to the site of the disease; keeping an eye on it and the communicability factor by drawing analogies from other communicable disease, he speculated analytically both about the living nature of the '*materia morbis*' and water being its chief carrier (in a literal sense) through the faecal-oral route. Snow's contribution gave both the etiological and epidemiological investigation pertaining to cholera a firmer foundation and fillip.

It is generally understood that Snow 'saved the germ theory of cholera and catalyzed it further'[45] which 'culminated in the discovery of *comma bacillus* by Robert Koch in 1884'.[46] In his own days, Snow's theory was not accepted and he died a premature death in 1858. Much before Snow wrote his pamphlet on cholera in 1854, in an evidence to a Parliamentary inquiry in 1848–1849, he had drawn attention towards the dangers of attaching water closets to antiquated sewers that allowed leakage into surrounding water courses, thereby becoming the cause of epidemics. After his Soho investigation, he established the fact that water companies which drew water from the polluted section of the Thames caused more cholera mortality among the users, than water companies drew water from the unpolluted section of the river.[47]

However, Snow's findings in the above regard were not heeded to by the Parliamentary Committee appointed to inquire into the 1854 cholera epidemic. The committee clung to the prevailing 'miasmatic theory'.[48] Gradually, Snow's theory found converts from among his opponents. A very prominent member of the 1854 committee of inquiry, William Farr, statistician to the Registrar-General, talked of the earlier committee's error of not heeding to Snow's water-borne theory. Himself convinced of Snow's theory, while investigating London's final cholera epidemic of 1866,[49] Farr was 'thus prepared to scrutinize the water supply... and, despite denials by water company officials, (he) traced the source of epidemics to open ponds, tainted by sewage from a nearby river which were being used as emergency reserves. This practice was stopped and the epidemic ceased'.[50] Farr was revising his earlier anti-contagionist stance regarding cholera communicability and he mocked at his own earlier held conviction as, in his opinion, 'only a very robust scientific witness would have dared to drink a glass of water of the (river) Lea'.[51] Sir John Simon, who in Snow's lifetime had remained cold and aloof to his water-borne theory, described this theory in the 1870s as 'the most important truth yet acquired by medical science for the prevention of epidemic of cholera'.[52]

Cuningham's Obduracy Remains Intact

In contrast to the metropole where Farr got converted to Snow's theory, in the colony, his own disciple Bryden and Bryden's successor, J. M. Cuningham, not only remained stubbornly stuck to the 'miasmatic theory' and their anti-contagionist viewpoint, but even defended them as far as possible.

In the metropole the conversion from the air-borne theory to the water-borne theory had started from the 1860s. The 'weakness of the contagionists arose from their restricted epidemiological observations'[53] and their inablity to 'explain the occurrence of isolated cases where there was no proof of contact'.[54] Moreover, the fundamental pathology and site of the disease process in cholera and their possible linkages to epidemiological facts had not been very comprehensibly established before Snow. As alluded to earlier, Snow established the relationship between the etiological and epidemiological aspects of the disease. His epidemiological structure rested on a clear and sound understanding of the pathological process.[55]

The shift from the 'miasmatic theory' to the water-borne theory made the search and identification of that living '*materia morbis*' very important. And therefore, it is important now to stop our to and fro journey from the choleraic colony to the cholera stressed metropole so as to have a look at the 'colony under the microscope'. As already mentioned, the shift from 'miasmatism' to the water-borne theory was very late in the colony. Even Koch's theory of 1884 was not given its due immediately. Its acceptance had to await the retirement of J.M. Cuningham, who ironically, in his capacity as the Sanitary Commissioner of India, acted as the host for the German Cholera Commission led by Koch, just before the latter informed the world about the *vibrio cholerae* or the *comma bacillus*, as it was then called.

Colony under the Microscope

Till the mid 1880s, 'miasmaism' along with an idea of *'materia morbis'* coexisted, and was held by the colonial medical establishment as a validation of its anti-contagionist stance. Although there were a few individual rebels, they, instead of being heeded to, were castigated for holding a contrary opinion. The anti-contagionists thought that they could predict the outbreak of the disease in certain weather. The ecstasy of the attacking vibrios had an intimate link, they thought, with the disturbed state of the atmosphere. 'When the atmosphere is gloomy and clouds gather over head obstructing the sun's rays, but no shower comes within a day or two; we are sure that ecstasy of joy of the vibrio for devastation comes out. It appears to us that the period of their division comes then.'[56]

Koch, acting on the blueprint of Snow's water-borne theory, tried to establish the identity of the *'materia morbis'*. The isolation and bacteriological study of this *'materia morbis'* was only one element of his encompassing agenda. He strove like Snow to undertake a combined pathological, biological, and epidemiological program of enquiry. Koch's 'announcement of the isolation of the *comma bacillus* in February 1884, was not the first description of a vibrio'.[57] Many like Filippo Pacini in 1854 had characterized the cholera 'vibrion' and had also described the cholera symptoms in detail.

The novelty of Koch lay in the fact that he established the causal role of the vibrio by analytically moving from the 'sufficient' causality argument to the 'necessity' causality argument. In his investigations in Egypt and India, he found the microbe in the evacuations or in the small intestines of every cholera victim examined. As the *bacillus* could not be found in non-cholera deaths, i.e. in deaths caused by non-choleraic diarrhoea or intestinal disturbances, Koch first of all invoked the 'presence-absence' arguments. As all efforts to induce cholera in animals failed, he had to move from his 'presence-absence' argument in a different analytical direction. This became all the more necessary because the stress only on the 'presence' or the 'sufficiency' argument pertaining to the *bacillus* rendered it a weak and partial argument. 'The *bacillus* or microbe could, in fact, be but the concomitant to other factors present, any one (or several) of which might well be the true cause of the disease.'[58] Therefore, to make the argument sturdier, one had to move from the 'sufficiency' argument to the 'necessity' argument. This analytical step involving the shift from the 'sufficiency' to the 'necessity' argument was accomplished by Koch by focusing attention on the non-cholera sick and the healthy, where the presence of the *bacillus* was ***necessarily*** absent.

It was on the stength of the above lateral vision Koch could state that, 'the *vibrio cholerae* was the "necessary" cause of the disease because, in its absence or with other factors remaining the same (in so far as this is ever possible in biology), the disease, too, remained absent'.[59] Thus by underscoring the 'presence-absence' argument, Koch could provide a persuasive causal statement pertaining to the role of the vibrio in inducing cholera. I turn now to provide a brief family history of that 'villianous' vibrio as given by contemporary medical understanding.

Vibrio Cholerae: The Causative Organism of Cholera

As alluded to earlier, though *vibrio cholerae* was observed and scientifically marked, its causal role with finality was established by Koch in 1884. It was formerly called *vibrio comma, comma bacillus, spirillum cholerae asiatica.*

A member of the genus vibrio, it causes a number of important infectious syndromes. Ten human pathogens are currently recognized within the genus vibrio. Included are species associated primarily with gastro-intestinal illness and species associated primarily with soft tissue infection.[60] There are between 35 and 50 recognized species of vibrios that have nothing to do with cholera or diarrhoea.[61]

The anti-genic character of *vibrio cholerae* was demonstrated by Gardener and Venkatraman (1935). The species *vibrio cholerae* comprises a host of organisms classified on the basis of their somatic 'O' antigen. Those which agglutinate in 'O-group-I' antisera are called *'vibrio cholerae O-I'*. These exist in two bio-types, 'Classical' and *'El Tor'*, that are distinguished on the basis of a number of characteristics. Each bio-type is further subdivided into two sero types, termed Inaba and Ogawa.[62] The existence of these serological types was established by Kabeehima.[63]

With the established of the 'germ theory' and the advancement of bacteriological science, it is now held that a specific disease is caused by one species of bacteria however mild, severe, atypical the clinical picture, and however diverse its epidemiological factors. So any attempt to define cholera only on a clinical and epidemiological basis without regard to the specific species/organism will be regarded as incomplete from the public health perspective. It will be worthwhile to note that, this public health perspective incorporating the clinical, epidemiological, and bacteriological was being espoused by Mahendra Lal Sarkar at the turn of the twentieth century.[64] The modern Eurocentric definition of cholera lacks such a public health perspective, as has been pointed out at the beginning of this essay.

So cholera should be regarded as a disease which may occur in epidemic, endemic, and even in a sporadic form in which the whole range of symptoms come from the infections of the *vibrio cholerae* (Classical or *El Tor*). It was Hugh who showed that, from the taxonomic point of view, *El Tor* vibrios are solely a bio-type of *vibrio cholerae.*

General Characteristics of *Vibrio Cholerae*

Cholera vibrios are gram-negative rods, often occurring in comma shape, pleomorphic and resembling an 'S', and are non-capsulated. They have only one polar flagellum and are highly motile. They grow well between 30–40 degrees C, but less rapidly at lower temperature. The organisms grow better under aerobic than under anaerobic conditions. Alkalinity favours their multiplication. They easily reside in tidal rivers and bays. The organism has proven capable of establishing itself in inland water rather than in its classical niche of coastal salt water and has already become endemic in many such areas.

The Odd Cousin

The discussion will be incomplete without discussing 'non O-I vibrios'. Among the ten human pathogens within the genus vibrio, one in 'non-*O-I vibrio cholerae*'. This is so called because the vibrio is not agglutinated by 'O-I group' antisera prepared from Inaba and Ogawa sera-types. It does not imply that such vibrios cannot be agglutinated with sera prepared against their own antigens.[65] The 'non-*O-I vibrio cholerae*' are a heterogeneous group of organisms that are bio-chemically indistinguishable from '*O-I vibrio cholerae*', but fail to agglutinate in O-I antiserum.

Vibrio Cholerae: A Global Citizen

The *vibrio cholerae*, whose family history and identity have been alluded to in the above pages, was responsible for the various pandemics that occurred in the past. Though the number of pandemics are questionable due to the shifting focii of the disease and the time span accorded to it, we take this number to be seven, as has been mentioned in many medical textbooks. The first pandemic began in deltaic Bengal in 1814–1815 and lasted till 1823. It took Persia, Syria, Central Asia, and the Southern part of Russia within its ambit.

The second pandemic also started in India in 1826 and continued till 1837. Cholera revisited all the earlier lands which it had embraced in the first pandemic and took almost the entire Europe in its fold. In the east, China and Japan also came under its pestilential sway. The third pandemic lasted from 1846 to 1863, in which cholera revisited Europe and took both the Americas within its fold. The Far East or today's Southeast Asian countries were also invaded.

The fourth pandemic lasted from 1863 to 1879, when the Middle East, Europe and both the American continents fell under its sway. The fifth pandemic again began in India in 1879. It extended to Egypt and Europe in 1883. The disease reappeared in Russia and Europe in 1892. The sixth pandemic lasted from about 1898 to 1923. It was excessively disastrous for India in particular. Its reach extended to Burma, Malaya, Siam, China, Korea, Japan, and the Philippine Islands and also made its appearance in Persia, Syria, Turkey, and Russia.

With the exception of Russia, Europe has been relatively free from cholera since 1923. However, for the Asian countries, cholera is still considered a lurking danger. It is understood that we are living in the era of the seventh pandemic that started in 1961 and, though it has remained confined to Asia, is still ongoing.[66]

The largest number of cases and deaths due to cholera have been reported from India followed by the Philippines, Vietnam, Pakistan, Burma, Indonesia, Thailand, and Iran. In the period between 1961–1965, India alone was responsible for 73.9 per cent of the total world cases and 84.9 per cent of the total world deaths.[67] Even in the recent past, i.e. as late as 1993, there were 9,437 notified cases of cholera though the actual number may be much more inflated owing to the poor reporting about the disease from rural areas. Why is it that in rural areas, cholera appears even in advanced cities like Delhi, despite our entry into the 21st century? Quite recently, a news item in *The Hindustan Times* of the 17th May, 2002 reported that 'cholera and gastroenterities are taking a toll on Delhites, with more and more cases being reported'. As per the paper, the Municipal Corporation of Delhi puts the number of cholera cases at 228 and the number of gastroenterities cases as 17,534 till the 9th of May, 2002.[68]

Clinical Course

Both the above mentioned water-borne disease, i.e. cholera and gastroenteritis, display similar primary symptoms. They are both characteristically marked by loose motions and vomiting. The incubation period for cholera is one to three days and, at times, five to ten days. One of them is the typical, clinical cholera. The clinical course of cholera has been divided into several stages: 1. stage of premonitory diarrhoea; 2. stage of copious evacuations; 3. stage of collapse; 4. stage of reaction and 5. stage of uraemia.[69]

Mild forms which may never go beyond the first or the second stages represent 70 per cent to 95 per cent of the clinically manifest infections, and cholera is never suspected. A cholera epidemic is perhaps never anticipated before the typical cases occur because a few clinicians think of the possibility of a cholera infection when the disease is not officially reported in a country.[70] In an outbreak of every case of a 'classical' disease, there will be at least ten other cases of mild or asymptomatic infections.[71]

The patient becomes infective during the stage of incubation and remains so for a week or two after the convalescence. So, they are regarded as incubatory carriers. There are also post-convalescent carriers (when the convalescence is very short and in his apparent health, the patient happens to be a carrier). Besides these two, there are symptomless carriers, i.e., persons who do not show any clinical signs of the disease but who are excreting cholera vibrios.[72]

Antibiotic Treatment

When antibiotics were introduced in the treatment of infectious disease, there were great hopes that cholera would be among those that could be conquered with the aid of such agents, and so several invitro experiments were conducted which gave variable results. On the whole, invitro studies on vibrios gave favourable results. Soon, however, researchers had to concern themselves with the antibiotic resistant strains of the disease.[73] 'Almost since the beginning of the antibiotic era, bacterial resistance has been seen as the major obstacle to successful treatment. Hardly any group of antibiotics has been introduced into clinical practice to which some bacterium has not developed resistance.'[74]

In the context of the above fact, the Indian cholera situation becomes all the more alarming. In India, we have widespread use of antibiotics. This has led to drug resistant cholera. 'Strains of *vibrio cholerae* in India have become resistant to several antibiotics, and multi-drug resistance is increasing.'[75] Researchers of the National Institute of

Cholera and Enteric Disease in Calcutta who have conducted 'studies on *vibrio cholerae* strains isolated from patients in eastern India over the past six years show that the bacilli are resistant to several old as well as new antibiotics, including ampicillin, tetracycline, furazolidone, norfloxacin and ciprofloxacin'.[76] The Director of this institute, Dr. S. Bhattacharya has warned that 'our list of anti microbial agents still effective against cholera is shrinking and the emergency of resistance to specific antibiotics almost parallels the sequence in which the drugs were introduced in the market place'.[77]

Since we are in the seventh pandemic which started in 1961 and which continues today, the cases of cholera if not managed properly, can give rise to epidemics. India which does not have pure drinking water for a good part of the rural hinterland may have to relive the sufferings due to cholera epidemic. It is this concern which justifies our endeavour to look at the nineteenth century when cholera clouds hovered recurrently and yielded a rich harvest of death.

References

1. K. J. Isselbacher, E. Braunwald, J. D. Wilson, J. B. Martin, A. S. Fauci, D. L. Kasper (eds.), *Harrison's Principles of Internal Medicine*, vols. I and II, New York, New Delhi: Mc Graw (13th edition), 1994, p. 681.
2. *Ibid.*, p. 681.
3. *Ibid.*, p. 681.
4. 'EPIDEMIOLOGY: The study of the distribution and determinants of health-related states and events in populations, and the application of this study to the control of health problems. There have been many definition of epidemiology. In the past fifty years or so, the definition has broadened from concern with communicable disease epidemics to take in all phenomena related to health in populations. The *Oxford English Dictionary (OED)* gives as a definition: "That branch of medical science which treats of epidemics" and cites Parkin (1873) as a source. However, there was a 'London Epidemiological society' in the 1850s. The identity of the scholar who first used the word at that time has been lost. *Epidemiologia* appears in the title of a Spanish history of epidemics, *Epidemiologia espanola*, Madrid, 1802. Epidemics is much older. The word appears in Johnson's *Dictionary* (1755), and *OED* gives a citation dated 1603. The word was, of course, used by Hippocrates.' Taken from John M. Last (ed.), *A Dictionary of Epidemiology*, New York, Oxford, Toronto: Oxford University Press, 1983, pp. 32–33.
5. 'NOSOLOGY, NOSOGRAPHY: Classification of ill persons into groups, whatever the criteria for their classification, and agreement as to the boundaries of the groups, is called "nosology". The assignment of names to each disease entity in the group result in a nomenclature of disease entities, or nosography. (K. Faber, *Nosography in Modern Internal*

Medicine. New York: Hoeber, 1923).' Taken from John M. Last, (ed.) *A Dictionary of Epidemiology*, p. 71.

6. 'EPIDEMIC: [from the Greek *epi* (upon), *demos* (people)] The occurrence in a community or region of cases of an illness, specific health-related behaviour, or other health-related events clearly in excess of normal expectancy. The community or region, and the time period in which the cases occur, are specified precisely. The number of cases indicating the presence of an epidemic will vary according to the agent, size and type of population exposed, previous experience or lack of exposure to the disease, and time and place of occurrence; epidemicity is thus relative to usual frequency of the disease in the same area, among the specified population, at the same season of the year. A single case of a communicable disease long absent from a population or first invasion by a disease not previously recognized in that area requires immediate reporting and full field investigation; two cases of such a disease associated in time and place may be sufficient evidence to be considered an epidemic. The word may be used also to describe outbreaks of disease in animal or bird population.' Taken from John M. Last (ed.), *A Dictionary of Epidemiology*, p. 32.
7. Oscar Felsenfeld, *The Cholera Problem*, St. Louis, Missouri, USA: Warren H. Green Inc., 1967, p. 3.
8. Dion R. Bell, *Lecture Notes on Tropical Medicine*, Blackwell Scientific Publications, New Delhi: P. G. Publishing Pvt. Ltd. 1981, 1985, pp. 143–44.
9. 'ENDEMIC: The constant presence of a disease or infectious agent within a given geographical area or population group; may also refer to the usual prevalence of a given disease within such area or group.' Taken from John M. Last (ed.), *A Dictionary of Epidemiology*, p. 32. Sometimes, the term also indicates 'a disease of low morbidity that is constantly present in a human community, but clinically recognizable in only a few.' Taken from *Dorland's Pocket Medical Dictionary*, New Delhi & Calcutta: Oxford & IBH Publishing Co. Pvt. Ltd. 1995 (25th edition), p. 283.
10. M. A. Kamal, as quoted by Felsenfeld, in Oscar Felsenfeld's *The Cholera Problem*, p. 11.
11. R. Pollitzer, S. Swaroop and W. Burrows, *Cholera*, Geneva: World Health Organisation, Palais Des Nations, 1959, p. 52.
12. S. N. De, *Cholera: Its Pathology and Pathogenesis*, Edinburgh and London: Oliver and Boyd, 1961.
13. C. Macnamara, *A History of Asiatic Cholera*, London: Macmillan and Co, 1876.
14. R. Pollitzer, S. Swaroop and W. Burrows, *Cholera*, p. 14.
15. Oscar Felsenfeld, *The Cholera Problem*, pp. 4-5.
16. *Ibid.*, pp. 4-5.
17. Mahendra Lal Sarkar, *A Sketch of the Treatment of Cholera,* Calcutta: P. Sircar, Anglo Sanskrit Press, 1904 (2nd edition), p. 40.
18. *Ibid.*, p. 40.

19. *Ibid.*, p. 41.
20. *Ibid.*, p. 40.
21. *Ibid.*, p. 40.
22. *Ibid.*, pp. 40-41.
23. C. Macnamara, *A History of Asiatic Cholera*, London: Macmillan and Co, 1876 and Macpherson, *Annals of Cholera from the Earliest Period to the year 1817,* London: Ranken & Co., Durry House, 1872.
24. By juxtaposing the delineations by Macpherson and Macnamara, both contemporary historians of cholera in the nineteenth century, Dr. S. N. De, pathologist and bacteriologist, has demonstrated how one set of facts regarding the existence of cholera in European countries prior to 1817 was silenced so that credence to the Asiatic or more particularly Indian origin of cholera could be propagated and sustained. De allows the silent records to speak and the comparison of both the accounts makes De himself hypothesize a theory of 'local persistence of sub-clinical infection' which entails the possibility of endogenous recrudescence of cholera in Europe in the 1830s. Thus, De refutes the colonial construction of 'Asiatic' or Indian origin of cholera. See for further details S. N. De's *Cholera: Its Pathology and Pathogenesis,* Particularly the chapter 'Is Cholera Asiatic?' pp. 27-40.
25. In Sarkar's age, the dominant medicine's pharmacopea was slim; a few sheet anchor drugs were available and were administered in arbitrary doses. This was more true for an 'inscrutable malady'—cholera. It was this context which stimulated Sarkar to explore the therapeutic option of 'proven drugs' from homeopathy. For this 'blasphemous' veering towards homeopathic therapeutic option, Sarkar was ousted from the Calcutta chapter of the British Medical Association and was denied, for sometime, a position on the Faculty of Medicine of the Calcutta University.

    Strangely, Sarkar in his book on cholera remains impartial to both the pathies. He welcomed the homeopathic option for its reliance on 'proven drugs' as against the arbitrary practice of dominant medicine. But unlike Hahnemann and the later Hahnemmanians, Sarkar was not at all dismissive about the efficacies of knowledge of Bacteriology and Pathology in unravelling the causality of the mysterious disease. Rather, he wanted these emerging sub-disciplines of dominant medicine to be further strengthened. But his rights to be eclectic about theses matters were questioned by the dominant medical orthodoxy.
26. William Scott, *Report on the Epidemic Cholera as it has appeared in the territories of fort St. George. Drawn up by the order of the Government under the Superintendence of Medical Board,* Madras Asylum Press, 1824, p. ii.
27. *Ibid.*, p. ii.
28. Mark Harrison, *Public Health in British India: Anglo-Indian Preventive Medicine 1859–1914*, Cambridge: Cambridge University Press, 1994, p. 100, also see Arnold, 'Cholera and Colonialism' in *Past and Present*, No. 113, 1986, pp. 121-122.

29. T. W. Korner, *The Pleasures of Counting*, Cambridge University Press, 1996, pp. 3-4.
30. Geoffrey Gill, Sean Burrell, Jody Brown, 'Fear and Frustration—The Liverpool Riot of 1832' in *The Lancet*, vol. 358, July 21, 2001, p. 233. also see Norman Longmate, *King Cholera: The Biography of a Disease*, London: Hamish-Hamilton, 1966, pp. 24-25.
31. *Ibid.*, p. 233; Longmate, *King Cholera: The Biography of a Disease*, pp. 24-28.
32. Longmate, *King Cholera: The Biography of a Disease,* pp. 24-28.
33. Geoffrey Gill, Sean Burrell, Jody Brown, 'Fear and Frustration–The Liverpool Riot of 1832', p. 233.
34. *Ibid.*, pp. 233-237.
35. William Baly and William W. Gull, *Report on Epidemic Cholera drawn up at the desire of The Cholera Committee of The Royal College of Physicians*, London: John Churchill, 1854, p. 9.
36. S. N. De, *Cholera: Its Pathology and Pathogenesis,* p. 35.
37. Snow was in fact affirmative about this *'if'*. In his understanding, the disease which was communicated from person to person should be caused by 'some material' which passed from the sick to the healthy, and that it should have the property of increasing and multiplying in the systems of the persons it attacks. Snow drew analogy from other communicable diseases like syphilis, small-pox, and vaccinia where there *existed physical proof* of the increase of the morbid material when introduced within the human system. Snow extended this analogy to cholera. See B. W. Richardson, *Snow on Cholera being a reprint of Two Papers by John Snow, together with a Biographical Memoir,* Introduction by Wade Hampton Frost, New York, London: The Commonwealth Fund, 1936, pp. 14-15.
38. *Ibid.,* p. 15.
39. S. N. De, *Cholera: Its Pathology and Pathogenesis,* p. 9.
40. B. W. Richardson, *Snow on Cholera being a reprint of Two Papers by John Snow, together with a Biographical Memoir,* p. 22.
41. *Ibid.*, pp. 22-23.
42. T. W. Korner, *The Pleasures of Counting*, p. 5.
43. *Ibid.*, pp. 8-9. also see B. W. Richardson, *Snow on Cholera being a reprint of Two Papers by John Snow, together with a Biographical Memoir,* pp. 45-60.
44. *Ibid.*, p. 11, also see B. W. Richardson, *Snow on Cholera being a reprint of Two Papers by John Snow, together with a Biographical Memoir,* pp. 45-60.
45. S. N. De, *Cholera: Its Pathology and Pathogenesis,* p. 9.
46. *Ibid.*, p. 9.
47. Stephen Halliday, 'Death and Miasma in Victorian London: An Obstinate Belief', *The British Medical Journal*, vol. 323, 22nd to 29th December 2001, pp. 1469-1471.
48. T. W. Korner, *The Pleasures of Counting*, pp. 13-14.

49. Stephen Halliday, 'Death and Miasma in Victorian London: An Obstinate Belief', pp. 1469-1471.
50. T. W. Korner, *The Pleasures of Counting*, pp. 13-14.
51. Stephen Halliday, 'Death and Miasma in Victorian London: An Obstinate Belief', pp. 1469-1471.
52. Wade Hampton Forst, 'Introduction' in B. W. Richardson, *Snow on Cholera being a reprint of Two Papers by John Snow, together with a Biographical Memoir,* p. xix.
53. S. N. De, *Cholera: Its Pathology and Pathogenesis,* p. 9.
54. *Ibid.*, p. 9.
55. *Ibid.*, p. 9.
56. B. Dutt, *Why Cholera Requires Research,* Calcutta, 1932 (first edition), p. 35.
57. William Coleman, 'Koch's *Comma Bacillus*: The First Year' in *Bulletin of the History of Medicine*, vol. 61, no. 3, 1987.
58. *Ibid.*, p. 327.
59. *Ibid.*, p. 327.
60. K. J. Isselbacher, E. Braunwald, J. D. Wilson, J. B. Martin, A. S. Fauci, D. L. Kasper (ed.), *Harrison's Principles of Internal Medicine*, p. 683.
61. Oscar Felsenfeld, *The Cholera Problem*, p. 29.
62. K. J. Isselbacher *et. al.* (eds.), *Harrison's Principles of Internal Medicine*, p. 681.
63. R. Pollitzer, S. Swaroop and W. Burrows, *Cholera*, p. 222.
64. M. L. Sarkar, *A Sketch of the Treatment of Cholera,* p. 41–42.
65. Oscar Felsenfeld, *The Cholera Problem*, p. 29.
66. K. Park, *Park's Textbook of Preventive and Social Medicine,* Jaipur: Banarsidas Bhanot Publications, 1997, p. 163; also G. C. Shattuck, *Diease of the Tropics*, New York: Appleton-Century-Crofts, Inc., 1951, pp. 314-315.
67. K. C. Patnaik and P. N. Kapoor, *Statistical Review of Cholera Problem in India. With particular reference to Endemicity and Epidemicity,* Central Bureau of Health Intelligence, Ministry of Health and Family Planning, New Delhi, 1967, pp. 1-3.
68. *The Hindustan Times*, 17th May, 2002.
69. S. N. De, *Cholera: Its Pathology and Pathogenesis,* p. 1.
70. Oscar Felsenfeld, *The Cholera Problem*, p. 59.
71. D. R. Bell, *Lecture Notes on Tropical Medicine*, p. 145.
72. Oscar Felsenfeld, *The Cholera Problem*, pp. 60-61.
73. *Ibid.*, p. 94.
74. Selection from *British Medical Journal,* vol. 16, April 2000, p. 84. Also see *British Medical Journal,* vol. 320, 22 Jan. 2000, pp. 199-200.
75. Selection from *British Medical Journal,* vol. 17, March 2000, p. 28.
76. *Ibid.*, p. 28.
77. *Ibid.*, p. 28.

5

Calcutta Plague: Epidemic, Colonial Intervention and Indigenous Society 1898–1900

—Amal Das

Plague is an ancient disease of man. According to Vaid Kaviraj Vijayratna Sen, plague had been known to ancient Ayurveda as *'bradna'* and was caused by 'eating phlegm-producing and indigestible food, inhaling damp air and sleeping on damp beds'.[1] Thucydides has given us a tragic but brilliant episode of plague, which in 430 BC ravaged Athens and its population. In fact, he himself was its victim. The disease with all its scourges left an indelible memory on the minds of the Athenian people.[2] In England itself, the people were not unfamiliar with the word 'plague' and its deadly effect. 'a plague on both your houses' was a popular cry in Tudor England. The high mortality from plague, or '*black death*' as it was called was a terrible blow for the British empire. During colonial regime in India, this lethal disease reached its shore as a nightmare. The deadly effect of plague was so deeply felt by people of all ages and sex that one newspaper wrote on 8 April, 1899 'The word plague is even in the mouths of children'.[3] So that curse of plague horror had fallen both on the men of the cold countries like Europe as well as on the men of the warm countries like India.

Plague, although present in some parts of India during the nineteenth century, had first attracted the serious and alarming attention of the British Indian empire in the year 1896, when it broke out as an epidemic first in Bombay challenging the prosperity of one of British India's premier ports and administrative centres.[4] The crisis was further aggravated by the outbreak of plague epidemic in Calcutta two years later. This was a dangerous and threatening situation for the empire in India since Calcutta was at that time the seat of British capital in India and the main centre of all commercial and industrial activities. No disease in the colonial period created so much excitement, commotion and popular fury as plague did. The disease with a high rate of mortality and virulence was very massive in scale.

The paper will deal with the coming of the plague epidemic in Calcutta and its deadly outcome. It will examine only the epidemic's first, the most turbulent and serious phase, and not its long history. It is not an attempt at a comprehensive account of India's plague years. Although at the outset, the paper will tell, in brief, the beginning and movement of the lethal disease, the concern of the paper is to focus on the nature and implications of colonial medical intervention and the empire's plague policy and drastic measures. But the main thrust of the paper will be to study the disease as a focal point of social tension and indigenous popular outbursts that developed in urban areas. Of course, the plague with its political, social, economic, and demographic consequences deserves many different approaches and interpretations which the present paper will like to attempt.

I. Plague Epidemic—Its Beginning and Movement

No age group and sex escaped from this lethal disease. The people who had the misfortune to have a look at the dying plague patient stared horror-struck at the sight.[5] From a child of two and a half years to the very old, all were the victims of the disease.[6]

Official sources indicated that plague in Calcutta had its beginning in the month of April, 1898. The disease spread as an epidemic in Calcutta and the adjoining districts. Some died and many more were removed to hospitals. The first incident of plague that came to the notice of Cook, the health officer, happened in Kapalitala Lane near Bowbazar in central Calcutta. The day was a Sunday morning, the 17th of April, 1898. Cook, called up by the Inspector of police, Bowbazar, hurried to the spot accompanied by the police officer. There he saw the dead body of a man lying in a kutcha-built grocer's shop. The deceased was a young man of thirty and of good health. The origin of his infection could not be traced because he had not moved from Calcutta for quite some time. However, the history of the case is given below.[7]

> The deceased passed Thursday night at the house of a woman. On Friday morning, he returned home and went out as usual to sell ghee. He came back at 11.30 am somewhat earlier than usual and took his meals despite some pain in the groin and a feeling of uneasiness. But at 1 pm the pain was worse with a shivering. The fever turned severe and he was very restless and tossed about in

> his bed. He himself complained that his heart was bursting. On Saturday morning, he was unconscious till upto 10.30 am when he succumbed to death. On clinical examination, it was found that he had a left femoral bubo characteristic of a plague bubo. On post-mortem examination, made by Surgeon Major Gibbons, large extravasions of blood extending from the affected gland upwards and downwards and also small extravasions on the heart, and bowels were noticed which were very characteristics of plague.

Subsequent reports of plague cases received by Cook, proved that many more cases had already taken place which had been treated in the Medical College Hospital. These cases, as reported by Surgeon Colonel Bomford, the principal Medical Officer, were found to be true cases of plague after taking into consideration the clinical history in combination with the post-mortem appearances.[8]

From April 14th to 20th, the disease began to spread far and wide. Reports of plague cases were coming from Manicktola Hospital, Calcutta Medical College and Municipal Hospitals. Pusan, a child of two years and a half, Parbati, aged 26, the child's mother, Shaik Etwari, Kamini were cases of plague victims. The other worst victims of plague were the *doms*. Many among them who had assisted at the post-mortem examination of plague deceased, were attacked and then died. From April 20th to 30th, the disease began to spread further and a number of cases increased, the maximum number of cases happening on 24th April. Reports of plague cases were coming in large numbers throughout thc month of April. The official report shows that by the end of the month, the number of attacks in the city reached forty one which could be distributed as follows:

April 14th to 20th	-	7 Cases
April 21st to 27th	-	17 Cases
April 28th to 30th	-	17 Cases

The above statistics indicate that the outbreak was distinctively higher; the number of attacks reported in the second week being nearly two and half times more than the number of attacks in the first and the number of attacks in the three days at the end of the month being equal to the number in the preceding week.

From the statistics furnished officially upto the 2nd of July 1898 of plagues attacks and death, it is found that the total number of attacks upto that time stood at 190, or 0.027 per cent of the population. The number of mortality was 155 in 16 weeks, or 0.74 per cent per mile per annum. But after the official announcement that plague had entered into the city, the reported cases were noticeably fewer, probably for lack of knowledge on the part of the government due to concealment of cases by people. The following table gives the number of attacks and deaths from plague upto July 6, 1898.[9] This will provide an idea of the nature of plague attacks, mortality, and calamity.

	Male	*Female*	*Total*
Seizures	152	38	190
Death	126	29	155

II. Colonial Medical Intervention

The rapid spread of the disease and the increasing number of attacks and deaths perplexed the colonial state and its health department much more than other lethal diseases like cholera, malaria, and small-pox. Behind this lay several reasons.

Unlike malaria, cholera, and small-pox which were regarded as native diseases, plague was seen by the colonial rulers as an invading disease which had its root probably from Hongkong by sea-route.[10] So the state and its medical team were determined to resist it by any means before it could establish itself. Secondly, the disease had completely altered the demographic map of the city. Many died of plague and many more fled out of scare. The up-country labouring coolies fled to their native home.[11] Thirdly, European commercial and industrial magnates and their organizations like the Bengal Chamber of Commerce, the Indian Jute Mills' Association, Traders' Associations exerted tremendous pressure on the colonial empire and its health department since British economy in India was dangerously threatened with the outbreak of plague epidemic. The desertion of labourers completely paralysed trade and commerce. The loss incurred by the European commercial and industrial establishments was heavy. As *Amrita Bazar Patrika*, a contemporary local daily observed, 'trade, commerce and business of every description was dislocated'.[12] The Bengal Chamber of Commerce and the Indian Jute Mills' Association sent repeated letters to the Government of Bengal putting much stress on the impending economic danger. This apart, the economic pressure for prompt action was increased by the possibility of an European embargo on Indian trade unless the epidemic was speedily brought under control. Fourthly, no less significant was the pressure that came from the medical experts in Britain and India. They suggested appropriate prompt measures and their quick and thorough implementation to curb the disease. Fifthly, the protection of the health of the British army, the British administrators, and the European civil population in the British Indian empire from epidemic diseases persuaded the colonial state to pay more attention to the matter. Finally, plague had shattered the general life of the people of the city.

Worried by the development and pressed by the circumstances, the empire in India paid serious attention to the matter. It had to rely entirely upon its doctors and health department to tide over the crisis. European doctors, and the health department were empowered with full authority and responsibility for the first time in colonial history in India to deal with the very tough situation.[13] Although financial as well as political constraints discouraged the colonial state from a greater degree of medical intervention until late in the 19th century, there was, however, a substantial change in state attitudes soon after as the alarming situation demanded it.

In this connection, it may be mentioned that the tremendous development of public health system in Great Britain, the success in sanitary and environmental reforms, and the curbing of epidemics in Great Britain created pressure for similar campaigns in India. Western medical science expanded significantly in colonial India at a time when plague reached India towards the end of the 19th century. This expansion encouraged greater medical and government intervention to eradicate lethal diseases like plague, cholera, small-pox etc. The birth of medical institutions with high prospects, the development of distinctive worthy medical research in India, more particularly in tropical diseases, a grid of western-oriented hospitals, clinics, public health policies, the advances made by Louis Pasteur, Robert Koch and many others in the new science of bacteriology, the development of analytical treatment methods—all these created a confidence among British doctors and officials of the health department in India that epidemic diseases could be 'conquered' only through the application of western scientific knowledge and reason and not through indigenous system of medicine and treatment.

Despite such advances made by western medical science in colonial India, the medical department and its doctors took quite a long time to understand the etiology of plague disease. The role of rats in its transmission was still generally thought secondary to that of man. The part played by rats' fleas in spreading the disease was finally established in 1908. The human body including clothes, bedding, and habitations associated with it, were regarded as the disease's principal source of origin.

The colonial health department and the European doctors, being highly equipped with western medical knowledge, science, and reason, made an all-out attempt to stop the disease from spreading in the wider part of the city and around. They had to impose discipline in the entire medical system. The doctors began their task with the process of strictest observation of the suspected plague patients. The intention was to determine thoroughly the specific symptoms of attack by the method of clinical examination. The plague hospitals and clinics were brought under the strictest system of discipline through a series of measures. Registers were maintained with proper specifications and these were well circulated among the doctors. The regular meetings of doctors on an emergency basis to compare them, the transmission of their data to the government, the keeping of the records and statistics of attacks, cures, deaths were the main parts of the disciplinary process. The plague hospitals and clinics were transformed into great laboratories where thorough investigations were made.[14] Cases of Iswar Chandra Dey, Parbati, and Pusan were thoroughly examined. From post-mortem examination, clinical history, pathological, microscopical and cultural confirmation, the doctors came to the conclusion that they were genuine plague cases. The *doms* who assisted at the post-mortem of Iswar Chandra Dey, were segregated to Manicktola hospital for close observation.[15]

'A number of medical men closely observed Budri's case'—says a medical report. Hence the cases of Suku, Parbati, Iswar Chandra Dey, and *doms* were individually recorded and registered. The charts were regularly maintained and closely observed in order to watch the nature and symptoms of attack. The conflicting opinions of the doctors about a number of cases had been confirmed by such clinical examination. A physical examination was made to try to find the characteristic buboes or swellings. In dubious cases, post-mortems were used to search for internal evidences. This was evident from the following report of Dr. Cook.

> "Had it not been for the post-mortem appearances and typical plague cultures from Iswar Chunder Dey's case, I could not myself have said that Pusan, Parbutty and Budri were plague cases, though I should have regarded Parbutty's case as extremely suspicious. Of the other contacts, none developed plague, so they were discharged after ten days' segregation."[16]

Apart from these, a sign of medical efficiency and alertness was visibly seen in the wide range of publications of medical reports showing the analyses of plague symptoms, the circulation of a good number of medical bulletins, reports, gazettes, pamphlets, leaflets. Added to these, the medical department was entrusted with the task of protecting the general health of the public by the removal of the insanitary and filthy conditions to be found in towns and villages in the perspective of the outbreak of lethal diseases. The responsibility for health and sanitation was now taken away from the municipal councillors and given to small committees of European doctors, health officials, and civil servants.[17] In this way the control of the colonial medical department was rigidly enforced and kept under its grip. Never before had the medical department in colonial India exercised such a tremendous power and position over the indigenous population with a commanding voice.

III. Plague Policy of the Colonial Government: Preventive Measures

While Cook and other European doctors were concerned with the medical matter only, the colonial government was busy in formulating a plague policy and its effective implementation. To end diagnostic confusion and conflicting opinions of the doctors, the Lt. Governor, after considering Haffkine's positive affirmation of the cases of plague and the collective opinions of the practitioners, officially declared on 29th April 1898, the presence of plague as an epidemic.

The significant aspect of government's policy was the announcement of anti-plague measures under the Epidemic Diseases Act. One of such provisions was 'segregation'. If on enquiry it was found by the health officers that a fatal case of plague had occurred in the house or that any person therein was suffering from or infected with plague, he had the power to segregate the affected person to a hospital for immediate treatment. He was also empowered to remove other members of a plague-affected family and even all occupants of the neighbouring houses which were likely to be infected to a 'segregation camp' and detain them under observation for ten days.[18] Foucault's analogy between the prison and the hospital was most evident in these colonial measures such as hospitalization and segregation. The colonial government believed that such measures would offer better opportunities for isolation, observation, and control.

Another important provision was 'disinfection'. In a house where a case of plague had occurred, the Sub-Divisional Magistrate or Health Officer was given the power to take measures to disinfect and clean the house, to destroy bedding, clothes and other articles of similar nature and to improve the sanitary condition of the premises. The Sub-Divisional Magistrate might, on the report of the health officer, order the burning or destruction of any hut or other temporary structure if disinfection could not be satisfactorily effected. Otherwise, awarding of compensation to rebuild the structure that had been burnt or destroyed was considered.[19]

'Inoculation' was another significant provision of anti-plague measures. With regard to inoculation, it was said that inmates of an affected house could be given the option of being inoculated instead of being removed to an observation camp for the full period of inoculation. But after inoculation, it would be required to confine them to a segregation camp in the course of the inoculation under proper shelter and medical supervision.[20]

The anti-plague provisions thus empowered the government to detain and segregate plague suspects, to destroy property infected by the disease, to disinfect, evaluate, and even burn houses suspected of contamination. The government had even the power to prohibit fairs and festivals, examine road travellers, and rail passengers.

Additional Administrative Measures—Signs of Authority and Control

As plague was seen as an 'invading' disease by the British, special establishments were set up to tackle it. Medical officers, entrusted with the duties of inspection and enquiry for disinfection, house to house visit and inoculation, were appointed. The Plague Commission was entrusted with the duties to suggest appropriate measures for the improvement of sanitation and health of the people of Calcutta and its suburbs. While the administrative authority organized its forces, the commissioners were busy in forming vigilance committees in the district and ward committees in all the wards. Military officers were appointed to assist the district committees who were entrusted with the duties to detect plague cases. The government increased the strength of reserved armed forces in order to give effect to the plague regulations and the consequent danger arising out of the implementation of the government policy and plague measures.[21]

IV. Impact on Indigenous Society

(1) Rumours

As soon as plague was officially declared, rumours began to spread like wildfire and people who heard it, believed it at once and spread the tales to others and there were many to confirm the tales. Anxiety gradually extended down to the masses of the people. When Sir John Woodburn, the Lt. Governor of Bengal, held a meeting with doctors at the Eden Hospital to discuss the likelihood of an outbreak of plague in Calcutta, rumour rapidly spread. By noon the same day, 28th April, 1898, 'the excitement in the town was intense. In business houses and in bazaars, streets and bustees the question was discussed, had the dreaded Bombay plague come at last, were their houses going to be forcibly entered, and their wives and daughters torn away by British soldiers, was quarantine to be established, and were they all to be forcibly inoculated'.[21A]

Premankur Atarthi's memoir *Mahasthabir Jataka* depicted a typical case of plague rumour.[22]

> "One day the news spread that one woman arrived at the Howrah station by Bombay Mail and then started for Calcutta by hiring a carriage. When she came to Harrison Road in Central Calcutta, the carriage driver asked her, 'which place do you want to go?' The woman replied, 'don't you know me? I am the goddess of Plague. Then suddenly, she disappeared from the scene".

This rumour spread like wildfire and people cried out; 'Plague, everywhere plague, it's better to escape'. They believed that plague had invaded the city and the only way to save their life was to run away.[23] The rumours were mostly related to poisoning, inoculation, seizing and searching. Commonest of all rumours were those relating to the deliberate poisoning of Indians by doctors, hospital staff, and other colonial agencies. It was believed by the people that something was put to the noses of the patients in the white Bombay ambulance and that they died after swollowing it, also that there was a poisoned needle concealed in it which killed them. A rumour spread that the Queen desired to thin out her Indian subjects and so had given orders that they were to be inoculated with plague poison and thus to make them die a horrible death.

It was again rumoured that the Viceroy met a Yogi in some remote spot in the Himalayas and made compact with him to sacrifice two lakhs of lives to the goddess *Kali* to save the British Government of India. The British were suspected of trying to keep this bargain by distributing poisonous white powders and black pills and by giving lethal inoculations.[24] The most general idea was that government had found from the census and occurrence of recent famines, that the population was too large and consequently had given a sort of contract to the doctors to kill off so many lakhs.

This kind of rumour was limitless. If a man was questioned as to what he was afraid of, he replied that the ticcawallah would inject poison and he would at once die. This would be done because the hukum (order) from the Viceroy had gone out and the ticcawallah would carry out the order.[25]

It was further rumoured that the Viceroy was to come to Calcutta on the 15th of May, 1898, when men and women were to be forcibly inoculated; that the government was only waiting till a large proportion of the population had left, that the soldiers would be called out soon and inoculation enforced compulsorily, that the plague serum was being made from cows' blood. It was even rumoured later that the Queen had abdicated and that Gladstone had died of plague and that the emperor of Russia was marching to Calcutta.[26]

A similar kind of rumour among the urban poor could be shown from John Campbell Oman's presenting of rumour in connection with small-pox. The following was the kind of rumour that the author stated:

> "During the summer of 1878, when small-pox was going about Lahore, I was told by one of my domestic servants, not without a touch of suppressed feeling, that the *Sirkar* had given orders that the native women should all be vaccinated, not as usual, on the arm but on the breast."[27]

It is not my aim to measure the validity or absurdity of these rumours. But some significant elements come out of such rumours. First of all, the rumours prove that how widely the epidemic was discussed among the population. The rumours appear to take us appreciably closer to popular perceptions and responses than most other available sources. Secondly, the mode of popular discourses exhibits the atmosphere of fear and uncertainty generated by the plague measures and the colonial medical intervention. Thirdly, the significant element that emerges out of this kind of rumour was the deep distrust and strong hatred nurtured by the urban poor against colonial medical intervention and plague measures.

Under such serious condition, the rumours, whatsoever, got an easy access in the society with intense feeling. Although it was officially alleged that these rumours were set in circulation by *'badmashes'* (criminal elements) with the object of frightening people and getting an opportunity of looting them, a leading contemporary newspaper in its editorial, however, commented that the lower class people who spread the plague tales, could not be called *'badmashes'* for 'most of them are peaceful citizens—husbands and fathers who are never known to have ever broken in public peace'. Even one important official report had to comment that it was 'extraordinary how natives occupying a respectable position gave credence to the wildest and most improbable stories'.[28]

(2) Panic and Scare

By the end of April, 1898 when there was plague cry everywhere in Calcutta, the fear of plague and resentment for attempts made by government to effect 'plague regulations' were assuming very serious character. There was panic and scare throughout the city because the public had the feeling that the Government of Bengal would put them to the same severe treatment as in Bombay. The immediate sequel to this panic was the desertion of people from the city. A great number of people had already left the town on the 28th and 29th April due to the recrudescence of plague, and five hundred people had been refused tickets at Howrah station. But on the 30th April, the day when the plague was officially declared, there was a regular stampede by rail, river, and road. The people were unmindful of the excessive hardships suffered due to a sudden and unexpected migration of a whole family, including females, and little children. These included not only the urban poor, but even many respectable families who had never thought of walking in public streets without the male members or in closed carriages or palkies. They now made their way eagerly on foot to the station covered with thick veils. The fare demanded was exorbitant. In some cases, one rupee was charged for every minute. Howrah bridge was blocked. It was generally estimated in the town that from a quarter to one third of the population left. Many houses were vacant.[29]

There was large-scale desertion of mill labourers out of panic and plague scare. The reports of the special Inspectors of Factories hinted the intensity of scare and panic that existed among the mill labourers on both sides of the river. According to available reports, fear of the disease combined with segregation and inoculation disrupted the labour force in mills, particularly the mills in and around Calcutta.[30]

A letter received by the Government of Bengal from the Bengal Chamber of Commerce on 4th May, 1898, exhibited the inoculation scare and panic at its height:

> I am directed by the Committee of the Bengal Chamber of Commerce to represent to you the urgent necessity of notice being immediately given, in the most widespread manner possible, whether by handbills or by beat of drum that there is no intention on the part of the authorities to make inoculation compulsory. It is especially necessary that the notice should be conveyed in such a manner as to be plain to the most ignorant people, as there is still a widespread idea, erroneous of course, that Government are intending to introduce compulsory inoculation.[31]

The native newspapers were very prompt in publishing the fear and sentiments of the people. One of the contemporary leading Bengali dailies described the fear thus:

> You see people are running, men and women are running away for lives. Is a tiger after them? No, nothing of that kind. Is the monster of plague coming to eat them? No, of course, they have heard of

> plague patients, but not seen one. They are yet trying to flee but why? It is just to avoid Government policy.[32] (Translated into English)

A good instance of public fear from plague regulations and administrative measures could be shown from Tagore's '*Chaturanga*', composed in Bengali.

> In that year of the first outbreak of plague in Calcutta, people were panic-stricken and extremely anxious, not so much for the dread of the disease but for the coercions and persecutions that were inflicted upon them by the peons and orderlies who went about with their official badges on.[33] (Rendered into English)

(3) Reality of the Panic

Why were the masses so fearful of plague regulations and government policy than the disease itself? Some possible explanations may be put forward here.

The provision of segregation of plague patients or suspected ones into the segregation camp or to a hospital for a period of minimum ten days was the most significant issue. Under this provision, the above patients would be kept confined for ten days for observation and if, after ten days, they were found not developing any plague symptoms, they would be released. This meant a separation of a plague patient or a suspected one from the rest of the members of his family, from most near and dear ones. It would separate a husband from his wife and children or vice versa.

The provision which says that 'persons, found to be suffering from plague are, at their discretion, permitted to report to ward, caste or family hospitals, maintained by private contribution instead of being removed for segregation to the public hospitals', benefitted only the middle classes of the society since they had the resources to set apart a portion of their dwelling or garden houses under the restrictions for use as private hospitals for themselves and their families.[34]

So the provision of segregation was less harmful to the middle classes of people than it was the case with the urban poor. The latter were the worst victims of the regulations because they had neither the resources to set up family hospitals nor any vacant space in their dwelling huts to set apart for such purpose. Hence, the only course that was left for a poor plague patient was to remove him either to the public hospitals of Manicktalah, Marcus Square, Budge Budge or to a camp or ward hospitals of the government.

To the urban poor, compulsory segregation accompanied with ten days strictest observation and detention was a very painful measure as it completely changed the rhythm of his life and pattern of living. Generally, among the urban poor, a large number earned their bread as casual labourers on daily basis working in the mills, factories, workshops. Some of them were employed as carters, sweepers, scavengers, municipal and railway coolies. A section of the urban poor was also engaged in unproductive means of livelihood such as begging, prostitution etc.[35] To all of them, a day meant a day of earning. The consequence was much more acute and problematic for such a poor man's family in which the plague infected patient or a suspected one happened to become the only earning member for the whole family. So concealment of cases for fear of confinement or the attempt to run away from the town to avoid segregation was very common among these classes of people.[36] Instances are not lacking where poor people were expressing their bitter resentment against removal to the segregation camps or plague hospitals. The reaction of the municipal conservancy sweepers may be cited as an instance. They threatened to strike work in the evening of the 20th May, 1898 on the ground that they were underpaid and more exposed to plague than any other class, and if they were attacked with plague and removed to the segregation camps, their families would remain without food. Under the given situation, quarantine meant more than a severe penalty, almost a death penalty for these poor people. It brought about a complete disruption in urban poor's family life and his social activities.[37]

Though the British empire in India regarded their plague hospitals or the segregation camps as the most healthy place for treatment and sanitation, the natives looked upon them with deep distrust and contempt. They regarded the hospitals as the 'Temple of Yama', a house of horrors, the place of killing the people, and the ill-centres of death.[38] While the government regarded the Manicktala hospital as an excellent plague hospital, the common people held the view that 'Manicktollah is a golgatha of Calcutta, a place of burial', so to say of a man 'he's gone to Manicktollah' is equivalent to saying, 'he's gone to his last resting place'.[39] This was the kind of distrust and suspicion nurtured by the people about the plague hospitals and the western system of treatment. They wanted to be treated by their family physicians, *hakims*, *vaids*. They did not like any sort of help from the colonial government. Major H. E. Deane, special health officer, had himself heard that people used to say, 'what is the use of this bother, we must die some time, and what matter if we die of plague'?[40] The high mortality in the plague hospitals increased the suspicion of these classes. As a consequence, these people used all means for concealing cases and mobbing ambulance parties to prevent the plague officers from sending their friends and relatives to what they considered an undesirable place, a place of pollution, contaminated by blood and faeces.[41]

From a sanitary point of view, it cannot be denied that the provision of disinfection was necessary for a house or a hut. But it hit hardest the poorer people as they had no other place to live in. 'You are only doing this to worry us', said the poor man to the disinfecting officers when operations were carried out.[42] Why? The answer lies in their poverty, uncertainty and unsettlement of life.

The destruction of bedding, clothes, and other articles might not be a serious concern to the middle classes of the society as they had the resources to purchase those articles. But it really mattered to the poor people of the society. Data of their living conditions reveal that the full amount of their earnings was to be spent on buying food. Under such pathetic condition, the burning of bedding, clothes, and other small furniture on the plea of disinfection was a severe blow for them.

The destruction or burning of huts meant the complete displacement of their family. It brought uncertainty and disruption in their life. Of course, compensation was granted to the hut owner for the erection of new construction but that was a question of time which adversely affected their life. Added to this, there was however no guarantee that the hut owner would let his hut to the old occupier.

Disinfection in plague cases and suspected ones was compulsory. But the subalterns, hardest hit by the provision of disinfection, showed bitter resentment against it. Even instances of bitterness among high caste men were seen. A brahmin family which was attacked by a case of plague, was visited by the plague officers for disinfection. The members of the family did not believe that it was a genuine case of plague. After a great deal of persuasion, they agreed to disinfection but wanted ten days' rest for performing some religious ceremonies. But that was not allowed by the plague officers.[43]

The *doms* were in great disadvantage as a result of the government policy and plague measures. The provision that the beddings, clothes, contaminated by the deceased plague patient was to be burnt or destroyed, appeared as a direct encroachment on their traditional practice. It was a customary practice going on for a long time among the Hindus that the beddings and clothes of the deceased would not be burnt or destroyed but be given to the *doms*. But the plague measures had taken away their old practice.

So the *doms* who believed that this had now become their legitimate right by virtue of their traditional practice, took it as a deliberate attempt on the part of the colonial state to snatch away their right. In fact, they had their earnings by the sale of those beddings and clothes to the buyers. From the point of view of sanitation and health, the state was fully justified in its action since such practice helped the spread of the disease in the society. But to the poor *dom*, any such consideration was absolutely meaningless since this would stop his regular source of earning.

(4) Popular Resistance

Evidences hint that the popular resistance reflected through protests, strikes, and riots against colonial drastic plague measures was the actions of the subalterns of the society, irrespective of Hindus and Muslims. They comprised the municipal coolies, scavengers, sweepers, carters, butchers, menial servants, workshop and railway coolies, mill labourers who were the worst victims of the plague measures. Social tension was up and very intense among these classes of people. So, opposition to plague measures and western medical intervention was very strong among them.[44]

Since the beginning of May 1898, a series of disturbances, riots, and strikes occurred in Calcutta and neighbouring areas. On 30th April, the municipal coolies in the markets of Calcutta threatened to strike. On one occasion, an ambulance was burnt in Champatolla near College Street. Throughout the month of May, a series of riots took place. On 3rd May, from early morning, there was indication of a general outbreak throughout the city. Groups of excited mobs were seen collected along the sides of Circular Road, Cornwallis Street, Mechua Bazar, Chitpore Road etc., as if they were waiting for a signal for any riot that might break out in the city. A young Austrian was beaten to death. He was carrying a handbag, and was suspected of being an inoculator. A furious mob at Bhowanipore attacked a district Medical Officer, S. R. Laing who had to shoot in self-defence.

Simultaneously, the strikes spread among subalterns in the society. The workers and mill labourers, the butchers in the general markets, the conservancy coolies, the municipal conservancy sweepers started strikes at different dates out of panic and inoculation scare. Besides, there had been other strikes carried out by railway and shipping coolies against plague regulations.[45]

(5) Popular Consciousness

From these riots and strikes, some specific features emerged which were the signs of popular consciousness. One significant feature of these riots and strikes was the quick mobilization and unity of actions by the people. Whenever an inoculator was at sight, either near bustees, or in a street or near the factories and mills, the mob at once assembled together and showed greater unity and solidarity in driving him out. The unity and solidarity was so strong that it forced the government to stop vaccination on several occasions, at least temporarily.[46]

Another striking feature of the riots and strikes was swiftness in actions and the quick dispersal. A glaring instance of this, among others was a riot in the Messers Burn and Co. in Howrah. The employees of the concern attacked the government pleader, Rai Narsingha Dutta Bahadur who was suspected of being an inoculator as he tried to argue with them. They went further and destroyed a number of *Jhilmills* of various doors in the civil court where the pleader took shelter and failing to find him there, attacked the *peshkar* in the compound whose head was broken as a result of attack. The whole event was completed within less than fifteen minutes since the start and the most surprising thing was that the incident happened at a place from where the police lines were very close. When the police force went to the yard, they found all working as usual as if nothing had happened.[47]

In these kind of popular actions, the targets of attacks were aimed at the inoculation officers, police, government pleaders, *peshkars* and European. Soon the target did not exclude even men wearing European dress or using European hat. The mob nourished a bitter resentment against a hatman and the native government officials who dressed themselves like Europeans. To the labourers and thousands of Indian peasants, the 'hat' was a significant symbol of the whitemen constituting a different race. The difference between the nations of western Europe and the 'conquered people' in social structure, food, clothes, religion, decorative styles was accentuated by the difference in physical appearance. Several attacks were made during the riots on hatman.[48]

Not only European dress but European decorations too, were targets of attack by the infuriated mob. If any inoculator or government officials could not be traced, the target was at once pointed to European decoration. That was evident from the destruction of a number of *Jhilmills* on doors in the civil court by the mob when they chased the government pleader Rai Narasingha Dutta Bahadur.[49] All these elements focus on the nature of behavioural aspects of the subalterns. It marked an attitude of defiance which was to be viewed in the perspective of the growing popular consciousness and anti-imperialist attitude.

The common people had their own grievances against government policy and measures which developed from their perceptions and awareness of the situation. Their suspicion led them to believe that the alien government of 'white European' had no sympathy for the Indians. It was capricious in tone and temperament and had been toying with their life. A sense of awareness led them to believe that the state had, without any valid ground, encroached upon their religious, social, and individual rights.

That the ordinary people had developed some sense of *ijjat* (honour) and humiliation, was evident when they were subjected to strictest examination. The examination of rail passengers travelling to Calcutta via Khana junction had evoked strong protests. Passengers were ordered to alight and wait in lines after being segregated by sex. They had been publicity inspected by a European doctor.[50] It was insulting to them and the *ijjat* of the females, was at stake. It was only after a considerable protest against this that screens were provided for the examination of women and women doctors were found to conduct them. Sarat Chandra Chattopadhyay in his Bengali novel *Srikanta* narrated distinctly how the *ijjat* of his hero Srikanta and other passengers, both male and female, had been attacked when they had been examined by the white doctors at having to wait in lines before being allowed to move for Rangoon. The doctor publicly examined the secret and sensitive parts of the bodies of all, irrespective of sex. So freely, roughly, and unhesitantly did the doctor examine the bodies of all that, the author said that even a wooden doll would have cried out in protest.[51] The native newspapers were highly critical of this type of examination. In October, 1896, a European doctor in Calcutta aroused protest by insisting on examining the body of a *zenana* lady who had died from mumps on the suspicion that she might have had plague. He asked the male members to vacate the room and then, without permission, took a sample of blood for examination. 'If this is not high-handedness' commented *Hitavadi* on 30th October, 1896, 'nothing is'.[52]

V. Change in Government Policy — A Moderate Tone and Attitude

The Lt. Governor, forced by circumstances, announced several relaxations in plague regulations. In regard to the government policy of segregation, the Lt. Governor assured the people that 'Whenever segregation is necessary it will be carried out with the strictest regard to the feelings of human nature. No wife shall be separated from her husband, no husband from his family and the better classes will receive every encouragement in the arrangement of private hospitals in their own compounds or in garden-houses in the suburbs, to which they can remove themselves and their families in case of attack'. About the scheme of inoculation, the Lt. Governor assured the people saying, 'Inoculation, I repeat, will be pressed on nobody'. At the time, he stressed on the necessity of inoculation to fight with plague. He expressed his opinion about the importance of segregation and inoculation thus: 'The policy of segregation is a painful necessity, the policy of inoculation is at least and for the first time in the great battle with plague in India, a policy of hope'. 'I am told', he said further, 'large number of people are leaving Calcutta under the apprehension that quarantine is about to be established. They may be reassured that there is no such intention whatever'. The government had shown its liberal attitude by the modifications of the rules that the families which had been completely inoculated would now be exempted from inoculation even if plague attacked any member of the family. Although risk was involved in this kind of exemption yet the policy was accepted from the belief that the inoculated patient would have the very mildest from of attack, and would not be a material danger to his family or neighbours. The modified regulation also included the provision that no one would be declared plague-stricken without being seen by a competent medical officer, male or female deputed by the municipality and no person would be removed except on the order of a medical officer. There would be no forcible removal through police or the army. Further, no one would be separated from his or her family. If necessary, all would go together to a camp, where the *purdah* would be respected.[53]

That the government was desirous of coming to a compromise with a section of the Indians was evidently clear from the new provisions of the regulations. The modifications of rules did not satisfy all classes of people equally. The provisions of private hospitals, family hospitals, *purdah* system etc., benefitted only the middle classes of the society. The urban poor had gained nothing from such relaxations. To prevent large-scale discontent, the government finally realized that they should understand the minds of the people and there must be some sort of flexibility on some points. A letter that was sent to Lord Elgin, the Viceroy, on April, 29, 1898 by Sir A. P. MacDonnell, the Lt. Governor of the North-Western provinces expressed the fear of the government.

> "In the present state of public feeling in the country, I consider the danger of popular discontent and tumult to be a more serious evil than even the prolongation of the disease."[54]

To stop the discontent going on in large-scale among the urban poor, the government ultimately had to seek the help of the Indian middle classes. How the latter responded at this hour of crisis is a matter to be looked up.

VI. Attitude and Response of the Indian Middle Class

While the subalterns revolted against the government's plague regulations and inoculations system, the Indian middle class had shown its favourable responsive attitude. The government's claim to success in its inoculation policy was confined only to this class who were western educated professionals and occupied a respectable position in the indigenous society. This enlightened class came forward to make the British inoculation drive a success by voluntarily agreeing to be inoculated and encouraging some of their followers to do so.[55]

A few names and their significant role can be given as instances. On 1st May, 1898, the second day after the official announcement of plague and the opening of the inoculation campaign at the request of Babu Dwaraka Nath Ganguly, Assistant Secretary to the Indian Association and his wife, Kadambini Ganguli, Cook, the health officer, inoculated sixty-one members of the Brahmo Samaj at 13, Cornwallis Street, which included men, women, and children. This was the first contingent of the enlightened community that volunteered for inoculation. On the 2nd and 4th May, the students of the American College, an enlightened body of the indigenous society of nearly 100 members were inoculated on voluntary basis.[56]

Another native gentleman of social pre-eminence and high position who voluntarily agreed to be inoculated and set an example to others was Raja Binay Krishna Bahadur of Shovabazar who was inoculated at the Rajbari with the Maharani and other members of his family and friends, numbering sixty in all, on the 10th of May. But surprisingly enough, the raja did not risk asking his servants to be inoculated on account of the panic among their classes, in spite of the fact that he himself and his family were held in high respect and great confidence by his servants. As the latter were very much loyal and obedient to the raja and his family, they came in a body and asked why would they be deprived of the share of the benefit of the 'ticca'. The raja, by virtue of his position, dignity and power was subsequently successful in convincing many of his followers and his tenants to agree to inoculation. These included a brahmin *pandit* of high position and his wife, and also the residence of bustee lands which he owned, some of whom were scavengers.

Among the Mahomedans too, men of social pre-eminence and high position upon whom an appreciable section of the Muslim community had reposed their greatest confidence, came forward to take up inoculation and to set an example before their admires and followers. The first such Mahomedan gentlemen were the Hon'ble Maulavi Mahomed Yusuf Khan Bahadur and Munshi Abdul Ali, the two great advocates of government's plague policy and inoculation. Both were inoculated before a large gathering of their community, and explained the purpose of the inoculation to them. The ladies of their families were also inoculated. The result of this enlightened action was that the medical officers were repeatedly invited to the neighbourhood, at the instance of their leaders and patients and the plague officers inoculated nearly the whole of the Mahomedan population there, both rich and poor.[57]

Some of the European Companies by dint of their influence succeeded in bringing some of the natives into inoculation. Messrs. Anderson, Wright and Company succeeded in persuading Babu Bhojan Lal Lohea, to be inoculated with his family and he used his influence with other members of the community.[58]

The following two events would explain the difference of attitudes between the two sharply opposite classes in the society against the government policy. On Sunday, May 1, 1898, above one thousand educated Indian middle class assembled at a public meeting at Sovabazar to thank Sir John Woodburn for his generous plague policy. But the same plague policy that created a good impression upon the educated middle class, had persuaded a large number of municipal scavengers not only to strike and thousands of people to leave the city but hundreds of men to commit serious riots in different parts of the city too.[59]

VII. Observation and Conclusion

At the initial stage, the colonial state had adopted a very stern policy and was unconciliatory in its attitude with the Indian population in regard to the implementation of its drastic plague measures. It tried to tackle all opposition by applying coercion, power with arrogance and war-like military arrangements. The Indians were treated 'as mere beasts' with all the racial contempt.

As a sequel to the colonial plague policy, the Indian as an individual lost its right and control over its own body and health and the colonial state, instead, became the absolute and exclusive protector of the body and health of the Indian subjects. The omnipresence and omnipotence of the state became clearly manifested through its medical intervention with commanding power, its plague policy and preventive measures, its war-like administrative arrangements to enforce plague measures. At the early stage of plague history, this hegemonistic control of the British Indian empire worked well in indigeneous society. But with the passage of time, popular resistance against such control and drastic plague measures began to grow up which finally took a violent form. The movements, as stated, were clear evidences of popular consciousness which was reflected in their fight for protecting social, religious, cultural rights and practice, the sanctity of their bodies and *ijjat*. People's unity in mobilization, quickness in action, and strong collectivity and resistance finally forced the colonial state to change its rigid stand. It came to compromise with the educated Indian middle classes by modifying its plague policy and measures. This shifting in state's attitude was made in order to secure the assistance and cooperation of the Indian middle classes for the restoration of peace among the urban poor. The Lt. Governor announced several relaxations with regard to plague rules.

In view of the modifications of government policy, some comments may be made. Compromise to gain consensus often alternates with coercion in the establishment of hegemony. Thus it can be argued that the Lt Governor Woodburn was establishing hegemony by relaxing control and this relaxation was with regard to authoritarian plague measures. But evidence indicates that this relaxation did not satisfy all classes equally. While Sovabazar middle classes responded favourably to the government policy and cooperated with the latter in its immunization and sanitation policy, the urban poor, the mill coolies and the domestic servants reacted violently and took recourse to disturbances, strikes, and riots since the relaxation did neither improve their condition nor redress their grievances.

Secondly, as compared to other outbursts of this decade, it can be said that the reaction of the urban poor during Calcutta plague riots in 1898–1900 was sharply in contrast with the Talla riots that occured in Calcutta sometime in 1896–1897. The Talla riot was purely communal in character and both Hindus and Muslims fought against each other at the instigation of their community leaders.[60] In the plague riots, Hindus and Muslims combined together to oppose the plague rules. Here the target was the colonial state and its henchmen. The feeling of anti-colonial distrust, hatred was clearly evident in the plague riots. The subalterns demonstrated their solidarity and class consciousness in fighting against plague measures. Although the subaltern solidarity and class consciousness was frequently disturbed by disruptive tendencies such as communal, caste and sectarian conflicts, it should also not be forgotten that such fluidity happened to become one of the significant features of twentieth century Indian history, with community consciousness interpenetrating class and national consciousness. The plague episode was a clear indication of class and national consciousness of the poor ordinary people.

Finally, what happened to these violent plague reactions? Were they ephemeral and fragmentary? Certainly not. Throughout the colonial regime, 'protest movements' of the subalterns had developed a pattern of anti-colonialism in the surface of the main stream of nationalist politics. The episodes of the plague riots should not have been seen in isolation too. It was the symbol of protest by the Indian population against colonial policy of domination and subordination, its exploitation, arrogance, and policy of strong racism.

References

1. *Bangavasi* (Calcutta), 10th October, 1896
2. Thucydides, *The Peloponnesian War* (New York, 1954), pp. 109-113.
3. Hindustan, 8th April, 1899.
4. For Plague in Bombay, See David Arnold, 'Touching the Body: Perspectives on the Indian Plague, 1896–1900', in Ranajit Guha (ed.) *Subaltern Studies V*, OUP, PB edition, 1996, pp. 55-90.
5. J. N. Cook, 'Report on Plague in Calcutta' in *Report of the Epidemics of Plague in Calcutta during the years 1898–1899, 1899–1900 and upto 30th June, 1900* (Calcutta, 1900), p. 9.
6. J. N. Cook's, *op. cit.*, pp. 9-10.
7. *Ibid.*, pp. 4-8.
8. *Ibid.*, pp. 4-8; Green's Report in *Indian Medical Gazette,* pp. 5-6 (Calcutta, 1900).
9. *Ibid*, pp. 6-9, pp. 12-14.
10. *Ibid*, also see David Arnold, 'Touching the Body', pp. 59-60.
11. J. N. Cook, *op. cit*, pp. 10-14.
12. *Amrita Bazar Patrika*, 3rd May, 1898.
13. J. N. Cook, *op. cit*, pp. 8-10.
14. *Ibid.*, pp. 4-14.
15. *Ibid.*, p. 8.
16. *Ibid.*, p. 8.
17. *History and Proceedings of the Plague Commission, Bengal 1896–1898*; also see *Appendix V* of the above report for the sanitation of Howrah; also see J. N. Cook, *op. cit.*, pp. 10-15.
18. J. N. Cook, *op. cit*, pp. 10-12; also see *Report on the Plague_in India, 1896 and 1897* (Govt. of India)
19 *Ibid*, pp. 10-2.
20. *Ibid*, pp. 10-12.
21. Home (Police), July to December, 1898, Proceedings A., nos. 13-21; 56-64 (National Archives of India) (henceforth NAI).
21A. J. N. Cook, *op. cit.*, p. 10.
22. Premankur Atarthi, *Mahasthabir Jataka* (1st Part), (Calcutta, 1981), p. 46.
23. *Ibid*, p. 47.

24. J. N. Cook, *op. cit.*, p. 23; also see *Amrita Bazar Patrika*, 4th May, 1898, 9th November, 1898.
25. *Ibid.*, pp. 24-25.
26. Home (Public), June 1898, Progs B, nos. 91–92; (Letter from Secretary, Government of Bengal to the Secretary, to the Government of India, Home Deptt. Dt. 28th May, 1898) (NAI)
27. John Campbell Oman, *Cults, Customs and Superstitions of India*, (Delhi, 1972).
28. *Amrita Bazar Patrika*, 4th May, 1898 (Editorial Comment), J. N. Cook, *op. cit.*, p. 25.
29. J. N. Cook, *op. cit.*, pp. 10-11; *Amrita Bazar Patrika*, 3–4th May, 1898.
30. General (Miscellaneous), August, 1899, Progs. A, no. 23, 'Annual Report on the Working of the Indian Factories Act in Bengal for December, 1898'; Letter from C. A. Walsh, Special Inspector of Factories to the Secretary, to the Government of Bengal, Revenue Department (West Bengal State Archives; Henceforth WBSA); Also see General (Miscellaneous), August, 1899, Progs. A, no. 23, Letter from C. E. Buckland, Commissioner of the Presidency Division to the Secretary to the Govt. of West Bengal, General Department, Calcutta, the 25th May, 1899. (WBSA).
31. J. N. Cook, *op. cit.*, p. 24.
32. *Amrita Bazar Patrika*, 4th May, 1898 (Editorial Comment).
33. Rabindranath Tagore, *Chaturanga* (in Bengali), pp. 447-448.
34. 'A Compilation of Regulations issued by the Government of India and Local Governments in connection with Plague, Govt. of India', Home Deptt. (1899), pp. 84-105. Also see the Regulations of the Government stated in Chapter XVI, *Report on the Plague in India, 1896 and 1897* (Government of India) (Calcutta, 1900). Also see J. N. Cook, pp. 11-12.
35. *Census of India*, 1901, 1911, 1921 (Calcutta).
36. J. N. Cook, *op. cit.*, pp. 10-15.
37. Home (Public), June, 1898, Progs B, nos. 91–92; letter from Secretary, Government of Bengal to the Secretary, to the Government of India, Home Deptt., dt. 28th May, 1898, (NAI).
38. J. N. Cook, *op. cit.*, p. 15.
39. *Ibid.*
40. 'Report on Plague in Calcutta, June 1901 to June 1902', by Major H. E. Deane, Special Health Officer, in J. N. Cook, *op. cit.*, pp. 22-25.
41. J. N. Cook, *op. cit.*, pp. 13-15.
42. 'Report on Plague in Calcutta, June 1901 to June 1902', by Major H. E. Deane, Special Health Officer, in J. N. Cook, *op. cit.*, pp. 22-23.
43. *Ibid.*, pp. 13-14.
44. *Ibid.*, pp. 14-19, *Amrita Bazar Patrika*, 4th May, 1898. Judicial (Police), August, 1898, Progs A, nos. 14–19; August 1899; Progs A, nos. 106–111 (WBSA).

45. J. N. Cook, *op. cit.*, pp. 18-25; *Amrita Bazar Patrika*, 4th May, 1898. Judicial (Police), August 1898, Progs A, nos. 14–19; Para. 6–9. Judicial (Police) Progs B, September, 1898, (WBSA) (The details of the reports are not available as documents are lacking).
46. J. N. Cook, *op. cit.*, pp. 4, 18-19, Major Deane's Report in J. N. Cook, *op. cit.*, pp. 13-14.
47. *Amrita Bazar Patrika*, 4th May, 1898; Judicial (Police) August, 1898, Progs A, nos. 14–17 (WBSA).
48. Hats were particularly associated with Europeans from the early days of the British rule in India. A commonly used name for the Europeans was 'hatmen'. See Michael Edwards, *Glorious Sahibs*. (New York, 1968), p. 94; see Philip Mason, *Race Relations*. (Oxford University Press, 1970), p. 84. This feeling of bitter resentment against 'hatmen' was dominant during the later period of Champaran peasants' movement against the planters in 1917 where an old villager, after bitter experience about a Saheb, commented, 'All those who wear hats are alike'.
49. Judicial (Police), August, 1898, Progs, A, nos. 14–17, Para. 6–7 (WBSA).
50. David Arnold, *op. cit.*, p. 64.
51. Sarat Chandra Chattopadhyay, *Srikanta* (Calcutta, 1918, in Bengali), in *Collected Works*, pp. 17-18.
52. *Hitavadi,* 30th October, p. 1896.
53. J. N. Cook, *op. cit.,* pp. 12-13.
54. A Letter from Sir A. P. MacDonnel, the Lt. Governor of the North-Western Provinces, to Lord Elgin, the Viceroy on 29th April, 1898.
55. J. N. Cook, *op. cit.,* pp. 22-26.
56. *Ibid.*, p. 23.
57. *Ibid.*, p. 25.
58. *Ibid.*, p. 23-25.
59. *Ibid.*, p. 26.
60. For the Talla riots in Calcutta see Dipesh Chakraborty, 'Communal Riots and Labour-Bengal's Jute Mill Hands in the 1890's' in *Past and Present*, May, 1981. Ranajit Dasgupta, 'Material Conditions and behavioural aspects of the Calcutta working class, 1875–1899', Occasional paper, Centre for Studies in Social Sciences, Calcutta, 1979. Amal Das, *Urban Politics in an Industrial Area-Aspects of Municipal and Labour Politics in Howrah, West Bengal 1850–1928,* Calcutta, 1994.

6

Coping with Leprosy in 19th Century Colonial Bombay

—*Simkie Sarkar*

A Portuguese writer Heitor Da Silvera had referred to Bombay as the Island of the Good Life, but not for long. In the eighteenth century Grose wrote that, 'Bombay had long borne an infamous character for unhealthiness. It was commonly called the burying ground of the English'. Among many evils, it has been stated, that there is one great evil prevalent in this city, which one would not expect to find in an advanced city, that is, leprosy, in the most advanced and loathsome stage and a number of pauper lepers, wandering here, there and everywhere, to the great danger of the health of the population.[1]

The Disease

Leprosy is a disease of great antiquity or has always been held in superstitious dread and the leper considered 'unclean', and a social outcaste. The *Lepra Bacillus* was first observed by Hansen in 1874.[2] Though this was the first bacterial pathogen of man to be described, it remains one of the least understood. This is because it has not been possible to grow the bacillus in culture media.[3]

Leprosy attacks the skin and nerves and causes the skin to swell and become lumpy and discoloured. It is one of the most feared diseases because it damages the patient's appearance. Leprosy usually affects the peripheral (end) nerves near the surface of the face, arms, and legs. Nerve damage causes a loss of feeling in the skin.

Severe nerve damage may cause paralysis. The bacillus is rod-shaped 1/4000 inch long. Scientists believe the germ escapes from infected persons in discharges from nose and skin sores. It is possible that the germs enter the bodies of healthy persons, through small breaks or cuts in the skin.[4]

In India, as in other parts of the world, three forms of leprosy are met with, the tuberculated, the anaesthetic, and the mixed. In the first, the skin is primarily invaded by the leprous growth, afterwards the mucuous membranes and viscera. In the second form, the lesions occur chiefly in the peripheral nerves, while the third is simply a combination of the other two forms.[5]

Dr. Balachandra Krishna, at the end of a very able paper on 'Leprosy in Bombay in its Medical and State Aspects' sums up as follows:-

1. That leprosy is prevalent throughout India but satisfactory statistics are wanting to show both the increase and decrease.
2. That it is endemic.
3. That the weight of evidence is in favour of its hereditary transmission.
4. That of the three forms of the disease, the non-tuberculated or anaesthetic form is most prevalent in India.
5. That the weight of evidence is not in favour of the contagiousness of leprosy, generally and particularly of the anaesthetic and the tuberculated and mixed forms in their early stages, but there is some evidence in favour of the latter two being communicable in the ulcerating stage by inoculation of the pus on an abraded surface either directly from the patient or by the stained clothing or other articles contaminated by the secretions of the leprous sores.
6. That it is not communicable by aerial infection in the same way as small-pox or other exanthemata are.
7. Granting that the tuberculated or mixed forms are contagious in their later stages, still it does not follow that every case of leprosy, indiscriminately, is contagious.
8. That the diagnosis of the disease is not always easy, especially in the early stage.
9. That no satisfactory treatment of leprosy has yet been discovered.
10. That segregation of lepers has been found to exercise some wholesome check on the propagation of the disease but not to the extent of stamping it out.
11. That the present excitement or the scare which has taken possession of the public mind is groundless.
12. That a sober, quiet, unbiased and scientific investigation of the subject is an absolute necessity, which will help the medical profession and the state to grapple with the problem more effectively.[6]

Viewed in light of these conclusions, 'The Draft Leper Bill (Act 1895) circulated by the Government of India for the opinion of the local governments, seems to be a desirable measure, in so far that when it becomes an Act, it will serve pre-eminently to calm the public mind, which has been excited to the highest pitch, because it will be the means of removing vagrant lepers from the public gaze, but whether it will serve to stamp out the disease, I am not sure'.[7]

Fish Hypothesis

Interestingly, the view that leprosy was caused by 'fish', gained considerable importance through the weight of the authority of Mr. Jonathan Hutchinson who stated the fish hypotheses with great force at the 10th International Medical Congress at Berlin. Virchow stated that 'the more general use of bad fish very frequently coincides with endemic leprosy'. Dr. Liveing says that 'the combination however of milk and fish seems to have been considered especially favourable to the disease'.[8] Some members of the commission examined a large number of fish, fresh and dried, but with absolutely negative results. Dr. Arning has also never been able to find any leprosy bacilli in fish. But leprosy occurs among people of all caste and religion.[9]

Contagion

Again, there are conflicting views on the question of 'contagion'. U. Fluggs says that 'the diffusion of leprosy by contagion is exceedingly rare and evidently can only take place under special and predisposing favourable conditions'. A. Hansen, a contagionist expresses himself thus:- 'I do not know the way in which leprosy is communicated or transferred from a leper to a sound person but I am not inclined to believe it is done by a sort of inoculation; that there is wanted a very intimate intercourse and some defect in the integument of the infected'. R. Virchow believes that leprosy does not spread by contagion.[10]

Leprosy is not a highly contagious disease. At the same time, it is essential that lepers should be prevented from forming colonies in towns and cities and also from following trades and occupations that bring them into direct contact with the rest of the community or lead to the production or preparation of commodities, capable of carrying contagion. These objects can be attained by putting into force the provisions of the Leper Act of 1898, which provides for the segregation and medical treatment of pauper lepers and the control of lepers following certain callings. Under this Act, a pauper leper can be arrested by the police and after due examination before a medical officer and a magistrate, sent to a Leper Asylum, and there detained, unless a friend or relative undertakes to take proper care of him.[11]

Asylums

The first step towards the creation of a Leper Asylum in Bombay was taken by a Roman Catholic Bishop of Bombay in 1883, who requested the government to place at his disposal for five years, one of the old forts at Sion, Matunga, Sewri, or Varli together with a certain area of culturable land in the vicinity, with a view to converting it into the headquarters of a Leper Colony.[12] The request for some reason could not be granted and large numbers of lepers continued as before, to collect and ask alms in the crowded portions of the city. One band in particular, settled in 1889 around Nakhoda Tank on the Esplanade, between St. Xavier's College and Elphinstone High School, and were with difficulty dislodged.

The pressure of public opinion induced the government in 1890 to issue a notification declaring 'black leprosy' an infectious disease, dangerous to life and ordering that all lepers should be sent to the Edaljee Framji Albless Leper Home on Trombay Island or to the Dinshaw Maneckji Petit Leper Hospital in Ratnagiri. In fact, Sir Dinshaw Maneckji Petit offered the government one lakh of rupees for the erection on Trombay Island of a new asylum, the foundation stone being laid by H.R.H. the late Prince Albert Victor of Wales on the 25th March 1890. The Municipal Commissioner H. A. Ackworth followed his example and declared a public subscription, which by May 1892 amounted to one lakh, among the largest subscribers being H.H. the Gaekwar of Baroda, H.H. the Thakore Saheb of Bhavnagar, H.H. the Rao of Cutch, and H.H. the Agha Khan.[13]

The work of construction of the Matunga Asylum commenced in August 1890 and was completed in June 1891 at a cost of Rs. 63,000. By 1897, the Asylum was capable of accommodating 300 lepers, and in 1909, the Asylum could accommodate 350 persons and was in charge of a medical officer appointed by the Municipal Corporation, aided by a house surgeon and a leper school master. The average annual expenditure was Rs. 46,000. In 1904, the Ackworth Asylum was provided with a complete installation of X-rays and high frequency currents, which proved to be of considerable value to the treatment of the disease.[14] It was due to a very low allocation of funds in the government budget, that the indigenous people had to depend on philanthropists who endowed hospitals, dispensaries, and sanitary projects. David Arnold, in 'Medical Priorities and Practice in Nineteenth Century British India' remarks that the Government of India devolved most of the responsibility of health to the poor and inexperienced local authorities.

Treatment

As regards treatment of leprosy, experiments with Nastin-B were conducted and the name 'Nastine' was given by Dr. Deycke Pasha and

Dr. Reschad Bey, two physicians in the Imperial Ottoman Service. It is a fatty extracted from 14 days old culture of a species of Strepthothrix found in cases of leprosy. In 1905, these investigations found that when pure cultures of Strepthothrix were applied by way of injection to sufferers of leprosy, they affected a far reaching improvement and retrogression of the symptoms and was a destructive influence on the excitor of leprosy.[15] But Nastine injections could not cure severe, advanced cases. Nastine-B is a combination of Nastine with Benzoylchloride dissolved in olive oil.

It must be mentioned, that the oils of India were considered effective. Dr. George Watt mentions the oils which have been used in the treatment of leprosy. Dr. Vandyke Carter writes about the oils of groundnut, cashewnut, gurjun oil, chaulmogra, and kowti oil. Of these, the 'chaulmogra oil' was very beneficial and effective. Dr. Carter says that the longer the oil is used, the more favourable the result, both in degree and permanence. But the disease is never eradicated.[16]

Mr. Sakhram Arjun, who was in charge of the ward for incurables in the Jamsetjee Jeejeebhoy Hospital, Bombay gives his opinion of the value of 'chaulmogra oil' as follows:-

> Under the prolonged and continued use of this oil, the progress of the disease is arrested, the skin becomes soft and supple, the discolorations vanish, the different morbid sensations leave the patient, the mental turpitude passes away, the impaired sensibility is completely or partially restored, the ulcers heal and cicatrise, though ever prone to break out again and the general nutrition of the tissues improves, patients crippled before being known to walk about unassisted and to gain in strength and weight.[17]

Dr. Bhau Daji Lad Parsekar, dedicated his time to trying out all kinds of treatment on leprosy patients. It is an accepted fact that colonial medical policy privileged the needs of Europeans and the military. They were least concerned about the plight of lepers. There is the same indifference as in other matters of insanitation, dirt, and lack of hygiene. At the end of 1866, Dr. Bhau Daji had reported to Captain Jacob that 'my medicine can cure all the patients suffering from leprosy, but since they are all poor, the medicine has to be given free of charge'. The paper *Native Opinion*, published a year after, a letter from the famous Sanskrit Pandit Bal Shastri Dev Tonkedar, who claimed that he was completely cured from the dreadful disease by Dr. Bhau Daji. In the same year arrangements were made in the Rustomji Jamshetji Charitable Hospital adjoining Sir J. J. Hospital, for giving free treatment, and Dr. Bhau Daji was put in charge of the special ward. Some of the patients, including

Europeans cured by him, narrated the experience and gave the detailed nature of the medicine, diet, etc.[18]

It was known that Dr. Bhau Daji had great faith in the well-known 'Gyncordia Odoratta' or 'chaulmogra oil', which he was using for leprosy and he had also administered one or two other drugs experimentally and kept it a secret, until he was sure it was the right cure. It was then stated that 'In leprosy, there is no protective specific vaccine. There is talk about BCG being a preventive, even against leprosy but the evidence is not yet convincing, the drug Sulphone, which is used for the treatment of leprosy, can act as a prophylactic, but one has to take it for quite a long time and regularly'.[20]

Conclusion

According to the Census Report of 1891, there were totally 1,26,244 lepers in India. The Leprosy Commission in 1891 stated that out of a population of almost 27 million in Bombay Presidency, the total number of lepers were 12,741.[21]

Hence, Radhika Ramasubban, in her pamphlet on 'Public Health and Medical Research in India', is right in stating that the British developed a distinctly colonial mode of healthcare, characterized by coercion, residential segregation, and neglect of the civilian indigenous population. In Europe, there had been 'Lazar Homes' for lepers, but the government in India, though composed mostly of Christians had never felt impelled to reduce the danger for the community, lurking in such uncontrolled movements of the lepers or the need for the relief of these pitiable sufferers. The only alternative left for the people was to turn to indigenous medicine, as in the case of leprosy.

References

1. *Gazeteer, Bombay City and Island*, vol. III, p. 164.
2. T. S. Krishnamurthy Iyer, *Leprosy in India*, p. 36.
3. R. Ananthnarayan and C. K. Jayaram Paniker, *A Textbook of Microbiology*, p. 356.
4. *World Book Encyclopaedia*, vol.12, p. 202.
5. Medical Files (MSA), *Report of the Leprosy Commission in India*, 1890–91, p. 2.
6. Medical Files (MSA), Wellesley Bailey, *The Lepers of our Indian Empire, Appendix B*, p. 235.
7. *Ibid*, p. 236.
8. Medical Files (MSA), *Report of the Leprosy Commission in India 1890–91*, p. 337.

9. *Ibid*, p. 338.
10. *Ibid*, pp. 283-285.
11. Medical Files (MSA), *Leprosy and its Control in the Bombay Presidency*, pp. 1-2.
12. *Gazeteer of Bombay City and Island*, vol. III, p.196.
13. *Ibid*, p. 197.
14. *Ibid*, p. 198.
15. Medical Files (MSA), *Report on Experiments with Nastin-B*, p. 1.
16. Medical Files (MSA), *Report of the Leprosy Commission in India, 1890–91*, p. 367.
17. *Ibid.*, p. 368.
18. G. M. Laud, *Dr. Bhau Daji Lad Parsekar*, p. 41.
19. *Ibid.*, p. 42.
20. R. D. Wardekar, *Leprosy, Everyone's Concern*, p. 11
21. *Gazetteer, Bombay City Island,* vol. III, p. 180.

7

Malaria in the Countryside in Colonial Bengal: Some Demographic Observations

—*Arabinda Samanta*

Diseases have always had a role in shaping the course of human history. Historians have been struck by the devastating impact of bacteriological invasions on society, all the way from Periclean Athens through black death in the fourteenth century in Europe to Sub-Saharan Africa in the twentieth century. However, in-depth studies of specific diseases have been less than adequate.[1] In recent years the history of disease and medicine has begun to receive scholarly attention. The role of disease and medicine in African, European, and North American societies is increasingly coming under close scrutiny. Historians have of late produced some important works on the history of infectious diseases, epidemics, and their demographic and biological consequences.[2] But unfortunately, despite the prevalence of epidemics in South and Southeast Asia, the literature on disease and medicine in these parts, still remains relatively scarce. India, for example has survived cholera, small-pox, plague, and malaria in epidemic form throughout the nineteenth and twentieth centuries. But except for a few monographs on some of the epidemics, we still lack a comprehensive account of the subject.[3] Again, Bengal, a vertiable disease laboratory, has not had a systematic campaign against any epidemic, nor a comprehensive account of its epidemic disease. As such, scholarly investigation into Bengal's journey through epidemic disaster continues to remain a desideratum. The present paper on malaria in the countryside in colonial Bengal is a modest attempt in that direction.

Malarial fever was, in fact, not an unknown phenomenon in Bengal. The Bengalis were acquainted with malaria even in the Vedic past. People did suffer from the fever, and the village *kaviraja* used to prescribe palliative drugs in individual cases. Unable to beat it with the medicine they had at their disposal, they gradually learnt to live with it. Malaria as such posed no threat to the community, for it never appeared with an epidemic virulence. But Bengal under British rule offers a different story altogether. The province experienced a spate of epidemic malaria throughout the late nineteenth and early twentieth centuries. It afflicted a greater number of people on a wider geographical scale. Worse still, it lingered longer over more than a century. Besides, malarial fever in Bengal was more than just an epidemic disaster. It became a phenomenon. Its compelling impact was kept alive in the collective memory of the people. It entered into the social psyche of Bengal. The phenomenon found its way well into the Bengal literary traditions—novels, dramas, poems, pamphlets, and anti-malaria advertisements. It held its sway on the Bengali cultural life for more than a century. Such a disease, endemic or epidemic, constitutes a tale which needs to be retold in its proper historical perspective.

1. Biography of the Epidemic

The epidemic fever first broke out at Muhammadpur in Jessore district sometime in the 1820s.[4] It broke out among a body of 500 to 700 convicts of Sitaram Ray's jail, working on a road from Jessore to Dacca. Within a short time, 150 of the prisoners died, and the native officers in charge fled.[5] The epidemic continued in Muhammadpur for about seven years; it remained in fact till about 1843 when it was reported to have disappeared. In 1846, it broke out again, and in the next two years spread over the entire district of Jessore. After a temporary cessation, the fever broke out again in 1845–54, and this time it began to spread westward to Nadia and 24–Parganas, where it finally took the shape of a severe epidemic which devastated these districts from 1857 to 1864.[6] It attacked Nadia district in 1832–33 and devastated Ula in 1856. It reached Chakda in 1857 and affected the villages on the east bank of the river Hooghly in 24–Parganas from 1859 to 1861. The epidemic crossed the river from Chakda to Triveni, Bansberia and the villages north of Bandel in 1857–59. The fever reached Pandua in 1862 and Dwarbasini in 1863, spread along the Kana Nadi in 1864.[7] It reached Kana Damodar in 1866 and the east bank of the Damodar in 1867. It took about ten years to cross the area lying between the Hooghly and the Damodar. It spread across Arambag thana on the east bank of the Darakeswar in 1868 and traversed Goghat thana during the next three years. The west bank of the Hooghly in Serampur subdivision was badly affected in 1871–73. Altogether the epidemic fever visited Hooghly district for about 20 years from 1857 to

1877. Burdwan district was first attacked in 1866. The epidemic spread from Pandua to the village of Ghose near Memari. It affected the district for about ten years. Ghatal in Midnapur district was attacked in 1868 and the ravages continued till 1877.[8] Almost all the districts of Bengal experienced the epidemic with varying degree of intensity. It started relaxing its grip in the 1880s. But the respite was short-lived. From the nineties till the outbreak of the Second World War, malaria fever became endemic in Bengal.

2. Problem of Mortality Estimate

Attempt to arrive at even a rough aggregate of fever death is, however, frustrated on several counts. In census reports, the term 'fevers' recorded a large number of deaths from many diseases whose predominant symptom was fever. The mortality returns of the village chowkidars show that at least two-thirds of all deaths were caused by 'fever' during British rule. Although the malarial group was the largest and the most important of all these, especially in the rural areas, it would be incorrect to attribute all these deaths to malaria. The census figures regarding malaria death therefore seem to be rather an overestimation. Even the investigations carried out by different contemporary malariologists point to the fact that census reports regarding the number of malaria deaths were often inflated. On the basis of reports of special enquiries into the working of dispensaries, Leslie, a noted malaria expert, estimated that in India about one-fourth of the recorded 'fever' deaths in an ordinary year were due to malaria.[9] Lurkis, another malariologist, argued that more than half the deaths associated with 'fever' were actually caused by malaria.[10] Hehir, still another noted malariologist, believed that of all the reported fever deaths, one-third to one-fifth might be attributed to malaria.[11] Fry, who had investigated the malarial fever in Bengal, observed that two-third of the deaths reported under the 'fever' head and classified as malaria had no connection with that disease at all.[12] Christopher, Sinton, and Covell who had conducted some important malaria survey throughout this country, unanimously agreed that of the total deaths attributed to 'fever', only from 30 to 50 per cent were actually due to malaria.[13]

Thus, one can see that the proportion of 'fever' deaths considered to be malarial varied considerably in investigations carried out by different experts in different parts of the country. For Bengal, however, the report of Captain Stewart and Lt. Proctor regarding the prevalence of malarial fever in the districts of Jessore, Nadia, and Murshidabad provides us an insight into a reasonable estimate of the malaria deaths.[14] In the three districts, the history of the illness was obtained from the relatives of 835 persons who died during 1905 and 1906, and whose deaths had been registered as 'fever' deaths. From the detailed study they had made, it appears that acute and chronic malaria together were responsible for about 36 per cent or over one-third of the deaths registered as 'fever'. But it is necessary to remember that persons who had earlier suffered from malaria were certainly predisposed to such diseases as phthisis, dysentery, and diarrhoea. Therefore, some of the deaths ascribed to these diseases were also related to malaria. Besides, one can notice from the study of Stewart and Proctor that the seasonal incidence of mortality began to rise with the onset of the rains, continued to increase through the autumn, and was heaviest in December. The figures for deaths under such heads as pneumonia, phthisis, dysentery, and diarrhoea, etc., also showed a marked increase during the malaria season. This cannot arguably be completely explained by their seasonal incidence.

During the malarious months from June to December, there were in Stewart and Proctor's report, 327 cases under heads other than malaria. Considering the weakening properties of malarial fever, one can perhaps argue that 25 per cent of the deaths from diseases other than malaria were primarily caused by impaired resistance due to that disease. So, to the 302 deaths due to acute and chronic malaria, one may add another 82 deaths (25 per cent of deaths computed from June to December due to causes other than malaria), i.e., 384 or above 45 per cent. Therefore, one can argue that at least 45 per cent of the deaths registered under the head 'fever' may be ascribed to malaria. This presumption also roughly approximates the findings of Dr. Leonard Rogers who was fortunate enough to lay hands on more than two thousand post-mortem records of the Calcutta Medical College in the first decade of the twentieth century.[15]

This presumption, however, does not apply to the mortality figures during the decades of sixties and seventies of the nineteenth century, when fever appeared as an epidemic. The census returns of this period do not appear to be sharply different from those supplied by the medical officers on tours to the affected areas. Thus, one can say that the mortality records of the epidemic years were not generally inflated. Dispensary dispatches during the epidemic years and particularly after 1880 cannot, however, be trusted as a correct index to the mortality from malaria. All malaria patients did not visit the fever dispensaries; there were some who generally avoided the fever dispensaries as they strongly disliked the bitter taste of quinine, the usual medicine for malaria.

3. Malaria and Mortality in the Districts

In view of these constraints, one can form only an impressionistic view of the magnitude of malaria mortality in the countryside. First, the districts of western Bengal can be surveyed. Dr Elliot, Civil Assistant Surgeon on special duty to enquire into the fever, visited 21 villages in Hooghly in 1862. He found that four-fifths of the population had been affected, and at least 20 per cent had died.[16] Early in 1863, Pellow, the Collector of Hooghly district wrote: 'To talk of decimation is seriously below the truth as applied to mortality in many, very many, of these villages. Hardly the tenth part is left alive'.[17] Thus by March 1863, the officials admitted of mortality in a few villages in the Hooghly district. Available reports in March 1863, show that of 84,451 people in Hooghly district, 25,298 fell sick of malaria and 12,676 died. In other words, nearly 16 per cent of the population in Hooghly district were swept away by the epidemic wave.[18] In March 1869, Dr. Smith wrote: 'The present state of the Hooghly district is alarming. The blighting influence of malaria is everywhere conspicuous, the people are subject to constant and excessive sickness of an insidious nature; their vigor is being sapped. Silent but sure depopulation on an alarming scale is going on.'[19] The appalling mortality, as Dr. Smith computed, amounted to one-third of the entire population.

Mortality was still greater in the Burdwan district. The medical officers of the district told Beverley, the Census Superintendent, that two-third of the people in the southern thana had fallen victim to the fever. In census papers a large number of houses were returned as uninhabited as the inmates had either died out or migrated between the period of numbering the houses and of taking the census.[20] Dr. Jackson, the Sanitary Commissioner, remarked on the depopulation of Kalna and Katoa subdivisions that in some large and close villages, entire households were reported to have been swept away. In some houses only one or two remained out of 20 persons. In one household, only one remained out of 17.[21]

The district of Birbhum was decadent until 1891 owing to the ravages of fever. Between 1872 and 1881, the population decreased by 7 per cent. Dr. Roy who had seen much of the Burdwan fever in the late seventies forewarned that the fever was making a steady progress towards Birbhum and Midnapur. He strongly believed that the mortality from fever had been steadily increasing for the last five years, and that the disease had progressed in a direction from south to north-east along the line of railroad.[22] The district of Midnapur witnessed a decline in population by 1 per cent between 1872 and 1881. The ravages of Burdwan fever caused an estimated mortality of a quarter of a million.[23]

Conditions during the opening decade of the twentieth century were not favourable to a further advance. 'Fever', to quote the opinion of the

Census Superintendent, 'the most important factor in the health of the district' was rife in the water-logged areas.[24] The district of Howrah too suffered heavily from fever, which had caused 50,000 deaths by 1881. But the census of that year indicates an increase of population by 6 per cent. This was possibly due to immigration. There can be little doubt that the fever was responsible for a large proportion of the recorded deaths. Computation of the period from 1891 to 1906 shows that out of an average death rate of 31.03 per mile, fever accounted for no less than 14.45 per mile or nearly half.[25] The district of Bankura, however, had a steady growth of population since the first census in 1872. The census of 1881 showed an increase of 7.6 per cent. But malaria took its toll on the eastern part of the district, and growth of population was seriously hampered. There was, however, some recovery, but census reports show that in 1891 the demographic growth amounted to a meager 2.7 per cent.[26]

Things did not improve much even in 1931. So far as the district of Burdwan was concerned, the Census of 1931 recorded some improvement in the rate of population at least in some parts of the district. In Burdwan district, the construction of the Damodar Canal and of an irrigation canal passing through Galsi, Bhatar, and Ausgram police stations had attracted a number of labourers who were recorded during the census enumeration. Many of them, however, presumably left these areas when the work was finished. This immigration, together with the natural increase due to excess of birth over death, may be considered as the reason of increase of population in Burdwan, Raina, Khandaghosh, Galsi, Bhatar, and Ausgram police stations.[27] In all the police stations of Asansol subdivision the increase was attributed by the local officers to the collieries and other industrial concerns which attracted an increasingly larger number of immigrants. It was only the Iron Industry In this district which had an uninterrupted period of prosperity during the decade, and the collieries suffered from a depression. The increase can therefore be accounted for by the immigrants, many of whom supplemented their earnings in the collieries by agriculture had not been immediately driven away by unfavorable economic conditions in the collieries, but had been able to remain in anticipation of improvement.[28] The Census of 1931 recorded an increase in population in the Birbhum district. The increase, however, could be explained by immigration into Rampurhat and Nalhati caused by a stimulus of industrial development and railway settlement. In Sainthia, Bolpur, and Ilambazar, the increase was due to trading activities and opening of several rice mills.[29]

The epidemic fever first attracted the attention of the government in 1861 and was reported by Dr. Elliot. Dr. Elliot observed that a peculiar type of fever was prevalent in Jessore for many years prior to its appearance in the district Nadia. This fever, Dr. Elliot reported, was called by the local people *jwar bikar* i.e., fever attended with delirium. From 1857 to 1860 the epidemic spread over the southern part of Nadia and the whole of Barasat in 24–Parganas. Moreover, Chakda, Kanchrapara, Naihati, Bhatpara, Ichapur, Barrackpur, Titagarh, and Kharda in 24–Parganas suffered more than usual in 1862.[30] Available information indicates that the fever was prevalent in the entire 24–Parganas district even in 1877. The mortality was even greater than that of 1876 by 0.17 per 1000 of people. The worst affected areas were Sonarpur, Barrackpur, and Dum Dum.[31]

The Nadia district recorded a decrease in population by 8 per cent again between 1911 and 1921. However, the population increased by 2.3 per cent between 1921 and 1931.[32] The district of Murshidabad too recorded a decrease. The decrease in Hariharpara was ascribed to malaria fever. Jiagang, where a decrease of 3.5 per cent was reported, witnessed a decline of the silk industry, and this possibly had led to a number of silk workers leaving the locality.[33] Jessore witnessed a decrease in population by 3 per cent between 1921 and 1931.[34] The decrease was particularly marked in Bongaon, Jhenida, and sadar division. In the west and central parts of the district, the offshoots from the Ganges had decayed, and water could no longer move freely. The result was that local trade and commerce were adversely affected. Land tended to go out of cultivation and subsequently were covered with jungles. In a country deprived of the arterial rivers in this way, the mosquitoes could thrive quite easily. Consequently, malaria prevailed and the effect of continued attacks of this disease left the people weak and listless.

The story was more or less the same in the districts of north Bengal, though of course, its virulence was not so pervasive as in other parts of the country. Between 1872 and 1891, the population of the district of Rajshahi was shown in the census reports as almost stationary, and in the next ten years, one notices a small increase of 1.6 per cent. During these thirty years the south and centre of the district were decadent. The thanas concerned sustained a population loss of 12.8 per cent. Fever continued in the district unabated in the opening decade of the twentieth century.[35] The Census of 1881 showed that the population of Dinajpur was practically stationary. Bourdillion, the Census Commissioner, remarked: 'Dinajpur had made no progress at all during the last nine years. This pitiable result is due only to the ravages of malarial fever for which this district has as evil a reputation as its neighbor Rangpur'.[36] In the Census of 1891 a slight increase of population was noticeable. The

Census of 1901, however, showed still further increase of population. Here again immigration from the west accounted for a large proportion of this increase.[37] The Census of 1931 recorded a decrease in population in the Rajshahi district by 4.6 per cent than the previous decade.[38]

Reports from east Bengal show that this part of the province was far from healthy, and the chief scourge of the people was malaria. The district of Dacca and Chittagong divisions which formed east Bengal suffered from malarial fever throughout the entire period of the present study. Malaria visited the Khulna district in an epidemic form sometime in 1868.[39] By 1886, the returns of the Dacca division show that 15,513 of its villages were invaded by fever against 14,861 in 1885.[40] No less than 1,19,170 succumbed to it in 1866 out of a population of 87,00,939 or at the rate of 13.69 per 1000.

Reports on health in east Bengal at the beginning of the twentieth century indicate that things had not changed substantially. Mortality from fever in 1900 continued unabated. Faridpur maintained a slightly reduced rate. Dr. Fink, the civil medical officer of Faridpur, recorded in 1900 that malarial fever attained its maximum intensity during the months of November and December, and continued to do its ravages till the rains properly set in.[41] The fever was not confined to any particular locality, but visited almost every household in the district. During the first decade of the twentieth century, malaria was extremely virulent in Chittagong. Between 1901 and 1910, Chittagong had the highest death rate from fever of all the districts in the division.[42]

Evidences adduced so far indicate that the population infected with malaria was remarkably large and that mortality due to this disease was enormous. It appears that at a rough estimate some thirty million of these people were infected with malaria and more than ten million suffered from the disease in an aggravated form in the first decade of the last century. The magnitude of the disease can be comprehended if one looks into the overall provincial situation. And one way of looking at its impact is possibly the number of malaria patients admitted or treated in the government hospitals or dispensaries. At the Special Endemic Dispensaries in the districts of Burdwan, Hooghly, Birbhum, and Midnapur no less than 9,44,717 persons were said to have been treated during 1873.[43] Report on the Charitable Dispensaries under Government of Bengal for the year 1876 points out that fever cases topped the list of the principal diseases causing admission.[44] Cholera, because of its suddenness, the rapidity with which it carried off its victims, the attention it excited, and the panic it spread, was considered probably the most dreaded of diseases. But an examination of the death-rate of the province will show that malaria fever ought to be rated as deadlier than cholera. Fever caused 74 per cent of the deaths and it was eight-fold more fatal than cholera. In 1878, 4,19,294 males and 3,23,593 females died of fever in the whole province. The total death rate from the disease was 12.38 per 1000 against 7.58 per 1000 on the previous five years' average. Available information show that the disease prevailed in all the districts of Bengal during 1878 and fever deaths were returned from every registration circle. It was prevalent in 1,23,340 villages out of a total number of 1,92,287 villages, or in about 64 per cent.[45]

4. Malaria and Its Impact on Demography

Though malaria fever attacked rich and poor alike, the great bulk of those who died belonged to the poorer classes. Dr. Jackson, the Sanitary Commissioner of Bengal, argued that the purely farinaceous character of the food had greatly increased the mortality. During the epidemic years milk was comparatively scarce, and thousands of lives had been lost for want of proper nourishment. 'Food', Dr. Jackson contended, 'if it could have been provided on enormous scale required, and if the people would have consented to receive it, would have saved far more lives than medicine has been able to preserve'.[46] The Magistrate of Burdwan gathered similar information. He wrote that 'the class visited most sevrely by the fever has been the lowest class... that of the worst fed, clothed and housed'.[47] Jogeswar Mukherjee, the Deputy Magistrate on Special Duty in connection with the Fever Enquiry, reported with 'tolerable accuracy' that the well-to-do cultivators who could save capital escaped with comparative immunity, while those who lived from hand to mouth, the masses of cultivators, agricultural labourers, weavers died without number.[48]

Poverty undoubtedly explains the heaviest tolls from the fever amongst the poorer labourers, who had no land and who worked as coolies or hired cultivators. Scholars like Benoy Bhusan Chaudhuri who investigated this phenomenon do admit it.[49] But the question is why was it so. The greater mortality among the poor was probably due to three reasons: one, their greater number, two, their inability to escape temporarily to more healthy places, and three, their inability to secure good medical attention, medicines, and diet appropriate to their ailment.

Almost all important reports pertaining to the question of mortality alluded to the phenomenon that the denser the population, the heavier the tolls. For instance, R. C. Mukherjee, Deputy Magistrate on Special Duty reported to Pellow, Magistrate of Hooghly in 1874: 'the districts of Hooghly and Burdwan have of late been so much overpopulated that the increased demand for houses and other accommodation has occasioned the occupation of all open ground and pasture lands by buildings, gardens and tanks...'.[50] Dr. Jackson argued in 1873 that it was most fatal where the population was densest.[51] Despite heavy mortality the poor people in general refused to emigrate to other parts of the country presumbly for two reasons: first, their pecuniary position, and second, emotional attachment to their ancestral home. Generally speaking, the male adults had but little objections to going out to other districts. They would leave their wives and children behind in the care of the head of the family, but nothing seemed to have induced them to permanently desert the family residence.

One can also probe the question of differential impact of the malarial fever among the Hindus and Muslims as also among the different caste groups among the Hindus. According to the Census Reports of 1872, there were in that year a little over 1,71,00,000 Hindus and nearly 1,67,00,000 Muslims in Bengal proper. In other words, the Hindus had a numerical preponderance over the Muslims in 1872. But this trend was reversed in the subsequent census. In the census figures for the year 1881, there were 1,83,96,117 Muslims as against 1,80,69,352 Hindus. In 1891, the numbers of the Hindus and the Muslims were 1,89,75,978 and 2,01,74,593 respectively. The Census Report of 1901 shows the Hindu population as being 2,01,91,082 and the Muslims 2,19,54,977. This steady decline of the Hindu population in Bengal had been discussed in contemporary journals and newspapers, the most important being the discourse of Kishori Lal Sarkar, a *vakil* of Calcutta High Court. Sarkar's views can be summarized as follows.[52] (1) Owing to the prevalence of malaria in Bengal, the rate of population growth both among the Hindus and the Muslims was falling off gradually. The phenomenon was striking when compared with the rate of growth at an all India level; (2) On an average, in the four natural divisions of Bengal, the Muslim population was falling off at a somewhat less accelerated rate compared to the Hindus; (3) This was because of the fact that in one of these divisions, viz., east Bengal which was inhabited mostly by the Muslims, there was comparatively less prevalence of malarial fever and the economic conditions were also more favourable; (4) If this division of east Bengal which was mostly in the occupation of the Muslims be excluded from calculation, it would be found that mainly owing to the malarial epidemic, the Hindus and the Muslims were actually sailing together down the stream of extinction at the same rate.

Nevertheless, the fact remains that more Hindus died of malarial fever than did the Muslims so far as the population of Bengal proper as a whole was concerned. This, however, does not mean that the Hindus as a rule were more susceptible to this ailment. Malaria did not favour any particular caste or a religious group. It was basically a function of economic condition of the people. In other words, relatively better off castes could resist malarial infection more than the poorer castes. Moreover, the castes which had to do outdoor work were less liable to malarial infection than the castes which by their occupation had to be confined to their houses. This can be proved by a micro-study done by Dr. Sarasilal Sarkar in 1912 in the town of Arambag, Hooghly district.[53] Dr. Sarkar, assistant surgeon, Howrah General Hospital, spent a large part of his leisure during his service at Arambag in making a spleen census of the children between 2 and 12 years of age. Dr. Sarkar's study shows that the *goalas* or the milkmen suffered least from malaria infection. This may be due to their habits of making smoke in their houses to drive out mosquitoes during the nights to save their cows from mosquito-bites. Again the *malakars* who made fancy articles and ornaments for idols and gods, and the carpenters suffered most severely not only because of their sedentary occupation, but also because they kept their houses dirty. Their dwelling rooms often being store-rooms for their manufactured articles, the nooks and crevices furnished the favourite resting places for mosquitoes.

Finally, one can also discuss the question of susceptibility of malaria infection to age group. As regards the age incidence of the fever deaths inquired into, Stewart and Proctor's study shows that large proportion, nearly half of all deaths due to acute malaria, occured in children under 5 years, and that about half of all the deaths due to acute and chronic malaria were under 10 years.[54] The large infant mortality due to malaria is not surprising because most of the cases went absolutely untreated. The difficulty in giving quinine to children owing to its bitter taste rendered it even less likely that they got sufficient treatment than in case of the adult. Again, of the adults, women in Bengal were probably more exposed to the bites of mosquitoes than their male counterparts. For, women in Bengal remained in the house for the most part of the day; they usually worked both in the early hours of the morning and late in the evening. As a result mortality rate from malaria might have been greater among the females than the men though of course we have no sufficient data to prove it conclusively.

References

1. Jones, however, was an important exception (L.H.S. Jones, *Malaria and Greek History*). He argued in 1909 that the Greeks who surrendered to the Roman legions were not the same who had fought off the Persian invaders, and the difference was primarily due to malaria.

2. To cite only a few, one can refer to David Arnold, (ed.), *Imperial Medicine and Indigenous Societies*, Oxford, 1989; GW Hartweg and K.D. Patterson (ed.), *Disease in African History: An Introductory Survey and Case Studies*, Durham NC, 1978; W. H. McNeil, *Plagues and Peoples*, Harmondsworth, 1979; D.Landy (ed.), *Culture, Disease and Healing: Studies in Medical Anthropology*, New York, 1977; A. W. Crosby, *Ecological Imperialism; The Biological Expansion of Europe, 900–1900*, Cambridge, 1986; Terence Ranger and Paul Slack (eds.), *Epidemics and Ideas: Essays on the Historical Perception of Pestilence*, Cambridge, 1992.
3. Ira Klein, 'Malaria and Mortality in Bengal, 1840-1920', in *Indian Economic and Social History Review*, vol. IX, June 1972; David Arnold, 'Cholera and Colonialism in British India' in *Past and Present*, no. 113, Nov. 1986; David Arnold, 'Touching the Body: Perspective on Indian Plague, 1896–1900' in *Selected Subaltern Studies* ed., Ranajit Guha *et al.* Oxford, 1988; R. W. Nicholas, 'The Goddess Sitala and Epidemic Smallpox in Bengal' in *Journal of Asian Studies*, vol. XLI, no. 1, November, 1981; David Arnold, *Colonizing the Body: State Medicine and Epidemic Disease in Nineteenth Century India*, Oxford, 1993.
4. M. A. Momen, *Final Report on the Survey and Settlement Operation in the District of Jessore, 1920–1924*, Calcutta, 1925, p.19.
5. L. S. S. O'Malley, *Bengal District Gazetteers*, Jessore, Calcutta, 1912, p. 61.
6. *Ibid.*
7. *Ibid.*
8. D. G. Crawford, *Hughli Medical Gazetteer*, Calcutta, 1903, p. 113.
9. *Proceedings of the Imperial Malaria Conference, Simla*, 1909, p. 3.
10. *Records of Malaria Survey of India*, vol. 1, no. 2, Calcutta, 1916, p. 141.
11. P. Hehir, *Malaria in India*, Oxford, 1927, p. 129.
12. A. B. Fry, *Second Report on Malaria in Bengal*, Calcutta, 1914, p. 111.
13. S. R. Christophers, J. A. Sinton, and G. Covell, 'How to do a Malaria Survey', in *Government of India Health Bulletin* no. 14, Malaria Bureau No. 6.
14. *Report of the Drainage Commitee, Bengal*, (Presidency Division), Calcutta, 1907, Appendix 1, p. XI.
15. Leonard Rogers, 'Gleanings from Calcutta Post-mortem Records', in *Indian Medical Gazette*, February 1914, p. 42.
16. *Supplement to Calcutta Gazette*, 18 April 1863, pp. 159-160.
17. *Ibid.*, p. 157.
18. 'Abstract statement of probable mortality of a few village in the Districs Hooghly, Barasat and Nuddea during the epidemics of 1860, 1861 and 1862'. *Proceedings of the Government of Bengal* (hereafter Progs. GOB), General Department (hereafter Genl. Dept.) March 1863, no. 58, p. 76, West Bengal State Archives (hereafter WBSA).

19. Report of D. B. Smith to the Secy to the GOB, in the Judicial Dept. Progs of the GOB, May 1869, Genl. Dept., Sanitation Branch (hereafter San Br.) no. 13, p. 17, WBSA.
20. From Rameschandra Mukherjee, Deputy Magistrate, Hooghly, to F. H. Pellow, Officiating Magistrate, Hooghly. Progs of the GOB. Genl. Dept., San. Br., Nov. 1870, no. 2, p. 94, WBSA.
21. *Ibid.*
22. Robert Harvey, *Tenth Annual Report of the Sanitary Commission for Bengal, 1877.* Appendix to the Progs of the GOB. Finance Dept. San. Br. August 1878, p. 51, WBSA.
23. *Census of India, 1911*, vol. V, part 1, p. 86.
24. *Ibid*, p. 86.
25. L. S. S. O'Malley, *Bengal District Gazetteers*, Howrah, Calcutta, 1909, p. 55.
26. *Census of India, 1911*, vol. V, part I, p. 85.
27. A. E. Porter, *Census of India, 1931*, vol. V, part I, Calcutta, 1933, p. 38.
28. *Ibid.*
29. *Ibid.*, para. 46.
30. Progs of the GOB, Genl. Dept., March 1863, no. 108, p. 61, WBSA.
31. Robert Harvey, *Tenth Annual Report of the Sanitary Commission for Bengal*, 1877, Calcutta, 1879. Progs of the GOB, August 1878, Finance Dept., San. Br. p. 52, para 171, WBSA.
32. *Census of India*, 1931, vol. V, part I, p. 41, para 53.
33. *Ibid.*, p. 44, para 54.
34. *Ibid.*
35. *Census of India*, 1911, vol. V, part I, p. 98.
36. Cited in F. W. Strong, *Eastern Bengal District Gazetteers*, Dinajpur, 1912, p. 31.
37. *Ibid.*
38. *Census of India*, 1931, vol. V, part I, p. 4, para 58.
39. Report of D. B. Smith to W. H. Ryland. Progs of the GOB, Pol. Dept. San. Br. February 1870, no. 16, pp. 13-17, WBSA.
40. R. Lidderdale, *Nineteenth Annual Report of the Sanitation Commissioner for Bengal for the year 1886.* Appendix to the Progs of the GOB, Judl. Dept., San. Br., December 1887, p. 16, WBSA.
41. H J Dyson, *Thirty-third Annual Report of the Sanitary Commissioner for Bengal, Year 1900.* Appendix to the Progs of the GOB, June 1901, Municipal Dept. San. Br., p. 72, WBSA.
42. *Census of India*, 1911, vol. V., part I, p. 114.
43. *Report of the Charitable Dispensaries for the year 1873.* Progs of the GOB, Med., Dept., San. Br, March 1875, p. 60, WBSA.
44. J. F. Beatson, *Report on the Charitable Dispensaries under the Government of Bengal for the year 1876*, Progs of the GOB, Genl. Dept., March 1878, p. 10, WBSA.

45. *Memorandum of the Army Sanitary Commissioner for Bengal for 1878*. Progs of the GOB, Med. and Mun. Dept., San., Br., May 1880, pp. 15-16. WBSA.
46. C. J. J. Jackson, *Sanitary Commissioner's Annual Report* for 1873, para. 376, p. 77.
47. Progs of the GOB, Genl. Dept., San. Br., Sept. 1875, para. 3, WBSA.
48. *Ibid*; para 4.
49. Benoy Bhusan Chaudhuri, 'Agricultural Production in Bengal, 1800–1900: Coexistence of Decline and Growth' in *Bengal Past and Present*, vol. 88, 1976, p. 16.
50. Vide D. G. Crawford, *op. cit.*, p. 140.
51. C. J. J. Jackson, *op. cit.*, para. 367, p. 76.
52. Kishori Lal Sarkar, *A Dying Race*: *How Dying,* Calcutta, 1913.
53. Sarasilal Sarkar, 'Investigation into the incidence of malaria in the town of Arambag, Hooghly district' in *The Indian Medical Gazetteer*, vol. XL VIII, September 1913, p. 343.
54. G. E. Sewart and A. H. Proctor, *op. cit.,* Appendix, p. XII.

8

Kala-azar Epidemics in India

—*Kaushik Roy Choudhury and*
Syamal Roy

Introduction

Since times immemorial, mankind has been plagued by epidemics. They came in different forms and swept through civilization in the form of outbreaks leaving a tale of devastation in their trail, often in catastrophic proportions. The curse of the gods, as epidemics were known in most early civilizations, brought a shudder of fear to every soul from kings to paupers. The curse spared none. However, definitive historical evidence of epidemics is rare. Innumerable references have been made to curses throughout ancient literature from across the globe, though little of these have ever been confirmed. After all, a term as broad as 'curse' could mean a lot of other things as well.

One of the earliest and best documented of epidemics is the outbreak of plague in Athens from 430 to 428 BC. We know for sure that it occurred and that it killed many people, irrespective of their social status or political affliation, and played a major role in upsetting the outcome of many a battle. It has been thoroughly documented in the *History of the Peloponnesian War* by Thucydides, the Greek philosopher.[1] Another such epidemic was the Justinac plague outbreak recorded by John Ephesus in his *Historia Ecclesiastica*.[2]

Though plague is the best known culprit of epidemics in ancient times, it was not alone. Ancient historical accounts refer to other epidemics that can today be identified as malaria, cholera, small-pox, influenza, leprosy, etc. Many of these diseases were fatal. One such disease that came in outbreaks of epidemic proportions and has so often been confused with malaria and other diseases is the dreaded *kala-azar*. It was almost always fatal.

Kala-azar Epidemics

Kala-azar epidemics probably occurred for centuries in parts of Mediterranean Europe and Africa, but there exists no good documentation of this. It was probably brought into the orient by the European traders shortly after the age of discoveries.[3] But once it entered, it made these parts of the world its home, especially the eastern parts of British India. In the years following 1858, when the British formally assumed power over the whole of India, the Government of Bengal became concerned with reports of an epidemic of quinine resistant fever in the district of Burdwan and Hoogly into 'a valley under shadow of death'.[4] From the beginning of 1860, the government in Calcutta received many reports of an epidemic fever afflicting the area of Burdwan which Sir Leonard Rogers later considered to be *kala-azar.* The earliest *kala-azar* epidemic that has been thoroughly recorded in this part of the world was in 1870 in Assam, as reported by Archibald. The disease was similar to malaria and killed many people, though it was not curable with the drugs that cured malaria. It was dubbed 'Sarkari Bimaari' by the locals who rather strongly believed that the officials of the Raj were somehow responsible for the disease. After a devastating spell, in the 1890s, the epidemic phase was gone from Assam, only to return fifteen years later. By then, it had already captured Burdwan (the named Burdwan fever), Calcutta (Dum Dum fever) and soon after, most of India. Ever since, there have been repeated epidemics in some part of the country or the other. The worst of these are described below.

Five years after the second epidemic in 1885, another outbreak started in Assam and lasted till 1900. It swept through the hilly regions of northeastern India and even covered parts of the plains below. The epidemic was so severe that it depopulated whole villages and reduced populations over large areas. In 1917, another epidemic started in Assam and Bengal, reached its height in about 1925 and then mysteriously subsided. By 1931, it disappeared almost.[5] In 1937, a new outbreak began in Bihar and like the 1890 epidemic, depopulated whole villages in its path.[6] More recently, a huge *kala-azar* outbreak swept through UP and Bihar in 1978.

The Discovery of the cause of *Kala-azar*

Till the end of 19th century, the cause of the disease bewildered medical men and laymen alike. Everything from germs to supernatural forces were suspected. At the turn of the century, although more people started to believe in the existence of a hitherto unknown germ causing the disease, none had been found. Sir Ronald Ross had just pinned down the culprit causing malaria and a fanatic search began to identify the germ for *kala-azar* as well. The break came in 1903 from two independent sources. Dr. William Leishman was a lieutenant with the British Indian Army and served as a physician in his regiment. During his service in India, he encountered numerous patients suffering from acute *kala-azar*. He was aware of Ronald Ross's work on malaria and studied blood samples under the microscope. He found strange bodies in the blood cells (later named Leishman bodies) and could demonstrate that these were actually germs.[7]

At around the same time, professor of physiology at the Madras University Medical College, Charles Donovan, an Irish physician who took part in the sanitary service of the British Crown in India, was also studying patients' samples and successfully identified a new parasite (germ) from samples of spleen.[8] Soon after, James Homer Wright, MD 1871–1928, described the first case of Leishmania infection in an Armenian patient in Boston.[9] Both Leishman and Donovan's findings were published in rapid succession and a controversy ensued as to who should be accredited with the discovery. Finally, towards the end of the same year, Sir Ronald Ross was asked to intervene. Sir Ross was an extremely respected and revered figure in those days and he came to a solution that hurt neither investigator. He accredited both Leishman and Donovan equally for the discovery and named the new parasite *Leishmania donovani.*[10]

Finding the germ was one thing, but knowing how it is transmitted is another ball game altogether. Ross had proven beyond doubt that mosquitoes carried malaria. Now everyone wondered what was it that carried the germ for *kala-azar*. Knowledge of the carrier (vector) would help in controlling the disease.

In 1907, Patton in India observed that in the gut of the bedbug, the germ for *kala-azar* could thrive and changed to a form that was highly infective for man. This was an unfortunate discovery, since it started investigators on a false trail in search for the transmitting agent and led to more than a decade of futile work. In fact, few problems in the science of parasitic diseases caused more fruitless effort, more blasted hopes, more false conclusions, and more unfounded speculation than the transmission of *kala-azar*.

In 1924 the *Kala-azar* Commission began work in Assam. This was led by Christophers, Shortt, and Barraud. Shortly before that Sinton had observed (and published) that the distribution of a certain sandfly in India coincided with the distribution of *kala-azar*. Meanwhile, working with the bedbug, Shortt and his colleagues in 1925 finally concluded that the bedbug had nothing to do with the transmission of *kala-azar*. Another suspect, fleas had recently been thrown out of court by Nicoll and Anderson in Italy. In the same year, 1924, Knowles, Napier, and Smith discovered that a high percentage of sandflies became infected when fed with blood from *kala-azar* patients. This was quickly confirmed by Shortt's group.

Then followed years of patient but largely fruitless effort to prove actual transmission by sandflies. In the course of hundreds of trials, four successful infections were obtained, all in hamsters (a small rodent, about the size of a rat). Transmission to human volunteers always failed.

In 1939, Smith, Halder, and Ahmed made an interesting discovery. They found that if sandflies after a bloodmeal from an infected person are fed on plant resins instead of additional blood, the germs in their gut grew immensely. When they tried to infect healthy hamsters with such sandflies, almost all the animals got infected.[11] This was confirmed using human volunteers by Swaminath, Shortt, and Anderson in 1942 in Assam.[12] Thus success came after twenty years of patience, perseverance, and sustained research.

Timely discovery of the drug *urea stibamine* by Sir U. N. Brahmachari[13] prevented the spread of the disease over other parts of Assam and Bengal, and thus saved these parts from the horrors. With the use of DDT to control malaria after World War II, there was a decline in the incidence of *kala-azar* due to destruction of the sandfly vector. With the cessation of DDT spraying, *kala-azar* started coming back. In the epidemic of *kala-azar* in north Bihar, some 70,000 to 1,00,000 attacks were estimated to have occurred between 1976 and 1977 with 4000 deaths. By 1992, *kala-azar* had widened its base to 39 districts in Bihar and affected 3 lakh people; bulk of the cases were unresponsive to the conventional treatment.[14]

Kala-azar today

Leishmaniasis is endemic to 82 countries (10 developed and 72 developing including 13 of the least developed countries)[15] and the World Health Organization (WHO) estimates an incidence of 12 million cases among 350 million at risk and an annual incidence of 6,00,000 cases.[16] Leishmaniasis is endemic to all countries of the New World (except Canada, Uruguay, and Chile), Mediterranean basin, Middle East, Southwest Asia, India, the newly independent states of former Soviet Central Asia and Transcaucasia, East Africa, and China. Despite its wide geographic distribution, human leishmaniasis is often very focal within an endemic area, leading to outbreaks of the disease.[17]

Today, several drugs are available in the market that can successfully cure *kala-azar*. However, there are problems associated with them. Either they have severe side effects, or require specialized facilities to administer or are simply too expensive for the poor. In India, although no longer in epidemic proportions, *kala-azar* still occurs, mainly in the states of Bihar and Uttar Pradesh, and the number of cases have been observed to be rising every year. Already it is in thousands.[18] Worse is the case in continental Africa and Latin America. Visceral Leishmaniasis (The technical name for *kala-azar*) has been recognized as a global problem by the World Health Organization. The situation gets even more alarming after confirmed reports that *kala-azar* patients have a tendency to get infected with HIV (The virus that causes AIDS).[19] This mutual gridlock between the germs of *kala-azar* and AIDS poses a serious threat before us. At present, the majority of cases of HIV-Visceral Leishmaniasis co-infection have been reported in the Mediterranean basin. As Magill has warned, the emergence of Visceral Leishmaniasis as a serious opportunistic infection in patients with AIDS in Europe has alarming implications for areas with endemic leishmaniasis, especially sub-Saharan Africa, Brazil, and the Indian subcontinent, where the prevalence of HIV infection is increasing.[20] Visceral Leishmaniasis has a prevalence of 7 to 17 per cent as a cause of fever of uncertain origin. Serologic studies in endemic areas suggest that L donovani infection may be asymptomatic. Asymptomatic latent infections have also been documented in HIV-infected patients. Dormant infection is believed to be five to ten times more frequent than *kala-azar*. Bearing this in mind, even in countries in which leishmaniasis is rare, a certain number of HIV-infected patients can be expected to acquire latent leishmaniasis during trips to endemic regions. Because of the severe immunologic impairment caused by HIV, this disease may be reactivated years after intial contact with the parasite, thus underscoring the importance of eliciting a complete travel history, especially in areas in which Leishmania is not so common.

The number of such simultaneous disease (called co-infection) is increasing rapidly and spreading like a wild fire. This co-infection has no known cure. If kept unchecked, it is sure to add another chapter in the epidemiology of *kala-azar*, perhaps the last one for humankind.

References

1. Thucydides, *History of the Peloponnesian War*, 428 BC.
2. John Ephesus, *Historia Ecclesiastica,* AD 525.

3. R.S. Desowitz, *The Malaria Capers*, W.W. Norton and Company, New York.
4. *U.N. Brahmachari and Perspective of Kala azar Research*. Indian Institute of Chemical Biology.
5. *Reports of the Indian Kala-azar Commission (1924–1932). No. 1, Indian Medical Research Memoir* 4; no. 2, *Ibid*, 25.
6. A.C. Chandler, C.P. Read, *Introduction to Parasitology*, John Wiley & Sons Inc, New York.
7. W.B. Leishman 'On the possibility of the occurrence of Trypanosomasis in India', *British Medical Journal* (May 30) 1903, p.1250 (hereafter *BMJ*)
8. C. Donovan 'On the possibility of the occurrence of Trypanosomasis in India', *BMJ* (July 11) 1903, p. 79.
9. R. E. Lee, R.H. Young, B. Castleman, James Homer Wright, A Biography of the Enigmatic Creator of the Wright Stain on the occasion of Its Centennial', *Am J Surg Pathol*, 26, 2002, pp. 88–96.
10. R. Ross, 'Further Notes on Leishman Bodies', *BMJ* (Nov. 28) 1903, p. 1401.
11. R. O. A. Smith, K. C. Halder, J. Ahmed, 'Transmission of *Kala-azar*', *Ind. Med. Gaz.* 75: 67; ed: *Ibid*; 97-98; Ind. *J. Med. Res.* 575 - 591; 29: 783–802.
12. C. S. Swaminath, H. E. Shoff, A. P. Anderson, 'Transmission of Indian *kala-azar* by the bites of Phlebotomas argentipes', *Ind J Med Res*, 1942, 30, p. 4703.
13. U. N. Brahmachari, 'Note on the history of the treatment of Kala-azar with Urea Stibamine', *J Trop Med Hyg*. (June 3), 1941, p. 67.
14. S. Sundar, 'Drug resistance in Indian visceral leishmaniasis'. *Trop Med Int Health*, 2001, 6, pp. 849-54. Erratum in: *Trop Med Int Health* 2002, 7, p. 293.
15. P. Desjeux, WHO/CTD International Document, The Leishmaniasis meeting of the interested parties on management and finalizing the control of tropical diseases other than malaria, CTD/MIP/Wp 93, 8, Geneva, Sep. 15, 1993.
16. World Health Organization Expert Committee, *Control of the Leishmaniases*, 1990.
17. K. D. Chatterjee, *Parasitology in Relation to Clinical Medicine*, Calcutta.
18. S. Sundar, M.Rai, 'Advances in the treatment of leishmaniasis', *Crr Opin Infect Dis*, 2002, 15, pp. 593-8.
19. P. Desjeux, and UNAIDS, *Leishmania and HIV in gridlock*, WHO, 1998.
20. A J. Magill, 'Epidemiology of the leishmaniases', *Dermatol Clin.*, 1995, 13, pp. 505–23.

9

Upendranath Brahmachari in Pursuit of *Kala-azar*

—Achintya Kumar Dutta

Introduction

The last decade of the 19th century upto the outbreak of the First World War may be described as a classic era in the history of 'tropical medicine'. During this period, remarkable researches in the disciplines of parasitology, entomology, and protozoology enriched medical science. It was a period when great importance was attached to the life cycles of parasites and their relationships with hosts and transmitters. It was also a time of optimism—faith abounded in the potential benefits of new discoveries.[1] The fatal and dreadful diseases in the tropics were considered conquerable. Research works on 'tropical medicine' were carried out both in Europe and the tropics. In India, the members of the Indian Medical Service studied tropical diseases and greatly contributed to their control. As in the case of other infective diseases, they struggled hard when *kala-azar* epidemic caused havoc and became a serious public health problem in late 19th century India. The most celebrated among them who worked on *kala-azar* and its remedy, were Rogers, Mackie, Hume, Castellani, James, Shortt, Napier, and Knowles. Along with them one should not forget to mention the name of an Indian medical scientist — Upendranath Brahmachari — who has earned fame for his legendary work on this disease. Brahmachari discovered the most efficacious drug for the treatment of *kala-azar*, named *urea stibamine* without which it might have been difficult for the British Indian Government to reduce the mortality due to this disease. This drug reinforced the fight for conquering this disease in India. The present article aims at focusing the efficacy of this drug and the contribution of Dr. Brahmachari to the conquest of this dreadful disease.

I

Kala-azar or 'Black Fever' is an infective disease caused by the protozoan parasite called *Leishman donavan body (Leishmania donovani)* which is inoculated into man by certain species of sand flies. It is characterized by fever of long duration sometimes acute or subacute, enlargement of the spleen and frequently also of liver, anaemia, and progressive emaciation. *Kala-azar* was highly endemic in India during the colonial period and had an adverse impact on the population and economic growth of the country due to its high mortality and morbidity rates. It could be a fatal disease with a mortality rate of more than 95 per cent. *Kala-azar* invaded a large part of eastern India and the worst affected areas were Assam, Bengal, and Bihar. It occurred also in Madras and certain parts of Orissa and the United Provinces. In India, *kala-azar* also broke out in epidemic form in Assam and Bengal where it occurred at intervals of 15 to 20 years lasting three to four years at a time.[2] Needless to say that this disease was not only confined to tropical regions. It was also prevalent in China, the Mediterranean basin, in European countries, such as Italy, Spain, Greece and in South America too. It became a global phenomenon in the 20th century.

Kala-azar was universally accepted as being a very severe and generally fatal disease. It became a matter of concern for the British Indian government since 1882 when a severe outbreak of this disease occurred in the Garo Hills in Assam. The disease spread steadily over a large area covering almost all the subdivisions of Assam including the tea gardens. From this date onwards, Assam faced two to three severe outbreaks of *kala-azar* epidemic during British rule.[3] The epidemic conditions were not limited to Assam, and serious outbreaks of epidemic *kala-azar* were co-existent in Bengal and Bihar.

In Assam, *kala-azar* had a more pernicious influence on public health than any other disease. It had adversely affected the growth of population and economic development. Of the people affected, about 90 to 95 per cent died. It had caused serious depopulation in the whole tracts of the Terai portions of Goalpara, Kamrup, and Nowgong districts, and had so greatly reduced the population of other parts that some of the tea gardens of Kamrup found it impossible to get more than a very small part of the labour they wanted from local sources.[4] Before the epidemic affected the district, they had more applicants than they could find employment, for, G. M. Giles in his report stated that the mortality from *kala-azar* was so serious that it was difficult to gain an exact idea of the absolute number of deaths it had caused.[5] It fact, *kala-azar* took a heavy toll of human lives in Assam. For instance, it caused the death of 63,874 persons between 1896 and 1900.[6] A painstaking study by T. C. McCombie Young in the early 1920s revealed that at a time when population growth was 15-20 per cent per decade, high mortality due to *kala-azar* had stilled not only the rise, but actually produced a decline in Assam.[7] Many villages had lost two-thirds of their population within a few years. There was a continuous drop in the population till 1921 due to *kala-azar* which seems to have retarded the natural growth of population.[8] Labour force was depleted by death and desertion, and working efficiency of the remaining labourers was impaired. Consequently, extensive areas in the affected districts had fallen out of cultivation and land had lost its value.[9] *Kala-azar* took such a deadly form in Assam that many areas were converted into veritable 'valleys of death'. In fact, Assam became a notorious centre of the terrible *kala-azar*. H. E. Shortt, Director of *Kala-azar* Commission, was of the opinion that in no other area of the world, with the possible exception of China, did it occur in the form of devastating epidemics.[10] The very name *kala-azar* struck such a terror in the hearts of the people of the affected parts that, when there was no effective treatment for it, the wretched sufferers from this disease had been turned out of the villages in which they lived and bandied about from one to another. No one was willing to admit them for fear of catching the disease themselves.[11] Thus, humane and social relationship of man was impaired.

Kala-azar attacked all classes, rich and poor, young and old, and all communities. But there was no effective treatment for it before 1915. The anti-*kala-azar* measures adopted before this date were limited to the use of some non-specific drugs and evacuation and segregation of the uninfected people from one place to another. These measures were found to be unsuccessful. The medical men deputed for anti-*kala-azar* works had also certain limitations in the diagnosis of the disease. Neither the cause of this disease nor the method of its spread was known to them. The majority of the physician regarded *kala-azar* as 'a bad form of malaria', notwithstanding its peculiar clinical features, its great fatality, the almost constant absence of malaria parasites from the blood, and the inefficiency of quinine treatment.[12] Well into the beginning of the 20th century confusion prevailed over the nature of this disease. However, from 1889–90 onwards, several investigations were carried on under the auspices of the British Indian Government to identify the disease and check its progress. Experts like G. M. Giles, Leonard Rogers, and Ronald Ross were sent to Assam to conduct investigations. But it remained elusive for a long time. It was in the year 1903 that the causative agent of the disease was discovered as a result of systematic efforts of William Boog Leishman and Charles Donovan. Leishman carried out his research in Great Britain and Donovan in India and they discovered the *kala-azar* parasite almost simultaneously but independently in two corners of the world.[13] Henceforth, the parasite has been known as 'Leishman-donovan body' (L D body) and the disease as *leishmania donovani*. By 1904, it was established that L D bodies were the causative agent of *kala-azar* that had already caused havoc in the eastern parts of the country. Thus, the confusion and controversy so far prevalent among the medical experts in the world came to an end. Until then no one seemed certain about the true nature of this sui generis disease and the same disease was known by different names e.g. Dum Dum fever, malarial *cachexia, kala-dukh, jwar vikar* and so forth.[14]

Though the parasite was identified, its remedy remained a mystery. Neither indigenous nor western drugs could prove to be effective to cure the disease. The role of modern medicine was still very limited in controlling *kala-azar*. The specific treatment for it was yet to come. Any dealings with *kala-azar* were found to be most trying experiences. The doctors used to visit the infected villages with no remedy to offer the unfortunate victims. The drugs, such as quinine, *thymol, leucocyte* increasing drugs, alkaloids, bone marrow and spleen extracts, and so on were given in the hope that they might possibly do some good. But these were of little effect and proved to be unsatisfactory.[15] Consequently, the ravages of *kala-azar* continued unabated. It was not before 1915 that modern medical technology found its success against it in India. In that year antimony was first introduced in the subcontinent in the form of *tarter emetic*. But greater success was achieved subsequently with organic compounds of antimony, especially after the discovery of the most efficacious drug—*urea stibamine*—in 1921, which heralded a new era in the history of 'tropical medicine'.

II

It is usually held that success in tropical medicine is mainly due to the work of western experts. There seems little doubt that members of the IMS greately contributed to the development of tropical medicine. Their research works and contributions have been widely acclaimed all over the world. But the contributions of Indian medical men belonging to subordinate grades have probably not been so emphatically recognized. In connection with the fight against *kala-azar*, one may unhesitatingly give special appreciation to the works of Upendranath Brahmachari for his discovery of *urea stibamine. Urea stibamine* was found by the medical men in all *kala-azar* areas of the world to be a very powerful therapeutic agent, and one of the best pentavalent antimonials without which it might have been difficult for the Government of India to rapidly check the mortality due to *kala-azar* in India.

Upendranath (1875–1946) was born in Jamalpur (Bihar) in 1875. His father Nilmani Brahmachari was a successful doctor in the Railways and had earned himself great reputation. Having completed his secondary education at Jamalpur, Upendranath obtained the degree of BA with honours in mathematics from Hooghly College in 1893. He had a very successful career as a student in the Calcutta Medical College. He obtained the degree of Doctor of Medicine in 1902. He was also keen to acquire knowledge in chemistry and achieved an M Sc degree in 1894 from the Presidency College, University of Calcutta. His knowledge in chemistry and mathematics perhaps stood him in great stead in his researches in the preparation of *urea stibamine*. He subsequently obtained a PhD degree in physiology from this university in 1904. After completing his MB degree, Brahmachari entered the Provincial Medical Service in 1898, served different medical institutions as teacher in medicine, and subsequently became professor of tropical medicine at Carmichael Medical College (presently R. G. Kar Medical College), Calcutta.[16] He spent the longest period of his service at Campbell Medical School, Calcutta (presently Sir Nilratan Sirkar Medical College and Hospital) where he discovered *urea stibamine*.

Brahmachari began to study *kala-azar* cases in the early years of his career at the Calcutta Medical College Hospital (CMCH), when all cases of enlarged spleen with anaemia, and a history of fever resembling that of malaria and coming from more or less malarious places used to be called *malarial chachexia*. He was struck by the frequent occurrence and worst prognosis of such cases. He started thinking over them when he found that they never showed any malaria parasites in the blood, that their fever could not be checked by quinine, that a very large number of them ended fatally, and many of them had *cancrum oris* and droppy.[17] It struck him that their cause was something that was not known. He further observed that the available drugs could not check the progress of the disease. Even he himself had tried quinine in small and large doses, fluorides and arsenic for *kala-azar* cases, but these were of no effect.[18] Needless to say that the *kala-azar* patients came in flocks for the treatment to the hospitals in Calcutta from different parts of Assam and Bengal. But the physicians were helpless. A large number of patients under Brahmachari's treatment at the Campbell Hospital died. Some left the hospital in a worse condition than at the time of admission.[19] None of the cases were benefited by the existing treatment. Brahmachari was moved by this phenomenon. Thereafter the problem of treatment of *kala-*

azar cases gripped his attention. Besides teaching, he spent a number of hours in his laboratory for its remedy, and after years of long and patient research succeeded in discovering the most effective drug, *urea stibamine*, in 1921 for its treatment.

There had been great pioneering workers before him in this line, notably Leonard Rogers, who first introduced antimony treatment in India (1915) in the form of *tarter emetic* for this disease. It is, however, known that Drs. Di-Christina and Caronia of Sicily used this treatment for *kala-azar* cases in the Mediterranean basin before Rogers introduced it in India and they obtained remarkable result.[20] The success of antimony treatment seems to have been reported even before that, when Brazilian doctor Gaspar Vianna used *tarter emetic* in the treatment of *dermal leishmaniasis* in South America in 1913.[21] But Rogers claimed that he had found out that remedy without previous knowledge of the works of Brazilian and Italian doctors. Whatever it may be, the conquest of *kala-azar* may be said to have begun with the introduction of the antimony treatment by Vianna, Di-Christina, and Caronia. This drug was also beginning to be used in India at the same time, and Rogers, Mackie, Hume, Castillani, and Brahmachari were the pioneers in this field in the treatment of Indian *kala-azar*.

As far as India was concerned, the introduction of antimony treatment was a great advance in the treatment of this disease. About 70 per cent of the cases could be curbed with this drug.[22] But it soon revealed certain defects. *Tarter emetic* had some serious toxic effects that was observed by Rogers himself, and also by Napier of Calcutta School of Tropical Medicine. It was replaced within a very short time by the better tolerated analogue, *sodium antimony tartrate*, which was the first in a succession of antimony derivatives to be tested in the treatment of *kala-azar* by the young Brahmachari who first used it in 1915.[23] But it was also not a very safe drug. In fact, antimony treatment for *kala-azar* cases was not satisfactory and it had certain disadvantages. Amongst those who underwent treatment with these drugs, the death rate was decidedly high. It is difficult to say how high it was —as the records on this point were very seldom obtained or, at any rate, reported, but in one of the large Calcutta hospitals the death rate amongst in-patients undergoing treatment with *antimony tartrates* during one year was 15 per cent and in the out-door department 25 per cent, and in well-conducted treatment centres in the mofussil, where conditions were probably less favourable, death-rates as high as 50 per cent had been reported.[24] In the campaign against the disease, the treatment had the disadvantage of being long and tedious. The treatment with tartrates extended over a period of 2 to 3 months during which an average of 30 injections had to be given for a complete cure.[25] The patients were tired of it and consequently a very large number of patients failed to complete the full course of treatment. There were certain very disagreeable symptoms associated with their administration, such as coughing, vomiting, and joint pains, which also encouraged patients to discontinue their treatment too early.[26] And, finally a certain percentage of cases showed no improvement when treated by these drugs. N. C. Kapur, Resident Physician of the Medical College Hospital, Calcutta observed in 1925 that a certain percentage of *kala-azar* was resistant to *tarter emetic*, or *sodium antimony tartrate*. When he used *urea stibamine* in those cases he found remarkable results.[27] Dr. J. Dodds Price, Medical Officer, tea estates, Salana, Assam also showed that cases of *kala-azar* showing little or no improvement with *sodium antimony tartrate* were subsequently cured by *urea stibamine*.[28] In other words, these drugs proved to be inefficacious in relapsing cases.

So, the antimony treatment could not become very successful in the fight against *kala-azar*. Treatment was found difficult to enforce in a state like Assam, which was then the hot-bed of *kala-azar*, as patients discontinued treatment altogether or continued very irregularly after a few injections. This irregularities made it very difficult to effect a complete cure.[29] Major T. D. Murrison, Director of Public Health, Assam once noticed that in spite of the regulations in force under the Epidemic Disease Act to compel the patients to undergo a complete course of treatment, campaign against the disease was greatly handicapped by the large number of patients who stopped treatment.[30] In 1924, out of 48,770 cases treated in Assam, 16,733 stopped treatment before the completion of their course; the ratio is about 33 per cent.[31] So the uncured patients could become dangerous to others.

Though many were prepared to be satisfied with this treatment, Brahmachari was not contended with these drugs and mode of treatment. He felt that to overcome this difficulty a more efficacious drug would be necessary which would take a much shorter time to effect a complete cure. With this end in view, Brahmachari continued his research on the chemotherapy of antimonial compounds. Between the years of 1915–1921, he carried out many experiments in a small laboratory attached to the Campbell Medical School in Calcutta. He first synthesized several new inorganic antimonials and achieved some treatment success with colloidal metalic antimony.[32] But dissatisfied with these results he turned his attention to organic aromatic antimonials. In 1920, shortly after being financed by the Indian Research Fund Association for carrying out researches into the treatment of *kala-azar*, he had almost reached his target when he prepared some of the organic compounds of antimony in his laboratory. Finally, early in 1921, Brahmachari produced the first organic antimonial (stibalinic acid with urea) to achieve wide acceptance as a treatment for human *leishmaniasis.*[33] With a brilliant background of mathematics and chemistry, extraordinary talents for clinical observation and imaginative genius, Brahmachari experimented with various salts, prepared several compounds, and tested them on animals (guineapig, rats) and in selected instances on man. Ultimately led by the knowledge that urea in combination with certain drugs reduces the pain on injection, he synthesized urea salt and prepared urea compound. This compound was named *urea stibamine*. In this discovery he is said to have been greatly inspired by the work of Paul Ehrlich on the development of organic arsenical *atoxyl* for the treatment of African sleeping seekness.[34]

III

Having obtained remarkable results in a number of cases, Brahmachari reported the therapeutic value of this drug and how he prepared it in renowned medical journals.[35] He was then a teacher of medicine at Campbell Medical School, Calcutta. He acknowledged the assistance of his staff in the research. They were Niharranjan Chatterjee, Saradacharan Chaudhury, Dr. Pramathanath Ghosh, and Sub-Asstt. Surgeon, Bibhuti Bhusan Maity.[36] Brahmachari also acknowledged the inspiration received in his research from Sir Patrick Manson who once wrote to him: 'Go on in your efforts to get an antimony compound that can be used as an intramascular injection or better still as a drug that can be administered by the mouth'.[37] Brahmachari concluded that *urea stibamine* was useful in *kala-azar* cases and much safer than the existing drugs. He also asserted that the resistant cases of *kala-azar* which were non-responsive to other drugs were cured by *urea sibamine.*[38]

The story of *urea sibamine* is itself worthy of recording as a dramatic medical breakthrough. After Brahmachari had satisfied himself with preliminary trials that *urea stibamine* could be used as an ideal drug, the compound was sent to other physicians of different institutions for its application in the treatment of *kala-azar*. At the request of Colonel E. D. W. Greig, Government Director of Medical Research, Brahmachari supplied samples of some of his products including *urea stibamine* to H. E. Shortt, the then Officer-in-Charge, *Kala-azar* Enquiry, Assam for trial at the Special *Kala-azar* Hospital in Shillong, the then capital of Assam. Of these products, Brahmachari said, '*urea stibamine* has been found useful in the treatment of *kala-azar*'.[39] As soon as the drug was tried in

Shillong (1922) by Shortt and Ram Taran Sen (In-charge, Special *Kala-azar* Hospital, Shillong), the results in the first few cases showed such an astonishing advance on those obtained with the older preparations that a larger supply was called for and supplied by Brahmachari and further experimentation carries out.[40] Shortt found it so effective that cases could be treated and cured by about eight doses instead of taking many weeks or even months, and with unpredictable results. In other words, a short course cured 90 per cent of all cases where previously 90 per cent of untreated cases died.[41] He also noted that the results were actually better than those claimed by Dr. Brahmachari himself.[42] On the basis of experience and results gained from the series of cases in Shillong, Shortt and Sen concluded in 1924 that *urea stibamine* proved to be superior to any of the other antimony preparation in general use and the most efficient drug for the treatment of Indian *kala azar*.[43] Shortt recommended its trial in certain approved centres in endemic areas.

The medical profession in and around Calcutta, also used this drug and recognized its value. Actual records of a large number of cases in the wards of the Calcutta Medical College Hospitals, under different physicians in 1923 showed that the disease was radically cured in three weeks by *urea stibamine*.[44] In fact, reports of remarkable results by this drug gradually came from every corner. Apart from Shortt and Sen, S. R. Christophers, Director of *Kala-azar* Commission, medical officers of the tea estates in Assam, and also the Government of Assam reported from their experience in this state about its remarkable efficacy.[45] Government of Assam quickly introduced it in certain hospitals and treatment centres for *kala-azar* cases. The governing body of the Indian Research Fund Association also recognized its therapeutic value from their reports. In Calcutta, its value was recognized by the physicians of the Calcutta Medical College Hospitals and successive superintendents of the Calcutta European Presidency General Hospitals.[46] In these institutions it was extensively used with the most satisfactory results. Its reputation quickly spread all over Assam, Bengal, Bihar and Orissa, and to more distant parts in India, such as Madras, Sanawar, Simla Hills, and others. Those who had tried this drug were convinced of the great advance made by its discovery in the treatment of *kala-azar*. Within a very short period after its discovery a number of papers on its successful use and remarkable results were published in some esteemed medical journals, where the value of this drug in curing *kala-azar* was emphasized.

Thus, *urea stibamine* proved to be specifically highly active in *kala-azar*. It shortened the course of treatment, occupying only two to three weeks to effect a complete cure, and was able to cure intractable cases which were resistant to antimony treatment. It was found to be a very stable, safe, and reliable drug and had no untoward complications. During the seven years from 1924, the doctors under the *Kala-azar* Commission treated some thousands of *kala-azar* cases with *urea stibamine,* and they saw thousands more treated in treatment centres. But they came across no cases of death directly attributable to this drug.[47]

From the economic point of view, there were certain advantages of its use for the government and also for the poor, miserable sufferers. Though *urea stibamine* was costlier than *tarter emetic* or *sodium antimonyl tartrate*, its use could easily save some money of the government. The extra cost of the drug in treating with *urea stibamine* as compared with the *tartrate* was Rs. 9-15-0, yet it could save Rs. 8-13-0 per (indoor) patient treated in diets alone, not to mention hospital accommodation, staff, and clothing.[48] For the patients could be cured by this drug in a much shorter period than the sodium salt, and consequently were released from the hospital quickly. So it would be economically sound to treat all indoor patients with *urea stibamine* in hospitals where competent medical officers were available. Therefore, for 1925, arrangements had been made to treat all resistant cases throughout the province of Assam by this drug in selected hospitals.[49] In the next year, mass free treatment with this drug was initiated by Government of Assam.

Thus Brahmachari's discovery opened a new vista of *kala-azar* treatment in India. E. W. C. Bradfield, an IMS officer, has rightly remarked that the modern treatment of *kala-azar* may be said to have commenced in 1922, with the introduction of *urea stibamine.*[50] Thanks to Shortt and Sen who established its use and opened the field for treatment by it in Assam. The intensive treatment carried on with this drug resulted in remarkable increase in cures and a more regular attendance of patients at treatment centres.[51] The number of 'stopped treatment' cases showed a tendency to decline, partly due to the shorter course of treatment by it, and also to other measurers including propaganda work adopted by the Public Health Department against this disease.[52] Quite a large number of patients were brought under successful treatment. They were cured and consequently mortality due to *kala-azar* reduced remarkably. This can be discerned from the following table.

Number of *kala-azar* cases treated and number of deaths due to it in Assam (quinquennial table)

Year	*No. of cases treated*	*No. of deaths*
1920	7188	2798
1925	60940	6365
1930	16430	953
1935	11100	845

Source: Annual Public Health Report of the Province of Assam, relevant years, relevant tables.

Urea stibamine thus became an established drug. It had successfully combated the enemy and saved the lives of innumerable victims. During the period 1923–1933, no less than 328,591 persons had been brought under treatment in Assam and nearly 3.25 lakhs of valuable lives had been saved.[53] In 1933, the Director of Public Health, Assam noted that '*urea stibamine* was our mainstay in the treatment of *kala-azar*'.[54] Prior to the antimonials, upto 95 per cent of sufferers had perished and death rate was also high with antimony treatment (upto 25 per cent), whereas the mortality rate was reduced in 1925 to 10 per cent and by 1936 to just over 7 per cent.[55] The treatment with this drug was confined not only to Assam; it was also used in other parts of northeast India. Short remarked, 'This was a dramatic curative success in tropical medicine and *urea stibamine* became the routine treatment in India with its many thousands of cases'.[56] Brahmachari's discovery was also appreciated by Sir John Kerr, once Governor of Assam, who was very hopeful about the complete control of this disease in Assam. Though some other drugs like *von Hayden* 471 (known as *stibosan*), *stiburea,* and *neostibosan* were put on the market subsequent to the introduction of *urea stibamine* and as a result of its success, none of them could replace it. For some time experiments with *neostibosan* were conducted side by side with *urea stibamine*, but it was of little effect. The patient treated with *neostibosan* showed very little improvement even at the conclusion of a course of treatment.[57] Though it was claimed in certain cases that *neostibosan* and *stiburea* were superior to *urea stibamine*, observations did not confirm it. However, their use was subsequently discontinued.[58] These drugs, some of which produced some disagreeable symptoms after administration, were not so efficacious as *urea stibamine.*

IV

It thus appears from the aforesaid historical account that Upendranath Brahmachari discovered the ideal drug for conquering one of the lethal diseases in India. Brahmachari's discovery may be considered as one of the greatest achievements in the history of medical science. Yet, all white physicians and officials were not ready to recognize it. Leonard Rogers, the celebrated IMS officer, had never tried *urea stibamine* and attempted to belittle its efficacy by highlighting the curative value of the other drug, *stibosan.*[59] It appears that Rogers' research on *kala-azar* was superseded by Brahmachari, a doctor belonging to the subordinate medical service. It seems to have hurt his pride and prestige. A conservative and Victorian gentleman of a landed family, Rogers was unable to welcome the achievement of a non-IMS Indian medical scientist. He failed to extend his support for the benefit of Indian medical men in general in any really constructive manner.[60] He could not break out of the paternalism which characterized the late Victorian era in which he had begun his imperial service.[61] L. E. Napier, another IMS officer, also tried to reduce the worth of *urea stibamine*. In his letter to Rogers, dated. 7 February, 1924, Napier wrote from Calcutta School of Tropical Medicine, 'Shortt appears to have had very good luck with *urea stibamine*. We have been given samples very grudgingly and have tried it on a number of cases with mixed success. The first case that I treated did very well but subsequent cases have not done as well and to one case I gave 20 injections amounting to 4 grams without effecting a cure'.[62] Napier said that *stibosan* was the most stable compound and it was more rapid in its action even than *urea stibamine*.[63] He further added in 1929 that *urea stibamine* had been used very extensively in India in the treatment of *kala-azar* and yielded good results, but most of the reports published on it were entirely unsatisfactory.[64] What is amazing is that, Roger's work, to Napier and Knowles (IMS), on *kala-azar* was much more impressive than that of Brahmachari.

Sir Arthur Dash, who acted temporarily as the Secretary to the Government of Bengal in the Medical Department in 1927, did not honour the spectacular achievement of Brahmachari. He stated in his memoirs that Brahmachari's assertion that he had invented a better drug for *kala-azar* cases and put it on the market at a much lower price than *stibamine*, a drug discovered by the School of Tropical Medicine, Calcutta (which was under the control of the British members of the IMS), was nothing but an attempt to attack the monopoly of the 'IMS ring'.[65] He said that the IMS ring had the medical skill, the qualifications, and the experience on their side. The IMS officers, British and Indian, not in the ring and all the Indian physicians and surgeons not in the IMS, lurked enviously and disconsolately outside the ring and they clutched eagerly at any pretext for attacking the monopoly of the 'IMS ring'.[66] He ridiculously described Brahmachari as a 'prophet' among them. Dash had a very inferior notion of the Indian doctor's ability and calibre. What is more, he was perhaps not fully aware of what *kala-azar* was and had little idea about the efficacy of *urea stibamine*.[67]

To minimize his work on this ground is nothing but an attempt to denigrate his contribution and marginalize Indian medical scientists. Upendranath's research was not guided by any ill motive. Brahmachari worked hard to provide relief to the *kala-azar* sufferers. He felt for them and devoted himself to give them a remedy. His response to the fight against this malign malady was spontaneous. Upendranath's discovery was in no way inferior to the discoveries of the medical scientists of the west, say discoveries of Pasteur, Koch, Laveran, or of Ross. It was the fruit of his physical and intellectual efforts. He had reacted in the most useful manner to the needs and problems of the time, endeavouring to be a worthy representative of the age and generation.

Upendranath's discovery of *urea stibamine* was not accidental nor was it an easy task. It became the subject of research for many years. This was a self-imposed work and he carried it out with single-minded devotion and dogged tenacity. Though funded by Indian Research Fund Association, Brahmachari had to work under great difficulties. No proper laboratory facilities were available to him at the time and he had to carry on his researches in a small room without a water tap or gas point and lighted by a kerosene lamp at night, and often in the midst of troubles and difficulties from many quarters.[68]

Brahmachari made an unforgettable impression by freely supplying *urea stibamine* to the *Kala-azar* Commission in Assam for the treatment of the disease for quite a long time. This Commission used, throughout the seven years of its existence, one drug only in the routine treatment of *kala-azar, viz., urea stibamine* and this drug was ungrudgingly supplied by him. The Director of *Kala-azar* Commission states, 'We have been greatly indebted to the generosity of Dr. U. N. Brahmachari of Calcutta, who first prepared *urea stibamine*, for an unfailing free supply of this drug during a period of seven years'.[69]

Upendranath Brahmachari was a genuine friend of India. He had a special blend of cognitive skill and extraordinary clinical interest. These combined attributes led him to discover Post-*kala-azar* Dermal Leishmanoid (PKDL), a skin lesion that developed in certain *kala-azar* patients after completion of antimonial treatment and apparent cure. Apart from *kala-azar* research, Brahmachari had also contributed to other areas of medical importance, such as malaria, filariasis, diabetes, leprosy and meningitis, and haematological disorders. All these focus upon his skill, talent, and qualities. Brahmachari's successful researches on *kala-azar* and his discoveries seem to have proved that India was capable of producing excellent scientists. He devoted himself to the promotion of medical science in the service of mankind. His discovery of *urea stibamine* considerably helped the government in controlling and combating *kala-azar* in India, and saved the people from the horror of this dreadful disease. It is really a matter of delight, as remarked by Sir Nilratan Sarkar, for every Indian to see that the British Indian Government depended upon one of our home-made products for the purpose of vanquishing one of our worst enemies. The medical profession should be proud of a talent like Upendranath Brahmachari.

Acknowledgement: I am thankful to the Commonwealth Scholarship Commission, UK for its support in carrying out my research at London which made this article possible.

References

1. Helen Joy Power, 'Sir Leonard Rogers FRS (1860–1962): Tropical Medicine in the Indian Medical Service', Ph.D. thesis, University of London, 1993, p. 9 (hereafter *Ph.D. thesis*).
2. T. H. Davey and W. P. H. Lightbody, *The Control of Disease in the Tropics,* London, 1965, p. 141.
3. H. E. Shortt, 'Recent Researches on *kala-azar* in India', *Transaction of the Royal Society of Tropical Medicine & Hygiene*, vol. XXXIX, no. 1, September 1945, pp. 13–29.
4. Leonard Rogers, *Report of an Investigation of the Epidemic of Malaria Fever in Assam or Kala-azar*, Shillong, 1897, p. 129 (hereafter *Report of Epidemic in Assam*).
5. *A Report of an Investigation into the Causes of the Disease Known in Assam as Kala-azar and Beri-Beri* by G. M. Giles, Shillong, 1890, p. 19.
6. *Annual Sanitary Report of the Province of Eastern Bengal and Assam for the Year 1905*, p. 9 (hereafter *ASR*).
7. For details see, *Kala-azar in Assam an Account of the Preventive Operations, 1910 to 1923* and *Notes on the Epidemiology of the Disease in Assam and India* by T. C. McCombie Young, London, 1924, pp. 6 - 11.
8. *Assam Secretariat Proceedings, Revenue Department, Revenue Branch*, December 1931, Progs. no. 273 (hereafter *Assam Progs.*).
9. Leonard Rogers, *Reports of Epidemic in Assam*, p. 132.
10. The British Library, Oriental and India Office Collection, Mss/EUR, *In the Days of the Raj and After, Doctor, Soldier, Scientist, Sikari* by H. E. Shortt, p. 70 (hereafter Mss / EUR, Shortt's papers.).
11. Leonard Rogers, *Report of Epidemic in Assam,* p. 129.
12. Philip D. Marsden, 'The Discovery of Urea Stibamine', *Revista Da Sociedade Brasileira De Medicina Tropical*, vol. 19, 1996, p. 115; Philip H. Manson Bahr (ed.), *Manson's Tropical Diseases*, London, 1921, p. 148.
13. For details see, Achintya Kumar Dutta, 'The Pursuit of *Kala-azar* and Upendranath Brahmachari', *History*, vol. III, no. 1, 2000, University of Burdwan, pp. 48-60.
14. 'The Conquest of *Kala-azar*' in *Science and Culture*, vol. V, no. 10, April 1940, p. 622.
15. Patrick Manson, *Tropical Diseases a Manual of the Diseases of Warm Climates*, London, 1903, p. 275; Philip H. Manson Bahr (ed.), *op. cit.*, p. 157.
16. For details about Brahmachari's biography, see Arun Kumar Chakraborty, *Chikitsa Bijnane Aviskar O Kolkata* (in Bengali), Calcutta, 1989, p. 63;

Kalpana De, *Baijnanikder Jeevani O Aviskar* (in Bengali), Calcutta, 1998 (second edition), pp. 96-97.

17. Upendranath Brahmachari, *Gleanings from My Research: Kala-azar, Its Chemotherapy*, vol. I, University of Calcutta, 1940, p. 253 (hereafter *Gleanings from My Research*).
18. *Ibid.*, p.259
19. *Ibid.*, p.259
20. *Ibid.*, p.442
21. *Tropical Diseases Bulletin*, vol. 5, no. 5, January 15, 1915–June 15, 1915, London, p. 269. Following the publication by Gaspar Vianna of cases of dermal leishmaniasis in South America successfully treated by intravenous injections of *tarter emetic*, Di-Christina and Caronia experimented with this treatment in cases of infantile *kala-azar*. The results they obtained were so encouraging that they were led to publish a note in *Tropical Diseases Bulletin* in the hope that others would give the method a trial.
22. P. C. Sengupta, 'History of *kala-azar* in India', *The Indian Medical Gazette* (hereafter *IMG*), vol. LXXXII, 1947, p. 283
23. Wallace Peters, 'The Treatment of *Kala-azar* — New Approaches to an Old Problem', *Indian Journal of Medical Research* (hereafter *Ind. J. Med. Res.*), 7 (suppl), January 1981, pp. 1–18.
24. 'The Treatment of *Kala-azar*'. *IMG*, December 1928 (editorial), p. 707.
25. *Ibid.*, p. 707; *Annual Public Health Report of the Province of Assam for the Year 1923*, p. 11 (hereafter *Health Report of Assam*).
26. *IMG*, December 1928 (editorial), p. 707.
27. N. C. Kapur, 'Observation on the Treatment of *Kala-azar* with Urea Stibamine in the Medical Outpatient Department of the Medical College Holpitals, Calcutta', *IMG*, vol. LX, May 1925, pp. 206–210.
28. J. Dodds Price, 'Cases of *Kala-azar* showing little or no Improvement with Sodium Antimony Tartrate, Subsequently Cured by *Urea stibamine*', *IMG*, vol. LIX, 1924, p. 464.
29. *Health Report of Assam for 1923*, p. 11.
30. *Ibid.*, p. 16.
31. *Ibid.*, p. 15.
32. Philip D. Marsden, *op. cit.*, p. 115.
33. *Ibid.*, p. 115.
34. *Ibid.*, p. 115; Wallace Peters, *op. cit.*, p. 2.
35. For detailes see U. N. Brahmachari, 'Chemotherapy of Antimonial Compounds in *Kala-azar* Infection' pt. I, *Ind. J. Med. Res.*, no. 2, October 1921, pp. 492-522.
36. *Ibid.*, p. 521.
37. U. N. Brahmachari, 'Chemotherapy of Antimonial Compounds in *Kala-azar* Infection' pt. IX, *IJMR,* vol. XI, no. 2, October 1923, pp. 405-410.
38. U. N. Brahmachari, 'Chemotherapy of Antimonial Compounds in *Kala-azar* Infection' pt. IX, *IJMR,* vol. XI, no. 4, April 1924, pp. 1205-1217.

39. *Indian Medical Research Memoirs No. 25: Reports of the Kala-azar Commission, India, Report No. II (1926–1930)*, Calcutta, 1932, p. 47 (hereafter *Kala-azar Comm. Report II*).
40. *Ibid.*, p. 47.
41. Mss/EUR Shortt's Papers, p. 73.
42. 'A Note on the Use of Urea Stibamine' by H. E. Shortt in *Ind. J. Med. Res.*, vol. XI, no. 2, October 1923, p. 403.
43. H. E. Shortt & Ram Taran Sen, 'Urea Stibamine in the Treatment of *Kala-azar*', *Ind. J. Med. Res.*, vol. XI, no. 2, October 1923, pp. 653–659; and 'Final Report on the Use of Urea Stibamine', *Indian Journal of Tropical Medicine*, vol. XII, no. 2, October 1924, pp. 335–336.
44. 'Conquest of *Kala-azar*' in *Science and Culture*, p. 531.
45. Upendranath Brahmachari, *A Treatise on Kala-azar*, London, 1928, p. 125.
46. *Ibid.*, p. 125.
47. *Kala-azar Comm. Report II*, p. 3.
48. *Health Report of Assam for 1924*, p. 16.
49. *Ibid.*, p. 16.
50. E. W. C. Bradfield, *An Indian Medical Review*, Delhi, 1938, p. 206.
51. *Health Report of Assam for 1927*, p. 16; *Triennial Report on the Working of the Dispensaries in Assam for the Years 1926, 1927 & 1928*, p. 5
52. *Health Report of Assam for 1925*, p. 14.
53. Upendranath Brahmachari, *Gleanings from My Research*, p. 458; *Health Report of Assam for 1933*, p. 20.
54. Upendranath Brahmachari, *Gleanings from My Research*, p. 458.
55. Wallace Peters, *op. cit.*, p. 3.
56. Mss/EUR, Shortt's Papers, p. 73.
57. L. E. Napier, *The Principle and Practice of Tropical Medicine*, Calcutta 1933, p. 169.
58. *Health Report of Assam for 1933*, p. 20; Upendranath Brahmachari, *Gleanings from My Research*, p. 444.
59. Arun Chakraborty, *op. cit.*, p. 64; Leonard Rogers, *Recent Advances in Tropical Medicine*, London, 1928, pp. 26-27.
60. Helen Power, 'The Calcutta School of Tropical Medicine: Institutionalizing Medical Research in the Periphery', *Medical History*, vol. 40, 1996, London, pp. 197–214; and *Ph.D. thesis*, pp. 14-15.
61. Helen Power, *op. cit.*, in *Medical History*, p. 214.
62. Wellcome Institute Library: PP/ROG/C1/1–88: Roger's papers, original letter from L. E. Napier to Leonard Rogers, dt. 7th February, 1924.
63. L. E. Napier, 'The Pentavalent Compounds of Antimony in the Treatment of *Kala-azar*', pt. IV, *Ind. J. Med. Res.*, vol. XVI, no. 4, April 1929, p. 901.
64. L. E. Napier, *A Handbook for Students and Practitioners*, OUP, 1927, pp. 164-165; Leonard Rogers, *Recent Advances in Tropical Medicine*, p. 27.

65. The British members of the IMS who held in their grip all the most lucrative medical and surgical posts in Calcutta and dominated the Indian Medical Service have been described as 'IMS ring' by Sir Arthur Dash. See Mss/EUR: The Memories of Sir Arthur Dash, pt. 3, p. 5 (at OIOC, the British Library).
66. *Ibid.*
67. Dash regarded that *kala-azar* and black water fever are one and same disease, see the The Memoires of Arthur Dash, pt. 2, p. 43.
68. 'Conquest of *Kala-azar*' in *Science and Culture*, p. 529.
69. *Kala-azar Comm. Report II*, p. 3. Brahmachari set up in his residential complex the 'Brahmachari Research Institute' in 1924 from his private means where *urea stibamine* and some other drugs were manufactured—see Arun Kumar Chakraborty, *op. cit.*, p. 65.

Western Medicine

10

Emergence of Western Medical Institutions in India, 1822–1911

—Anil Kumar

Concern for health has been an important feature of all historical processes, and more so in a process like colonization which involved aggression, intrusion, and imposition of one's will upon another. Every naval despatch from Europe had a surgeon on it, and he not only looked after the sick on board and land but was the first to report on the flora, fauna, and resources of the new territory. He was a surgeon-naturalist, and adventure-scientist in true sense! The medical training that he had (especially from Edinburgh) was different and made him feel superior while encountering other medical practices. Epistemologically, the system that he represented was not very dissimilar to that of the east, and some of them did show respect to the latter. But this was gradually lost in the victorious march of the colonizers' army. Gradual assimilation or synthesis was not on their agenda. Absolute supremacy of the one and total subjugation of the other characterized the Victorian imperialism for which the colonial medical men worked, and that is the reason their work, however noble and pioneering, can best be understood in terms of 'colonial medicine'.

Preservation of European health in new and 'hostile' lands was colonial medicine's first responsibility. Gradually the colonial doctors developed into a cultural force. They began defining or redefining what they saw in the colonies in terms of their own training and perceptions. Their work encompassed not only the understanding and possible conquest of new diseases but also the extension of western cultural values to the non-western world. Imperialism both as impulse and as attitude, required the operation of a set of skills and rules which European medicine undoubtedly complemented. As Franz Fanon put it, in the colonial context going to see the doctor, the administrator, the constable or the mayor became identical moves.[1]

During the 18th century, colonial medicine was wrapped in legendary adventures and medical geography in some scientific sense, but in the Victorian era it graduated into an organized colonial effort. Though the name given to it was tropical medicine, there was hardly anything tropical about it, apart from the fact that it operated in a tropical environment. Most of the so-called tropical diseases (except scala ringworm which thrived only in the tropical climes), which the tropical doctors dealt with, were to be found in Europe as well. Cholera, plague and small-pox, Europe had known for centuries. What distinguished them in a tropical climate was their intensity and ferocity. Very organized efforts were needed to combat it. In the 'settler' colonies where the Europeans had found a permanent home, medical discourse took the language of practical public health and professional advancement. But this was not to be so in classic colonies like India, Nigeria, or Congo where it worked as an appendage of the army and spoke the idiom of political and cultural superiority. Settler colonies were the extension of the European culture itself. In other places, both physical and cultural encounters took place in which the prevailing epistome and system had to be defeated and subordinated. So the prevalent Indian medical practices received more opprobrium than it deserved. Condemnation was easier but finding the cause of and a solution to the prevalent diseases was something different and difficult. So the blame was put on the climate; heat and humidity became the major obsessions of the tropical 'miasmatic' medicine. Miasma held its sway till Pasteur arrived.

The last quarter of the 19th century saw new breakthroughs. This was the era of bacteriology and parasitology. Search had begun for the microbes and the medium (the vector), and the tropical soil was found to be rich in both. What had begun as medical geography now became tropical medicine. A new discipline was ushered in with new specializations like helminthology, protozoology, and medical entomology. Parasitology gave many colonizers a sense of purpose and a practical programme. The microscope supplanted the sword, and the martial spirit gave place to the research habit in some limited sense.[2]

Yet, the fact remains that whether it were the early miasmatic theories of the 18th century or the tropical medicine of the 19th century, both were determined and influenced by the colonial conditions and imperatives; hence the use and relevance of the term 'colonial medicine'. Colonial medicine received the full political and military backing of the empire as its operations started with military conquests.

The earliest need for Indian helpers and assistants arose when the British medical officers began to treat the rank and file of regiments besides their brethren in various settlements and factories. They were called by different names such as 'native dressers' (Madras), 'country doctors', 'black doctors' (Bengal), and 'black assistants and 'apothecaries' (Bombay).[3] Later they were more popularly known as 'native doctors' and, by 1812, two of them were ordered to be attached to each regiment and one or more to each civil station. They were placed under 'Subordinate Military or Civil Medical Department' and termed as third class servants.[4]

Native Medical Institution

After 1812, a pressing need was increasingly felt to train the native doctors on a more scientific and systematic basis than the present method of teaching through the hospital or personal apprenticeships. Consequently, the Medical Board, impressed with the Orientalists' discoveries of richness and greatness of Sanskrit language and the availability of excellent treatises of Ayurvedic medicine, placed before the government in 1822 the proposal of establishing a novel medical institution where western as well as indigenous medical sciences would be taught side by side.[5]

Nomenclatured as the Native Medical Institution (NMI), it became functional in June 1823 with 20 students with a monthly stipend of Rs.8/– for a three year course in vernacular languages. At about the same time, Sanskrit medical classes were started at the Calcutta Sanskrit College where the works of Charak, Susruta and other Indian writers were studied along with the translated works in Urdu. Likewise, Urdu classes with the treatises on Unani were started at the Calcutta Madarsa.[6]

For clinical teaching, the students were required to attend the important hospitals of Calcutta. Dissection of the human body was not, however, performed and the only practical information given on the subject was obtained from the dissection of lower animals and from post-mortem examination at the General Hospital which the students were permitted to witness.[7] After qualifying the students were required to serve the army or civil department for 15 years on a salary or Rs. 20 per month, and an extra Rs. 5 when on field-service.[8]

John Tytler succeeded Surgeon Bretton as superintendent of the NMI in November 1830. Tytler was a noted Orientalist and during his tenure many vernacular translations appeared. Moreover, a small 30 bed hospital, for practical training was set up in August 1831, and was attached to the Sanskrit College. The hospital was largely the product of liberal donations made by Babu Ram Commul Sen.[9] All along, Tytler espoused the cause of medical education through vernacular languages. He regarded them rich enough to incorporate western medical learning and hence disapproved and opposed any imposition of English language till 1835 when he finally had to succumb.[10]

The Calcutta NMI was the first teaching institution of its kind in British India. Though the foremost objective of the government was to train a class of native doctors in Western medical system for military and civil requirements, an attempt at carrying forward the indigenous medical systems along with it, added a novel feature to British medical and educational policy. With the abolition of the NMI, for nearly a period of 85 years, the cause of rejuvenating and promoting the indigenous medical system was lost till the constitution of the provincial governments under the Act of 1919.[11]

Calcutta Medical College

In accordance with the recommendations of the Medical Commission, Bentinck, in January 1835, issued an order abolishing the NMI. Along with this the medical classes conducted at Calcutta Sanskrit College and Calcutta Madarsa were also discontinued. The same order sanctioned the foundation of Calcutta Medical College (CMC) from 1 February 1835.[12] The books and other equipment of the abolished Institution were made over to the new Medical College and Madhusudan Gupta, the 'Vaidya Professor' at the Institution along with his two assistants at the Sanskrit College, were transferred to the new medical college. Assistant Surgeon M. J. Bramley was appointed Superintendent (later designated as Principal), and Assistant Surgeon H. H. Goodeve as his only assistant to teach full time at the college. Later, during the same year, Assistant Surgeon W. B. O'Shaughnessy was appointed professor of chemistry and materia-medica.[13]

Initially, thus, with a three-member teaching staff, the Medical College started to train a group of 50 students in western medicine in English on monthly stipends ranging from Rs. 7 to Rs. 12, according to their seniority and merits. On leaving college, the native graduates were to be employed as sub-assistant surgeons (SASs), in the discharge of the duties of medical attendant in large dispensaries established in different parts of the country, on salaries ranging from Rs. 60 to Rs. 100 per month. They were, however, not compelled to enter government service and were free to establish themselves for private practice wherever they pleased. The first batch of students to secure the Diploma of Medicine and Surgery in 1838 consisted of Uma Charan Seth, Dwarkanath Gupta, Raj Kristo Dey, and Nobin Chunder Mitter. These four students were soon appointed as SAS to the hospitals at Dacca, Murshidabad, Patna, and Chittagong respectively at Rs. 100 per month.[14]

The native response towards the Anglicists' victory in the 'language controversy' and changeover to western medical education through the medium of English was simply enthralling. Raja Rammohan Roy, the leader of the newly emerged Hindu bhadralok, had been clamouring for the instruction of European sciences since long. He held it to be the panacea for many of the ills of traditional Hindu society. Babu Radhakanta Deb went a step further and publicly advocated the need for female medical education at a time when Hindu orthodoxy was not prepared even to drop *suttee* from its social practices. Not only this, he gave his wholehearted assistance to the popularization of vaccination in Bengal.[15]

The Calcutta Medical College gradually rose in public esteem and many prominent citizens of Calcutta began to attend the college lectures as amateurs, and contributed significantly in popularizing it among the lay public. Next, many rich and leading Calcuttans donated liberally to the Medical College and construction of hospitals. Further, many prizes and scholarships were instituted by them for students showing excellent performance in various branches of medicine. Within two years, the Brahmanical taboos associated with touching a dead body were thrown aside and increasing numbers of brahmin and Baidya youths were seen eagerly dissecting the human body with all calm and composure.[16] It is true that Madhusudan Gupta was the first modern Indian to touch and dissect a cadaver, but his feat was unduly exaggerated and publicized as demolisher of 'national and traditional prejudices'. In fact, western medical education became so popular that within a span of eight years, the government was compelled to open the entry of free students (non-stipendiary) in 1843 and to paying students in 1858, with an entrance fee of Rs. 5 per month during the course of their study in the College.[17]

The English class or the primary class at CMC was constituted in 1835 with 50 foundation pupils without any distinction of caste or religion, with the ability to read and write English and Bengali, or English and Hindustani aged between 14 and 20 years. The course was to last for three years at the end of which they had to pass an examination conducted by the examination committee of the College.[18] After completing the course they were given a diploma in medicine and surgery by the college, till Calcutta University was founded in 1857 which granted the degree of MD (Doctor of Medicine) and LMS (Licentiate in Medicine and Surgery). The degree of MB (Bachelor of Medicine) was added later on in 1860. Likewise, the duration of study was raised to four (1840) and later to five years (1845), and the minimum qualification for admission raised to Matriculation (1857) and later to the Fine Arts (FA) in 1860.

At the same time, in 1835, a secondary or military class was formed for the instruction of native doctors in the vernacular medium. Fifty young men, of whom it was required to be able to read or write their own language, were entertained on a monthly allowance of Rs. 5. Besides Madhusudan Gupta and Navakrishna Gupta, Sibchandur Kurmkar (October, 1839), Nobin Chunder Mitter (December, 1839), and Prossuna Coomar Mitter (March, 1843) were added to the faculty of the teaching staff. The military class, thus, was totally manned by Indian teachers. In 1843, Madhusudan Gupta was made superintendent and thus given independent charge of the military class. The course of instruction, however, differed from that of the original NMI in as much as the subjects were practically taught by aid of the dissecting room, the laboratory, and the hospital.[19] The two-tier medical education became three-tier when the Bengali vernacular class was opened in 1852 to fill the subordinate echelons of district and mofussil hospitals.

Medical education for the native doctors in Bengali vernacular was introduced in the academic session of 1852–1853. Need for such a class was long felt and public opinion in its favour was expressed through contemporary newspapers and journals. Besides meeting the requirements of the junior ranks of the growing number of civil stations, jails, tea plantations and mining and later railway establishments, the native doctors were deemed to be better interpreters and popularizers of European sciences among the masses than the elite graduates of the English class. An editorial of a medical journal commented:

> The natives by birth, become English by long education and do not willingly either speak or write Bengali ... whatever facilities of thought and language, the Sub-assistant surgeons possess, they invest in an English dress and have little more communication with the people of the land than European medical officers, perhaps less, because in some instances they are despised.[20]

By the mid 1850s, the CMC stood on solid foundations of the basic infrastructure of anatomical museum, chemical laboratory, an expanding library, with a sprawling hospital taking concrete shape due to the diligent efforts of European and Indian medical men and the government, encouraged and aided by an enthusiastic public and philanthropic elite of Bengal. The management of the Medical College and Hospital rested in the principal and the college council, composed of all the professors and was placed under the immediate control of the Director of Public Instructions (DPI).[21] By 1873, the total strength of the three categories of students rose to 1,226 compared to 50 of 1835 and the CMC earned the distinction of being one of the largest teaching institutions in the world in the field of medicine.[22]

Out of 1,226 students in the CMC in 1872–1873, the Bengali class alone accounted for 635 students, of which 421 were paying students. As the infrastructural facilities were gradually found to be inadequate and as more and more students were getting ready to pay for their education, the government decided to shift the vernacular schools of the Medical Colleges to new locations as well as to open new medical schools, giving proper weightage to geographical and linguistic considerations. Thus in November 1873, the Bengali licentiate class of the CMC was transferred to a newly constructed Campbell Medical School at Sealdah. In 1874, two more schools were opened, one at Patna named Temple Medical School and another at Dacca named Dacca Medical School. The Medical School at Patna started with a civil Hindustani class to which the military class of the CMC was transferred in 1875. In 1876, a medical school was opened at Cuttack to cater to the needs of the Oriya speaking people. Marathi and Gujarati licentiate classes were similarly separated from the Grant Medical College, Bombay and were shifted to Poona and Ahmedabad in 1878 respectively. Also from Madras Medical College, which carried on teaching for different courses exclusively in English throughout, the English licentiate class of hospital assistants was transferred to Royapuram in 1908.[23]

As in Bengal, the medical schools and colleges in Bombay and Madras presidencies after passing through the process of trial and error too concrete shapes by 1845 and 1850 respectively. In Bombay, the utilitarian Governor Elphinstone founded a medical school in 1826 with a loftier objective of educating the native youths to a workable knowledge of the European system, and then sending them into the district to serve and help the diseased masses. This experiment, however, flopped after six years when the government pleaded financial constraints and the acute difficulties encountered in translating the English texts into Marathi and Gujarati.[24]

After the death of Robert Grant in 1838 who had shown a keen interest in this project, his friends and liberal gentry of Bombay exhibited exemplary courage to establish a medical college in 1845 through public subscription and government aid. In the honour of Grant, it was named Grant Medical College. Next, a grand hospital was constructed in close proximity of the college, largely a creation of the munificence of a native Parsee gentleman Sir Jamsetjee Jejeebhoy and named after him. Later on, a score of other wealthy Parsees came forward and established a network of hospitals throughout Bombay. Thus, by way of private munificence, Bombay left Bengal and Madras far behind.[25]

However, on two counts Madras left the other presidencies far behind. First, it taught all the three classes of MB licentiates for the military and the hospital assistants in English language alone. No vernacularization or provincialization was ever encouraged and attempted. Second, when female entry into medical education was debarred all over the world, the Madras Medical College took the lead by opening its gate to them in 1875.[26]

Emergence of Different Kinds of Hospitals

Various types of hospitals came into existence by the mid 19th century which can be placed under four broad categories. First and foremost of these were the 'military hospitals' meant for the treatment and rehabilitation of the soldiers and sailors of the Company. The military hospitals, again, were of two types, temporary and regular. Temporary or camp hospitals were an immediate and urgent arrangement in some old and ruined buildings for medical aid to the soldiers near the battlefields. Once the war was over such hospitals were either abolished or shifted to newer war zones. Regular military hospitals were established within the confines of the cantonments or stable military stations, and were well-staffed and well-regulated. The second category comprised all such hospitals either at the metropolis or the district headquarters which exclusively attended on the European civilians. The third category comprised the general hospitals meant for all including the natives. In the fourth and last category came the charitable hospitals and dispensaries which were mostly the outcome of native efforts and were maintained by public subscriptions. However, few of the prominent charitable hospitals received government aid as well. The first three categories of hospitals were mainly financed and maintained by the government.[27]

Besides this system of graded hospitals, the British set up temporary lunatic asylums wherever the Europeans resided in sizable numbers. It offered quite a good business to few of the surgeons, as initially such mental asylums were put to private management by such people who had a place, time, and inclination to take upon this risky venture in lieu of fees given either by the government for its servants or by the relatives of the patients. Some of these asylums were later on taken over by the government, and by the 1850s, few of them were operating in almost every province of British India.[28]

Another set of hospitals to meet the requirements of chronic and contagious diseases like leprosy, tuberculosis, and different kinds of fevers came up from time to time in the form of leper asylums, TB sanatoriums, and fever-hospitals respectively. Also, to check and mitigate the ravages of epidemic or killer diseases like small-pox, cholera, malaria and plague, temporary hospitals were set up. They were abolished once the diseases subsided. However, in the endemic areas, they were granted a longer existence.[29]

Lastly, by the end of the 19th century, lock-hospitals were set up within the premises of most of the European regiments to protect European soldiers from venereal diseases. In the lock-hospitals, Indian women were subjected to periodical medical examination. If found healthy they were certified to carry on prostitution with the soldiers as usual, and if found infected, they were retained and treated at the hospitals; and if found to be incurable, they were expelled from the regimental or cantonment premises.[30]

Medical Organisation and Racial Discrimination

The colonial medical services in India took a discernible organizational shape by the end of the 19th century. Three distinct services, namely, covenanted, uncovenanted, and subordinate medical services, came to constitute the British medical organization. They were linked and ordered into a hierarchy, adroitly maintained and managed by well-formulated rules and regulations concerning qualifications, pay and privileges (like promotion, leave, allowances on special duties, and pension) and overall status of the incumbents of the respective services. Racial vanity ran through the nerve streams of the medical organization as the covenanated service was meant for the Europeans, the uncovenanted for the Eurasians and Anglo-Indians, the higher posts of subordinate military department like those of apothecaries and stewards for the local classes of Anglo-Indians and native Christians, and finally the lower rungs of subordinate department (both military and civil) for the Indians. The Indian medical graduates and licentiates had to suffer and withstand highly calculated racial discrimination. No amount of efficiency and experience could earn them approbation and elevation into the higher ranks of services. Various gradations were created from time to time within the subordinate department itself to contain the growing disaffections and discontent among this class of medical men.[31]

The Indian Medical Service (IMS) gained in status and importance immensely when Lord Cornwallis, in his bid to colour the top echelons of the Indian bureaucracy all white, burdened its members too with a covenant by his Regulations of 24th October 1788. Henceforward, the IMS men became covenanted or commissioned officers.[32] The IMS was purely a military service and its members serving in the civil department were only lent to it and they were liable to recall in times of war or other emergency.[33]

The civil surgeon of a district, the nucleus of medical administration in India, had to perform numerous and multifarious duties. At the district headquarter's hospital, he was supposed to attend to all difficult medical and surgical cases, the minor ones being taken care of by the Indian SASs. He had to visit daily the district jail of which he was often the superintendent. Next, he had to visit the police hospital and a very important part of his duties was to perform medico-legal post-mortems. Besides these, he was supposed to inspect all the dispensaries of his district four times a month. Again, he was also the ex-officio superintendent of vaccination and inspector of factories in his district. Lastly, by the close of the year he had to send an annual return of the aforesaid activities to the Inspector-General (IG) of hospitals. Thus, the works and experience of an IMS personnel as civil surgeon were extensive and varied benefiting him enormously in the long run. But that was not the case with the military surgeons. The pay was a little higher there but opportunities for professional excellence were very limited. There was no surgery worth its name and the whole professional work ended with the treatment of a few cases of fever, dysentery, blistered feet, or rheumatism. The medical officer, in this situation, was apt to become rusty and gradually lose his interest in the profession.[34]

The appointment of the natives of India as commissioned officers in the medical service was stricktly forbidden by the court. It was not until the introduction of competitive examination in 1855 that admission was thrown open to Indians.[35] Though few of the Indian graduates performed creditably like S. C. G. Chakarvarty (who topped the 1855 competition) and R. C. Chandra (who succeeded Chakravarty as Professor of Materia-Medica at the CMC), by 1905 only 5 per cent of the IMS men were Indians.[36] Several factors were responsible for this. Since the entrance examination was held in London, majority of the Indian graduates lacked financial resources. Next, travel outside India was considered by many Hindus as polluting, entailing the loss of caste. Even till the 1880s, Indian newspapers such as the *Hindu Patriot* continued to discourage travel abroad.[37] Racial discrimination was the other most important deterrent to the Indian aspirants.

The Indian students were often found equal to the best in Europe by European professors and administrators themselves, but equality in matters of pay, promotion, pension etc., was considered to be a ridiculous proposition.[38] The desire of the native SAS for independent charge of even minor civil surgency was regarded to be too ambitious and premature. The government believed that in the medical, as in all other departments, native agency was of the English value when it was vigilantly superintended. It held firmly that they were seldom efficient when placed in civil station at a distance from immediate superintendence.[39] The Indian SASs were discriminated even against apothecaries who held a lower degree (that of licentiate against the Indians' LMS or MB), but were often given independent charge of the minor civil stations and drew a salary of Rs. 250 per month as against Rs. 150 by the Indian graduates.[40]

In 1848, two Indian doctors, Bholanath Bose and Mutty Lal Seal returned from England with a recommendation from the court to be absorbed in suitable positions. The Council of Education found them qualified for a professorship at the CMC. But the Government of Bengal decried that 'to give the natives such high assignments was likely to inflame the ambition of others'. So one was sent to the CMC Hospital and other to a dispensary.[41]

Banishing the diplomatic language of the past decades, the Commission on IMS in its report in 1866 came out ruthlessly against the 'soaring ambitions' of the native SASs who in its view might be possessing excellent education but not the professional or the moral qualifications necessary for the charge of civil stations. The Commission quoted the Lt. Governor of the Punjab who could not repress the horrid contempt while commenting that to offer an English lady the services of a native SAS would, in fact, be virtually to deny her medical attendance altogether.[42] The prospect of attendance on European ladies by the Indian doctors was, thus, brightfully looked upon as too degrading and humiliating. To crown it all, even insane Europeans hated to be attended on by the native physicians however highly qualified.[43] Obviously the question at stake was not that of professionalism but that of racialism; racial arrogance was a hard nut to crack.

To draw parallels from other scientific disciplines, Acharya P. C. Ray had to wallow under a provincial service whereas men fresh from college landed in imperial service, simply because they were Europeans.[44] J. C. Bose could earn worldwide fame and a CIE but not parity in pay scales with the Europeans till 1903.[45] During the 1890s, the average remuneration worked out at Rs. 667 for each European and Rs. 36 for each Indian.[46]

This 'apartheid' in medical and other scientific disciplines repeatedly rankled the Indian psyche and in the last quarter of the 19th century Indians started reacting against it. The birth of Indian National Congress and sprouting of professional associations gave vent and impetus to the dormant fightback. M. L. Sarkar, K. L. Dey, P. N. Bose, and P. C. Ray were among the first scholars promising to fight for adequate reward and respect to the native scientific community.[47]

Emergence of Medical Research Institutions

Of all the medical disciplines, medical research was slowest to grow. Whatever researches that we find by way of studies into the causation, prevention, and cure of the numerous diseases encountered by the British in India till the close of the 19th century were mainly the products of personal interest rather than the products of any systematic products of the government's research policy. Few British physicians like W. Ainslie, Charles Horehead, N. C. Macnamara and others contributed to the medical knowledge on India through their own dedication and resources.[48]

The Government of India as well as the home government, in fact, were so reluctant and apathetic to research projects that the very few IMS men who took initiative for research on their own, were denied to avail of whatever meagre opportunities that came their way. A case in point is that of N. C. Macnamara of the Bengal Medical Service. He was interested in the investigation of cholera causation right from the 1860s. He found that the rice-water like stools of cholera were infective when swallowed, and that a number of persons who by accident drank a portion of the watery cholera stool developed the disease within a day or two. He was convinced that some sort of intestinal bacillus caused the disease and carried out further experimentations on animals during the course of which he contracted the disease and was forced to retire to England in 1876. But he did not lose interest and studied bacteriology under Koch at Berlin at his own expense. In February 1883, he requested the India Office to depute him to Egypt, where cholera had recently broken out to work on its bacteriology. This request was squashed, yet eight months later Koch was given every facility for his investigations in Egypt. Later Macnamara complained bitterly: 'The Secretary of State's refusal to accept my offer crushed any hopes I had of completing my life's work'.[49]

The year 1883 marked a major breakthrough in scientific investigation into disease causation. A German Commission led by Robert Koch discovered the cholera 'Comma' bacillus in Egypt and visited Calcutta in the same year to confirm his discovery. Koch's discovery was a significant contribution to the germ theory of disease causation which had emerged in western Europe in the 1860s; the studies like his and those of Louis Pasteur helped in firmly establishing the theory in the 1870s and 1880s. This modern scientific revolution in medicine challenged and ultimately triumphed over the earlier miasmatic theory.[50]

The detection and isolation of different germs causing different diseases thus led to the emergence of a new scientific discipline called bacteriology. While the whole world was hailing the new science, the British Empire was slumbering. Two factors finally forced it in the 1890s to break the slumber. First, it felt rudely shaken when the editor of the *British Medical Journal*, E. Hart severely castigated the IMS at the first Indian Medical Congress held at Calcutta in 1894 for having neglected to lay the basis for scientific exploitation of the largest disease laboratory in the British empire. He remarked bitterly:

> A pestilence breaks out in an important colony. The local physicians display ... unlimited courage and devotion to duty; but the scientific part of the work has to be done for us by the outsider .... Run over some of the names associated with the discoveries and judge—Cholera, Koch; Leprosy, Hansen; Malaria, Laveran; Dysentery, Losech; Liver-abcess, Kartulis; Endemic Haemataria, Bilharz; and latest of all, Plague, Kitasato.[51]

The second and more important factor to spur the Government of India into action was the sudden outbreak and rapid spread of plague in Bombay threatening to disrupt the entire trade, commerce, and administration of the country besides striking hard on its imperial prestige. Pardy Lukis claimed that what cholera did for sanitation in England 60 years ago, plague did for medical research in India.[52]

W. M. Haffkine was the first successful bacteriologist to work on the problem of cholera and in the preparation of cholera inoculation. Later he succeeded in 1896 in preparing plague inoculation as well and thus saved millions of lives through his works. Hankin organized a Bacteriological laboratory at Agra in 1900 with government funding. In 1899, the Plague Research Laboratory under Haffkine's charge was established in Bombay (later renamed Haffkine Institute in 1926). Central Research Laboratory at Kasauli was opened in 1906 and later Pasteur Institutes were set up at Coonoor (1906) and Shillong (1910).[53]

Thus, during the first decade of the 20th century we find lots of bacteriological activities in India but these were chiefly confined to the bulk production of sera and vaccines. The most important objective of fostering scientific research in tropical diseases was held back at the metropolis itself. Two schools of tropical medicine were founded at London and Liverpool in 1898, but none in India where the much scandalized tropical diseases thrived unbounded. However, one positive outcome of the spurt of bacteriological activities in the 1900s was the realization of the need of creating some kind of a co-ordinating and monitoring central body. This historic need finally found expression in 1911 with the creation of Indian Research Fund Association (IRFA). This was, in fact, the first concrete step of the Governmen of India to put countrywide medical research on an organized basis. The IRFA's aims were, 'to initiate, aid, develop and co-ordinate medical aid and scientific research in India and to assist institutions for the study of diseases, their prevention, causation and remedy'.[54]

The institutional evolution of the inter-dependent aspects of colonial medicine, viz. educational infrastructure, network of hospitals and dispensaries, hierachical medical services, and medical research was flaunted incessantly by the British throughout the colonial rule as evidences of the 'superiority of race' and as 'sites' of easing the 'white man's burden'. Bringing the much advanced, rational, modern, cosmopolitan medicine to the land of the sick and fallen, was interpreted as divine deliverance. To claim legitimacy for the empire they drew an image of benign, benevolent, and humanitarian state as colonial medicine, supposedly, cured diseases and reduced pain and suffering in India. A close look at the 19th century medical history of India, however, gives a contrary picture.[55]

Although imperialism and humanism were historical realities, they were not parallel phenomena. While imperialism had been a continuous process in British India, humanism was just an occassional intruder. Colonial medicine did not mean altruism, it meant uncanny imperialism par excellence.[56] Western medical institutions could achieve very little for the sake of the teeming millions of India. They merely served the military and civil populace of the empire, a tiny class of collaborators, and the few Indian urban elite. The overwhelming majority of the Indian masses still depended on the practitioners of 'folk medicine'[57] and on the hybrid quacks of both the indigenous as well as alien medical systems. The circumstantial and perchance advantage drawn by the poor and destitutes from the hospitals and dispensaries established in the cities cannot be generalized as 'subaltern-oriented' health policy as the vast rural masses of India still remained uncharted and left to worry about themselves. Colonial medicine singularly failed to make the transition from state medicine to public health.[58]

References

1. Quoted in R. Mac Leod and M. Lewis (eds.), *Disease, Medicine and Empire: Perspectives of Western Medicine and the Experience of European Expansion*, London, 1988., p. 3.
2. W. Anderson, '"Where Every Prospect Pleases and only Man is Vile": Laboratory Medicine as Colonial Discourse', *Critical Inquiry*, vol. 18, Spring 1992, pp. 506-29.

3. W. J. Buchanan, 'The Introduction and Spread of Western Medical Science in India', *Calcutta Review,* no. 278, 1914, p. 436.
4. J. Harrison, *The Origin and Progress of the Bengal Medical College,* Calcutta, 1857, p. 2.
5. The Hospital Board established in May 1786 for each presidency for overall administration of the presidential medical establishment was rechristened as Medical Board in May 1796 and functioned with this name till 1858 when the office of the Director-General came into being; National Archives of India (hereafter NAI), Home, Medical, 29 May, 1796. 'Regulations in Respect of the Military Hospitals in India'.
6. W. C. B. Eatwell, *On the Rise and Progress of Rational Medical Education in Bengal,* Calcutta, 1860, pp. 17-31.
7. *Ibid.*
8. *Ibid.*
9. Ram Commul Sen was a noted philanthropist of his age and contemporary of other Calcutta luminaries like Raja Rammohan Roy, Dwarkanath Tagore, and Radhakanta Deb. Besides, he was the grandfather of famous social reformer Keshav Chandra Sen. He was appointed as member (and only Indian) by W. Bentinck on the Medical Commission to enquire about the achievements and utility of the NMI; D. G. Crawford, *A History of the Indian Medical Service,* vol. II, London, 1914, pp. 153-59.
10. N. H. Keshwani, 'Medical Education in India since Ancient Times', in C. D. O' Malley, (ed.), *The History of Medical Education,* California, 1968, p. 324.
11. *Report of the Committee on Indigenous System of Medicine,* Madras, 1923, p. 12.
12. *Report of the Medical College of Bengal, 1839,* Calcutta, 1839, pp. 1-9.
13. *Ibid.*
14. *Ibid.*
15. *Indian Journal of Medical Science* vol. 1, no. 2, Feb. 1834, Calcutta, p. 63.
16. *Report of the Director of Public Instruction (hereafter DPI Report) Bengal, 1850 51,* Calcutta, 1851, p. 82.
17. *DPI Report, Bengal, 1857–58,* Calcutta 1858, p. 212.
18. *General Report of Public Instruction, Bengal, 1842–43* p. 86.
19. J. Harrison, *op. cit.* p. 6.
20. *The Indian Register of Medical Science,* vol. 1, Calcutta, 1848, p. 332.
21. *DPI Report, Bengal, 1855–56,* p. 125.
22. *DPI Report, Bengal, 1874–75,* p. 85.
23. E. W. C. Bradfield, 'Medical Education in India' in Bradfield (ed.), *An Indian Medical Review,* Delhi, 1938, p. 111.
24. NAI, Home, Pub., 18 July 1838, no. 18 k.w.

25. *Report, Board of Education, 1847–48,* Bombay, 1846. Besides J. J., Other eminent Parsees who tried to emulate him were Cowasji Jehangir, Pestonji Hormusji Cama, Bomanji Edelji, Bai Maltibai, Sir Dinshaw Petit and scores of other philanthrophists.
26. Keshwani, *op. cit.* p. 330.
27. D. M. Muir, 'Notes on the Origin of the Presidency General Hospital Calcutta', *Indian Medical Gazette* (hereafter *IMG*), vol. 38, no. 1, 1903, p. 3.
28. D. G. Crawford, 'Notes on the Early Hospitals of Calcutta', *IMG*, vol. 38, no. 1, 1903, pp. 6-8.
29. *Ibid.*
30. K. Ballhatchet, *Race, Sex and Class under the Raj,* London, 1980, pp. 10-11.
31. NAI, Home, Medical, 4 July 1901, nos. 102–14. The pay and prospects of the native doctors or hospital assistants was improved to some extent in 1901 on the basis of the length of service. This was, however, too little and too late. The grades and pay were to be as follows:

Fourth grade, under 5 years' service	-	Rs. 25;
Third grade, 5 to 10 years' service	-	Rs. 35;
Second grade, 10 to 15 years' service	-	Rs. 45;
First grade, 16 to 20 years' service	-	Rs. 55;
Senior grade, above 20 years' service	-	Rs. 70.

32. *Minutes and Regulations of Bengal Council, 20 October,* 1788.
33. Crawford, *History of IMS*, vol. 2, pp. 340-48.
34. *Ibid.*, p. 351.
35. Crawford, *op.cit.,* vol. 1, p. 502.
36. R. Jeffrey, 'Recognizing India's Doctors: The Institutionalization of Medical Dependency (1918–39)' *Modern Asian Studies,* vol. 13, no. 2, 1979, p. 310.
37. M. Harrison, *Public Health in British India: Anglo-Indian Preventive Medicine,* New Delhi, 1994, p. 26.
38. *Report of the Commission on IMS,* Calcutta, 1866, p. 11. J. Prinsep, DPI, Bengal, wrote to Prof. W. B. O'Shaughnessy after examining the chemistry students of CMC: 'All the essays are extremely creditable. I do not think that in Europe any class of chemical pupils would be found capable of passing a better examination'.
39. NAI, Home, Public, 21 August 1847, no. 40.
40. E. Edlin, (ed.), *The Indian Register of Medical Science,* vol. 1, Calcutta, 1848, p. 511.
41. NAI, Home, Pub., 29 April 1848, no. 10.
42. *Report of the Commission on IMS*, p. 2.
43. 'Report on the Asylum for European Insane Patients at Bhowanipore, 1856–57', *Selections from the Records of the Bengal Government,* no. XXVIII, Calcutta, 1858, p. 14.

44. G. K. Gokhale, 'The Employment of Indians in the Public Services', *Speeches,* Madras, 1911, p. 448.
45. NAI, Home, Education, October 1903, nos. 49–50.
46. J. G. Godard, *Racial Supremacy: Being Studies in Imperialism,* Edinburgh, 1905, p. 267.
47. D. Kumar, 'Racial Discrimination and Science in 19th Century India', *The Indian Economic and Social History Review*, vol. XIX, no. 1, p. 74.
48. O. P. Jaggi, *Epidemics And Other Tropical Diseases*, vol. 12, Delhi, 1979, pp. 1-80. Earliest study on cholera was made by W. Ainslie in *Observations on the Cholera Morbus of India*, London, 1825. Charles Morehead, Principal of Grant Medical College, Bombay gave vivid accounts of Indian diseases in *Clinical Researches on Diseases in India*, 2 vols., London, 1856. N. C. Macnamara wrote his magnum opus, *A History of Asiatic Cholera*, London, 1876.
49. L. Rogers, 'A Tragedy: How Surgeon-Major N. C. Macnamara was Deprived of Priority in the Discovery of the Causative Organism of Cholera', *Transactions of the Royal Society of Tropical Medicine and Hygiene*, vol. 43, no. 4, 1950, pp. 375–400.
50. R. Ramasubban, 'Public Health and Medical Research in India: Their Origins Under the Impact of British Colonial Policy', *SAREC Report*, Stockholm, 1982, pp. 21–24.
51. E. Hart, *The Medical Profession in India*, Calcutta, 1894, pp. 73-74.
52. C. G. Pandit and K. Someswara Rao, 'Indian Research Fund Association and Indian Council of Medical Research, 1911–1961', in *Fifty Years of Progress*, New Delhi, 1961, pp. 2–10.
53. *Ibid.*
54. V. R. Khanolkar, *Fifty Years of Science in India*, Calcutta, 1963, p. 3.
55. A. Kumar, *Medicine and the Raj: British Medical Policy in India* 1835–1911, New Delhi, 1998, pp. 216–225.
56. S. Chakravarty, *The Raj Syndrome*, New Delhi, 1991, p. 202.
57. S. Kakkar, *Shamans, Mystics and Doctors*, Delhi 1972, pp. 271-278.
58. D. Arnold, *Colonizing the Body: State Medicine and Epidemic Disease in Nineteenth Century India*, Delhi, 1993, p. 3.

11

'Colony' Under a Microscope: The Medical Works of W. M. Haffkine

—Deepak Kumar

> It is far not the richest states, as it is not the richest individuals, who contribute mostly to the advance of knowledge. The Greek communities did definitely far more than the Roman empire ... In our times the small German dukedoms are doing infinitely far more for promoting science than the immense British Empire ever did. The power of producing scientists, investigators, thinkers, lays not in the amount of money representing the budget of a state, but in the manner in which teachers are valued, honoured and encouraged by general sympathy and cooperation.
>
> ***W. M. Haffkine in 1896***[1]

> Scientific research requires on the part of the workers an endless amount of effort. It is only in appearance that such effort may present itself as spontaneous. In reality, the origin will always be traced—apart from the pleasure derived from successful thinking—to the charm of communicating new findings to one's fellow creatures, to the prospect of sympathy and approval ... Those engaged in the application of knowledge are prone to overlook the requirements of the gradual development of ideas, the impossibility of reaching practical goals without a number of intermediary stages being passed and are tempted to insist on the exclusion of studies of which they do not see the importance in their practice, or for which there does not appear to them to be a demand.
>
> ***W. M. Haffkine in 1900***[2]

When Waldemar Haffkine (1860–1930) expressed the above views, bacteriological researches were about to give medical science a new turn, a process in which Haffkine himself played a significant part at least in the context of British India. The newly emergent germ theory of disease, and the efforts to combat epidemics through new scientific methods held exciting possibilities. Of course, behind this emergence of a 'scientific' speciality there were political and economic considerations as dictated by the colonial imperatives, yet it did involve scientific exertions of a very high order.[3] The new scientific 'soldiers' discovered and tinkered with 'colonies' of microbes under their microscopes and to prove the efficacy and utility of their work, the 'play' shifted to the real colonies. Haffkine pioneered new methods to combat cholera and plague in India during the 1890s with mixed results. He was partly successful and partly not. He was determined to take the 'latest' in medical science to the people, and tried to do it at a pace never attempted before, even at the risk of irking the colonial bureaucracy. He dared to lecture even the mightiest in the land (Lord Curzon, for example as quoted above) on the requirements of scientific research, 'the charm of communicating new findings', and the necessity to 'conceive things beyond the immediate and temporary requirements of individuals or professions'. For him real development lay not in 'the budget of a state', but in 'the manner in which teachers (researchers) are valued, honoured and encouraged ....' How relevant and appropriate were such views for a colonial administration? One spark, and Haffkine had to leave India in disgrace. The present paper proposes to analyse the ups and downs in Haffkine's research career in India and through it try to capture the dynamics of medical research and preventive medicine in a colonial set-up.

George Bornside and Ilana Lowy have published comprehensive articles on Haffkine as a scientist and his work on the anti-cholera vaccine. While Bornside treats Haffkine as the architect of controlled field-trials, Lowy relates Haffkine's experiments to the larger questions of how a new laboratory-oriented procedure was to be introduced into medical practice, and how 'useful' and 'reliable' the use of animal models could be in studies of human disease.[4] But they leave out Haffkine as 'a man of action', his social views, his plague work, and his complex relations with the British officials in India (where he spent 22 years). My endeavour will be to bring the two together. The sources, as in Lowy's article, are directly from the horse's mouth, i.e. the Haffkine Papers, herein explored in its 'totality', and supplemented by the papers of Lord Curzon whose viceroyalty saw medical 'manoeuvres' at its peak. Recourse to private papers is useful, as it allows the actors to 'define themselves' (a la Latour).

Background: Personal and Scientific

Waldemar Haffkine was born in Odessa on March 15, 1860, of Jewish parents. His mother died when he was barely seven, and a sense of insecurity was to haunt him perhaps forever. He recorded it in moving terms later in 1899 on a voyage from India to England.[5] He attended the Gymnasium in Berdiansk and then the Imperial Novorossisk University in Odessa. The campus life influenced him in several ways. He joined a populist-socialist revolutionary group called *Narodnaia Volia* (Will of the People) and was even rounded up by the imperial police on some occasions. His political initiation made him a compulsive anti-establishment person and strengthened his resolve to work for society. But at the same time he would not abandon the Jewish traditions which he had inherited. Even under adverse circumstances he would not feel shy of disclosing his Jewish identity. In socialist ideas perhaps he had found a vindication of Jewish brotherhood. Both co-existed in him. Haffkine had become a favourite student of Elie Metchnikoff (a zoologist and later Nobel Prize-winner) who imbued him with a strong urge to devote his life to science. But the assassination of the Russian Czar Alexander II in 1881 led to an unprecedented academic repression. Metchnikoff himself resigned. Haffkine along with 95 students petitioned in his support and was expelled from the university. Luckily by that time he had completed his doctoral work in zoology and so was allowed to take his degree two years later in 1884.

Haffkine's revolutionary inclination gradually gave place to his dedication to science and he turned his attention to the 'biological front'.[6] His first research position was at the Odessa Natural History Museum where he worked till 1888 and published five important papers on the hereditary characteristics of unicellular organisms. Metchnikoff remained his guiding star. Meanwhile, Metchnikoff had established a bacteriological institute in Odessa, perhaps the first outside Paris. But the increasing demands for 'practical results', hostility of his fellow-medical-men and violent political conditions, made him emigrate to Paris in 1888. Soon Haffkine followed suit. He first settled in Geneva, teaching physiology at a medical school and the next year sought an appointment at the Pasteur Institute in Paris. With both Pasteur and Metchnikoff in Paris, the keen researcher in Haffkine could not have imagined a better place. With no position vacant, even an assistant librarianship was acceptable to him. Outside his library hours, he was permitted to use the laboratory facilities for research.

Hopes for a 'Golden Statue'

Now began the most innovative and fascinating stage in Haffkine's career. For some time, in line with his earlier interest in unicellular organism, he continued to work on the protozoan *Paramecium* and the results were published in the *Annales de 1' Institut Pasteur* in 1890. In collaboration with Metchnikoff, he worked also on the typhoid bacillus and was able to grow it in the watery content of the rabbit's eye. Around this time he felt interested more in devising methods to combat a disease than studying the disease per se and its etiology alone. He now wanted to perfect a prophylactic vaccine. Luckily for him, a senior colleague Alexander Yersine decided to leave the Pasteur Institute for field work in Indo-China, and his post as *preparateur* was given to Haffkine. The stage was thus set for full-time academic work. Its *vibrio* had already been discovered by Koch, the famous German bacteriologist in 1884. Several bacteriologists of the time were also working on cholera as it was a major health hazard. Haffkine set for himself the task of first growing the *cholera vibrio* in suitable laboratory animals and then develop a vaccine. In doing so, he was deeply influenced by both Pasteur's philosophy and methods. Haffkine's first *Cahier de Cholera* (dt. September 10, 1890) begins with two quotations from Pasteur; one saying that 'public utility and the interests of humanity enable the most repugnant work', and the second explained that 'hypotheses are merely invitations for experimentation'.[7] Haffkine was to follow it in letter and spirit. Later in India, he was convinced of (almost obsessed with) his work as 'public utility', but he could not convince others. There could be no other Pasteur. The methods followed were similar in some ways. Pasteur used to take down his observations on an experiment in his note books and once so entered they became for Pasteur 'incontestable truths'. Haffkine also got into the habit of maintaining meticulous note books. One night he hurriedly woke up Alexander Yersine to witness a change he was trying to induce in his experiments, and thought that it had become a 'scientific fact' once demonstrated to 'a qualified observer'.[8] Alas, it was not to be so. Nevertheless, he was lucky to have Pasteur's support and constant encouragement. Then he had there his former teacher Metchnikoff and Emile Roux (Pasteur's successor as director of the Institute) who supported and criticized him as the occasion demanded.

Haffkine's first task was to grow the cholera microbes in laboratory animals. The acidity of the stomach were inimical to the microbes, so he tried to grow them in a serum and injected a large quantity to a rabbit. It died but the bacillus could not be located in its intestines. Haffkine found himself in a blind alley. After several attempts he could locate the bacillus in the liver of another experimented rabbit. Thus, bile appeared as the ideal medium to grow the bacillus, but even this could not succeed in inducing a cholera-like disease in rabbits. Almost a year (October 1890–October 1891) passed in these trials with little success in sight. In his cholera notebook no. IV he quoted from Pasteur's earlier (1868) article, 'it is only by subtle, well-planned, and persistent experiments that one can force Nature to reveal a secret'.[9] Here was a faithful student inching his way. The master too had full faith in him. In November 1891, Pasteur introduced him to the visiting prince of Siam as 'the person who is now very near, nearest of all, to this (cholera vaccine) discovery'. The prince told Haffkine, if you find a remedy against cholera, Siam will erect a statue for you, to which Pasteur added, 'a golden statue'![10] The following month Haffkine succeeded in isolating the microbes from a rabbit intestine. But other experimented rabbits gave different results. Some died quickly, some after several days, and some even survived. So the quest for a 'fixed microbe' and 'reproducible result' continued.

Haffkine was not alone in this race. Earlier, in 1885, Nicati (1850–1931) and Rietsch (1848–1905) had succeeded in introducing the microbes directly into the intestine of rabbits. In Spain, Ferran (1852–1929) had experimented with *cholera vibrio* and even claimed to have developed a vaccine in 1885 which several bacteriologists rejected as a 'pre-Jennerian method of variolization'. To make a liquid of freshly-cultivated microbes was of course possible, but the goal was to obtain a 'calibrated' and 'effective' vaccine. A German bacteriologist Pfeiffer had meanwhile succeeded in growing the bacillus in the peritoneal cavity of guinea pigs. Haffkine's attention to this method was drawn by his 'critical' Director, Emile Roux. Haffkine's was now set on a new course and soon he moved ahead of Pfeiffer. By striking the right calibration and the right temperature, he was able to obtain *vibrio exalte* (i.e., a highly virulent form) in March 1892. Unlike his earlier experiments on rabbits, the new strain could kill the guinea pigs within a fixed and known period of time. The next step was to attenuate the germs. This devitalization could be done through the use of heat or chloroform. The guinea pigs thus inoculated could later survive an injection of virulent germs. Another problem was which type of injection would suit most. It could be intraperitoneal, intramuscular, or subcutaneous. Haffkine found the last most effective. A subcutaneous injection of the attenuated germs seemed to provide the required immunity against a subsequent lethal dose of the *exalte vibrios*. On July 9, 1892, Haffkine presented these results before the Paris Biological Society. The next week he confirmed that doves and rabbits also responded favourably to this method. The Society members were impressed but some questions still remained. The doses had to be quantified and then came the million-dollar question—can results obtained on laboratory animals be applied to human beings? How reliable the animal models could be?

Human Experiments

By now Haffkine had succeeded in 'fixing the cholera virus in a well-defined strength', and could decrease or increase its virulence with certainty. By this 'double discovery' Haffkine, could demonstrate as 'conclusively' as Pasteur had done against anthrax (a fatal cattle disease), that his vaccine would protect animals against cholera.[11] Would it do the same to humans? To test, Haffkine injected himself with attenuated microbes on July 18, 1892, and six days later with the exalted ones. He suffered pain at the injection site and temperature but nothing more. On July 30, he reported to the Paris Biological Society that his vaccines were totally safe for humans. Subsequently, more persons were vaccinated and they responded well. One of them was E. H. Hankin who was soon to go to India as a bacteriologist and who was to support Haffkine in India in several ways. Hankin published his observations on Haffkine's method in the *British Medical Journal.*[12] He gave a detailed account of the vaccine preparation and his own experience of being inoculated. But he also raised doubts that the conditions of infection 'that obtain in Nature' and that created in the laboratory must be 'widely different'. How, then, can one success in producing immunity against 'laboratory infection' of a guinea-pig guarantee immunity against 'natural infection' of a human being? Moreover, there existed several distinct varieties of the cholera microbe. Will immunity against one of them confer immunity against another? Then would this method confer a permanent immunity?[13] There were no certain answers. Hankin advised for 'further experiments on animals' before a definite conclusion could be reached. But convinced of its utility and that too, without any side-effects on human beings, Haffkine now wanted vaccinations on a large scale, and thereby prove his point 'statistically' as well. He looked to Siam and Russia but received no encouraging response. Russian officials had not forgotten his 'narodinic' past. Lord Dufferin, a former Viceroy of India, was then in Paris as the British ambassador. He recommended Haffkine to the authorities in London. In March 1893 Haffkine arrived in Calcutta.

During April 1893 to July 1895 anti-cholera vaccinations were given to 294 British officers, 3,206 British soldiers, 6,629 Indian soldiers, 869 civil Europeans, and 31,056 natives of India from the North West Provinces to the tea-gardens in Assam.[14] He used 'exclusively living', yet 'fixed' cholera virus. In Spain, Ferran had inoculated 'vibrios collected from cholera patients'; in India Haffkine was using a 'vaccine' on the lines of Jenner and Pasteur. Indians had used variolization (in which virus came directly from the infected person) against small-pox for a long time. What Haffkine now offered was virus at 'a given and fixed state of virulence' with the same safety and measurement as Jenner's calf-lymph or Pasteur's rabies emulsions. The dose, however, remained a problem. Initially Haffkine used 1/20 of a standard culture as a dose for an adult person but later a higher dose was found to provide a more lasting protection. His new testing grounds were the army cantonments, the tea-gardens, the jails, the pilgrim-routes to Haridwar, and the slums in Calcutta. In these places, cholera-epidemic would break out at regular intervals. But the results were mixed and varied when doses differed or when it was administered before the cholera outbreak or during the outbreak. The second attack of cholera even on an inoculated person was often found fatal. Some results were very favourable. In certain localities in Calcutta (where cholera existed all the time) several families were selected; half of its members were inoculated and half were not. They were observed for 450 days and it was found that the inoculated members had 17 times fewer deaths and 19 times fewer cases than the non-inoculated members of the same house.[15] In the Cachar tea-gardens, the 2,976 uninoculated had 60 deaths while inoculated 2,381 had 4 deaths. The jail in Gaya gave the following results:[16]

	Inoculated		*Uninoculated*	
	Cases	*Deaths*	*Cases*	*Deaths*
During the first five days after inoculation	5	4	7	5
During three days after the first inoculation	3	1	5	3
After eight days from first inoculation and thereafter	nil	nil	8	2
Total	8	5	20	10

In early 1896, W. J. Simpson (1855–1931), then the Health Officer of Calcutta, submitted an enthusiastic report asking for the continuation of vaccination on a permanent basis and reporting that the people came forward for these vaccinations voluntarily and without any pressure. He reported also that in his recent visit to Berlin professors Koch, Pfeiffer, and Kolle had confirmed the efficacy of Haffkine's method through their own experiments.[17] The Government of India responded by asking the different provinces to give Haffkine 'every facility in conducting his enquiries and work'. Recognizing the importance of the verification of results, every station visited by Haffkine was to be reported upon by a local medical committee consisting of two medical officers and a magistrate.[18] Even after he left Bengal for Bombay, cholera vaccinations were continued by the Indian assistant surgeons trained by him. One of them, Gopal Chandra Mukherjee reported on the growing 'faith of the people' and gave the following statistics on the success of the method: (See table on p.185)[19]

By this time Haffkine had every reason to feel satisfied. He had administered about 70,000 injections, inoculating more than 40,000 people. He prepared the vaccines 'while travelling by train, in the dusty passenger carriages, or at the railway stations, or else in rooms temporarily placed at my disposal and transformed for a day or two into a laboratory'.[20] Scientifically also he had not reached a dead-end. To fix the doses was a good challenge. In the course of his field-work, he developed a 'second' cholera vaccine which was 'kept at a fixed strength by passages through guinea-pigs, and devitalized by emulsification in a half per cent watery solution of carbolic acid'.[21] He also thought that his method could be applied *mutatis mutandis* to obtain a typhoid-prophylaxis and suggested it to the British bacteriologist A. E. Wright (who later won a Nobel Prize). In 1898, Wright visited India to study Haffkine's anti-plague inoculations and also test his inoculation for typhoid.[22] Haffkine maintained excellent communications with several medicalmen stationed in South Asia. Hayman Thornhill, a surgeon in Jaffna (Ceylon) was very much inspired by him. Thornhill defended him vigorously against sceptical remarks published by an anonymous doctor in a Ceylonese newspaper.[23] He was so much enthused by the anti-cholera vaccinations, that he looked to the serum technology for other diseases also. An anti-malarial serum, for example, it accomplished, 'would be the greatest boon ever conferred on the human race'.[24] At that time Ronald Ross (1857–1932) was about to discover in India the real cause of malaria. In 1897, Ross was quite frustrated at the attitude of the army medical authorities under whom he worked. Though Haffkine felt that the cause of his 'desolation' was 'imaginary', yet he wrote to the Surgeon General that Ross was 'a keen, earnest and therefore a very desirable worker'.[25] Till the turn of the century, it seems Haffkine was enjoying a high reputation and a very satisfactory career. This was to change in the wake of his plague works. Suspicion and discredit were not very far.

The Buboes in Bombay

The presence of the bubonic plague in India was announced publicly for the first time at a meeting of the Bombay Municipal Corporation at

Table of Results of anti-cholera Inoculations

Date	Place where Inoculations were performed	Incidence of Cholera previous to inoculation			Incidence of Cholera Subsequent to Inoculaton					
					Among Inoculated Persons			Among Uninoculated Persons		
		Population under observation	No. attacked	No. Died	Population under observation	No. Attacked	No. Died	Population	No. attacked	No. Died
14.4.97	Purulia	12130	219	143	338	2	..	237	49	26
2.7.94	Hazaribagh Town	16672	171	96	281	1	..	16672	282	223
15.7.97	Hazaribagh	976	26	19	180	..	..	770	14	12
21.7.97	Ranchi Jail	400	11	8	369	..	..	31	4	..
12.8.97	Daldali Ranchi	..	..	..	189	7	2	135	27	15
21.8.97	Ranchi Reserve Police	50	2	1	50	1	..	..	..	..
28.8.97	German Mission Ranchi	600	8	6	421	..	..	180	..	..
11.7.97	Deogarh	6163	96	43	111	1	1	?	17	8
	Total	36991	533	316	1939	12	3	18025	393	284

the end of September 1896. Haffkine's help was sought. His task was to prepare a suitable vaccine to ensure the immunity of the inoculated person from an attack, and if this failed at least to control the severity of the attack. Earlier in 1894, Yersin had discovered in Hong Kong the bubonic *pestes* and published his findings in the *Annales de l' Institute Pasteur*. He along with Calmette and Borrel found that it was possible to confer a certain amount of immunity against plague by the hypodermic injection of dead cultures of plague bacilli. Haffkine had the advantage of these developments and his own experience of cholera researches. Working at the Petit Laboratory of the Grant Medical College in Bombay, Haffkine observed what he termed 'a stalactite growth' of the bacilli when cultured in a nutrient broth. The bacilli had grown in long threads into the depth of the liquid. This was a new finding.[26] The toxins secreted by the 'stalactites' led to a luxuriant growth of the bacilli. To make the inoculation harmless the microbes were sterilized by heating. Unlike his anti-cholera serums in which 'living' (though 'fixed') viruses were used, his anti-plague vaccine was completely devitalized with no 'living' plague bacillus. The next step was to determine how much power it had to impart resistance against the disease. Would the resistance of the inoculated be reduced or increased? If the person was already incubating the plague, would it aggravate his condition or help him? How long would the immunity, if at all conferred, last? Then the amount of dose and severity of the reactions had to be tested. After a series of experiments on the laboratory animals, Haffkine first inoculated himself with the new vaccine in January 1897 (as he had done in Paris with his cholera vaccine).

The epidemic was there, and no time to lose. Soon various medical men and prominent citizens of Bombay were publicly inoculated with the new prophylaxis. The next test sites were the jails in Bombay and Dharwar where the tests were carried out with considerable success. In a village near Baroda, reeling under plague attack in early '98, thirty-five families were selected, of which 68 uninoculated had 27 cases with 26 deaths while the 71 inoculated reported 8 cases with only 3 deaths. This was a big reduction in mortality. The benefits were recognized. The task was now to perfect processes for turning out large and uniform quantities of the vaccine, mitigation of the reactions, and to devise means to ensure longer shelf-life of the prophylactic for distribution to distant areas. In the wake of the recurrent and larger plague outbreaks, the sanitary officials resorted to physical removal and segregation of the infected people. This was naturally resisted and led to numerous rumours and even riots. It was said that some 'sahib' had taken the poison out of a cobra and put it into the Bombay water-supply, causing plague,[27] and that those taking vaccines would grow horns.[28] Haffkine did not oppose the oppressive sanitary measures but did argue that the epidemics require 'specifics' and promptly administrable remedies. To talk of sanitation in the midst of an epidemic was like asking a patient 'to build for himself a new house or to dry up the marshy land', while he required a dose of quininc or other suitable medicine.[29] Every epidemic, he argued, had its own characteristics. In cases of rabies, small-pox or leprosy, the infection was basically in the patient. In such cases, isolation or segregation could help contain its further spread. But the bacilli of cholera, typhoid, or plague were different. Once brought, these multiplied quickly and enormously in nature. One would then need personal protection by means of a prophylactic treatment. The serums provided just that.

Such arguments, however, did not convince many. The Indian Medical Service (IMS) personnel were themselves sceptical, nor were they geared to the task. They invariably reported that the people were against inoculations. When plague broke out in Lonavali (near Bombay) in July 1897, Haffkine wanted to visit the place. The surgeon stationed there sent the standard reply of people's unwillingness. Still on arrival Haffkinc could vaccinate several hundreds. People were hesitant, but once convinced of the harmlessness of the remedy and its possible benefits, they came forward. It definitely required persuasive skills and perseverance for which an average health officer was hardly inclined or motivated. As Haffkine recalled later, 'whenever an enquiry is made as to the possibility of introducing preventive inoculation in a certain locality, the answer received from the best intentioned and the most experienced local authorities is invariably in the negative'.[30]

Haffkine took care of the religious feelings of the people; so the nutrient broth (or the bouillon) in which the bacillus was grown, was made of goat's meat, and not beef or pork. One of his assistants, Gibson succeeded in preparing even a vegetarian broth (made of wheat flour).[31] But out of professional jealousy, even doctors were spreading rumours. Curzon recalled that, at the height of the plague, a medical officer at Hyderabad deliberately stated that the serum had pig's blood in it.[32] Elgin, the preceding Viceroy, had also noted that professional jealousies were at work.[33] The Bombay Chamber of Commerce even adopted a motion condemning use of offensive material. Ironically, the maximum support that Haffkine received was from the Khoja Muslim community in Bombay. Their chief, H. H. the Agha Khan understood Haffkine's method perhaps better than some of the doctors! But all this confusion definitely made the senior civil officials nervous and wary of Haffkine's plans.

Elgin's advisers would insist on giving Haffkine every assistance, but 'not insist on the adoption of his method officially or as an alternative to segregation'.[34]

The virulence of the epidemic and the doubts raised over the methods to combat it, necessitated the institution of a commission of inquiry. The Indian Plague Commission was constituted in September 1898. One of its member was Almroth Wright who later perfected the anti-typhoid vaccine. Haffkine's method was put on trial and his data closely scrutinized. The first attack was on his method of standardization. It was found 'unsystematic', and the quantification of dose 'arbitrary'. The method of controlling the purity of the cultures by naked eye inspection was considered unscientific. The method of sterilization was seen as unsatisfactory and bottling hazardous. Out of a total of 125 bottles examined, 26 were found to contain bacterial impurities. Haffkine protested that these micro-organisms did not reduce the efficacy of the vaccine and were as harmless as 'those innumerable microbes that we eat and drink and breathe in our daily life'.[35] The Commission differed. It argued, and rightly so, that such impurities if introduced into the alimentary canal with food or drink were 'innocuous', but when injected into the sub-cutaneous tissues could well be harmful. It did not agree also with his suggestion that this vaccine protected not only against plague but against other diseases as well. The enormous statistical data presented before the Commission were pricked and several discrepencies were pointed out. In spite of these criticisms, the Commission agreed that this inoculation 'sensibly diminishes' the plague attack; it 'greatly diminishes' the death-rate among those inoculated, and though the protection conferred was not 'absolute', it certainly lasted some 'considerable' number of weeks, even months. The Commission fully recognized Haffkine's difficulties in Indian conditions, a semi-trained staff, an ill-equipped laboratory, 'the pressure of great urgency', and concluded that his work though not based on 'any new scientific principle', nevertheless was 'a great practical achievement in the region of preventive medicine'.[36]

The Intrigues

This was precisely the kind of report the Government of India had looked for. Before this Commission was appointed, one of the issues of concern was whether to include sensitive issues like 'the efficacy of quarantine and segregation' within the scope of its enquiry or not. With professional men as its members—'wholly ignorant of the country and its administration'—the officials decided not to take such risks. Otherwise, as the viceroy himself clarified:

> You might have this most dangerous dillemma, that a commission, which we ourselves desire should speak with an authority that the nations of Europe will respect, might condemn administrative measures which we know to be essential, or prescribe others which we are certain would bring about a revolution.[37]

So instead of segregation and other administrative measures, the focus fell on Haffkine's works. This was not all. There was a proposal to establish a National Health Institute or a Central Laboratory in India. Many did not want Haffkine to head such an institute. One of the members of the Plague Commission, A. Wright, 'having got a hint that he has a chance of this appointment, turned against Haffkine when the Commision was taking evidence, and put questions tending to discredit his work'.[38] Haffkine could sense the change in Wright's attitude (and later called his practices 'thievish and swindling').[39] Several IMS officials had deposed against Haffkine's arguments and statistics. Even his close associates like Bannerman, Gibson, and Liston whom he had brought from obscure field-stations, betrayed him in subtle ways.[40] Taking advantage of the criticisms of the Plague Commission the government proposed in October 1899 to hand over 'effective' charge of the Bombay laboratory to Bannerman and asked Haffkine to concentrate on scientific problems such as the standardization process. Haffkine was then away in England; he naturally panicked and lobbied with Lord Lister. The India Office took up the matter but Curzon remained unimpressed.[41] Though Haffkine was styled as 'Director-in-Chief', he remained worried over losing effective control of the laboratory to his deputy who was an IMS and had good rapport with the government. The day he returned to Bombay, he was served the notice: 'Major Barnerman will remain in charge of the Laboratory on Haffkine's return setting latter free for scientific work'. Haffkine protested but could do no more.[42]

One of the possible reasons, apart from the IMS factor, for the government's displeasure was the close relation that Haffkine had with some of the 'native' princes who wanted to establish a Pasteur Institute with Haffkine as its head. The idea was not new. In April 1893, some senior officials of the Punjab Government had proposed for such an institute.[43] Even a public appeal for funds was issued. But the Government of India was hesitant; it was not sure of the Pasteurian methods and people's reactions. As Haffkine's work progressed, and as the news of the success of certain bacteriological researches spread, the Rana of Dholpur and some more ruling chiefs decided to establish a Pasteur Institute as a commemoration of the Queen's Jubilee. The Rana wrote to Haffkine in glowing terms.[44] Funds had been raised privately; only government's permission was needed. The issue was raised in the House of Commons also, where it received evasive replies.[45] Elgin was sympathetic to the proposal but Curzon 'stopped' it. The Secretary of State agreed: 'I think you have acted very judiciously in extinguishing the Dholpur Jubilee Health Institute ... the risks attending its establishment seem to me too great to be worth encountering'.[46] But these risks were largely imaginary. It was not the deeply-religious and superstitious people of India but the Lord Bishop of Calcutta who made a 'representation' to the Viceroy against the proposed Pasteur Institute.[47]

At the turn of the century the plague showed no signs of abatement and the demand for the prophylaxis continued to grow. The need of a bigger laboratory was definitely there and some talk was still going on to open a central laboratory at Mukteswar. Haffkine still hoped to find a new appointment. In early 1901 he wrote to the government:

> Permit me to point out, in justification of the better terms which I begged for my proposed new appointment, that there are now in villages and in big manufacturing towns—attending to their daily avocations, contributing to the wealth of their employers, earning wages and paying Government and other taxes—at least 10,000 individuals who, but for the work which the Government were pleased to entrust me to carry out, would be today in their graves or their ashes have been scattered to the wind... If one considers the number of places where the inoculation has been done, the number of those inoculated in the most exposed areas (Bombay alone counting over 2,00,000 and Jullundher over 1,00,000), it will become evident that by further supporting bacteriological research and endowing an Institute like the one contemplated, Government will be diverting for that purpose some fraction of a farthing from the daily produce of the workers preserved to the country.[48]

Such a complicated outburst, however noble and valid, would not have endeared him to the government officials. Haffkine was inching towards self-destruction. Back in the Bombay Plague Laboratory, his relations with colleagues, especially Bannerman and Liston, continued to deteriorate.[49] This must have also affected the quality control of the vaccines. Some of the medical officers did notice the decanting and bottling being done in 'a slipshod manner'. One of the fears of the Plague Commission regarding contamination came true when, in November 1902, in the village of Mulkowal (Punjab) 19 out of 107 vaccinated persons developed tetanus and died.

In the Dock

The blame for this disaster was promptly put on Haffkine, the method of decanting in his laboratory and the changes he had recently introduced in his vaccine-preparation method (i.e., substitution of the broth-cultivation method by that of water-agar cultivation without carbolic acid). 'Haffkine ought to be hung for his folly', screamed Lord Curzon.[50] 'If this appealing catastrophe comes out, there will be an end to all inoculation in India, and the cause of science will be set back for a generation.'[51] Curzon gave his judgement when the incident had been barely reported and much before an enquiry could be held; 'Haffkine, in my opinion, deserves to be tried for his life'.[52] Now right from a junior IMS official in his own laboratory to the mighty Viceroy, Haffkine had a formidable array of 'enemies'.

An enquiry was duly held by three senior officials. After examining all the papers and the persons concerned, they held that the contamination was introduced before the deadly bottle no. 53 was opened at Mulkowal. How it was introduced could not be ascertained. The compounder accepted that he had dropped the forcep on the ground while trying to open the bottle.This was held by Haffkine as the source of infection and not the change in method. The change in the prophylactic method from broth to water-agar cultivation had the approval of the Pasteur Institute in Paris. In fact, this had become a standard practice and Haffkine had informed the Bombay Government about this change months before.[53] Haffkine's defence was that had the forcep been sterilized on flame after being picked from the ground, the tetanus contamination would not have taken place. There was nothing wrong with the vaccine because the same brew did not cause tetanus elsewhere. Had it been contaminated at the source, it would have given a foul smell at the time of opening, and the doctor who administered it testified that there was no foul smell. Moreover, by that time the tetanus toxin would have been so strong as to kill those vaccinated immediately. They died slowly. But these arguments were not acceptable to the inquiry committee which held the change in the preparation method, the absence of carbolic acid as a sterilizing agent, and the decanting process as the responsible factors.[54] The matter was later entrusted to the Lister Institute in London for its opinion which largely confirmed the findings of the enquiry committee but stopped short of blaming Haffkine. By this time some of his scientist friends in London, especially Ross and Simpson, had begun mobilizing opinion in favour of Haffkine. Subsequently the Lister Institute submitted three successive versions of its own opinion, 'couched in most guarded, even obscure wording'.[55]

Haffkine explained that his shift from broth to water-agar cultivation was 'Pasteurian' and was necessitated by the evergrowing number and urgency of the demands. In 1902, the demand for the vaccine had grown to more than 80,000 doses per day! Haffkine's office used to receive letters like this one:

> The people in this town are dying at the rate of 8 to 10 per day and I have daily calls from the population begging to be inoculated. I would take it as a personal favour if you will send as many doses of serum as you may be able to spare up to 2,000 ... if you can not supply immediately, will you write informing me when you may be able to do so, as the Deputy Commissioner in pressing.[56]

Haffkine's explanations could not convince the higher officials.[57] They now had a solid case to proceed upon. Bannerman saw in it a great chance to become the Director himself. Haffkine retaliated by entering adverse remarks in the confidential reports of Bannerman and Liston.[58] The government acted swiftly; the water-agar method was stopped, a new bottling system was introduced, the promotion of Haffkine which was under consideration from 1901 was cancelled, and finally he was removed from the laboratory.[59] The opposition to Haffkine was such that even the employment of a bacteriologist (Maynard, who had invented a new decanting process) was stopped because he was considered 'a strong supporter' of Haffkine.[60] Haffkine returned to England in disgust and disgrace.

His only hope of an 'academic' acquittal now rested upon his scientific friends like Ross, Simpson, and Hewlett who enjoyed high reputation and some authority in England. They rose to the occasion.[61] Ross had first-hand experience of the bureaucracy in India; he had once called the Government of India a 'mule' which would not move unless driven.[62] He wrote a series of letters to *The Times* and *The British Medical Journal*. Another influential journal published every bit of detail of the affair.[63] The India Office refused to institute another inquiry but felt compelled to issue a Parliamentary *Return of Papers* on the incident. Soon ten eminent bacteriologists signed a joint letter to *The Times*, asking for Haffkine's exoneration 'publicly'.[64] This was a great consolation for Haffkine. He exulted, 'Never probably has in the history of science known another *cause celebre* like the present one; and surely never has a cause united in a consensus of opinion a committee of experts of that eminence'.[65]

A Subdued Return

Officially, the Government of India never issued any statement exonerating Haffkine but decided to re-employ him. He had asked for the emoluments and status equal to the Director-General of the IMS. This was declined. The salary was to be the same what he got in 1896. He was asked to concentrate on research work only, no vaccination programme, and was given a small laboratory attached to the General Hospital in Calcutta. Haffkine waited. In November 1907, the India Office informed him that his re-employment did not involve any censure or punishment for the Mulkowal affair, and also acknowledged that 'an important body of scientific opinion' had exonerated him of any responsibility.[66] Haffkine now agreed to return with his wings firmly clipped. India Office was not that opposed to Haffkine as the IMS or a section of the Indian administration was. In fact, even at the height of the anti-Haffkine feeling after Mulkowal, the Secretary of State had written to Curzon:

> I should be sorry if you parted with Haffkine. He is a genius with a quite exceptional power of research. I think he will be so humiliated and depressed with the result of his own folly that you will find him for the future a more valuable servant, as he has to wipe out the discredit which will be for years to come attached to his murderous serum.[67]

Hamilton was right except that the strain to 'wipe out the discredit' drained Haffkine so much that he could hardly be a 'valuable servant' any more. Haffkine of the 1890s was lost forever.

On his return to Calcutta Haffkine resumed his work on anti-cholera inoculations. But soon in July 1908, all anti-cholera inoculations were stopped in view of a report published in the *Journal of American Medical Association* on the death of several people in Manila because of an accidental contamination of the cholera vaccine with a culture of plague bacilli. Haffkine was asked to explain his 'technique' and the 'precautions' adopted. Later the government agreed to lift the ban only after Haffkine accepted 'personal responsibility for all the vaccines used'.[68] Haffkine withdrew himself completely. During 1908–1915 he filled about 20 notebooks on the various experiments he conducted on sera, pus, agar, comma, etc.[69] But he did not seem to have made any scientific paper out of these. The spare time he spent reflecting upon the tides or soaring-birds and aerodynamics or solving Pythagorean theorem.[70] Occasionally he would write letters, clarifying his position, whenever his name was mentioned with Mulkowal.[71] On reaching the retirement age in 1915, Haffkine returned to Europe on a new 'mission'.

Return to Religion

In his student days, despite his socialist-*narodinik* inclinations and the mounting anti-Jewish feelings among the orthodox Russians, Haffkine was never shy or scared of disclosing his Jewish birth and upbringing. But he never showed or aired orthodox religious views while practising his science and craft. Even in the midst of 'crisis' he did not seek help from any Jewish political or business group.[72] It is not a mere coincidence that his religious propensities grew. Frustrations in career perhaps had a telling effect on him. He sought refuge in religion, and after retirement, assumed virtually a messianic role.

In early 1914, the small community of Shephardi (Baghdadi) Jews in Calcutta held a meeting, and claiming descendence from the Spanish Jews of the 15th century, asked for parity with the Europeans in education, etc. Haffkine refused to preside over such meetings and even warned them that this would be liked neither by the Indians nor the Europeans.[73] He wanted them to be helped and raised on voluntary and community basis, not through government succour. Community-conscious he definitely was. In 1916, he wrote, 'communities, even more than marriages, are made in heaven; but suitable lines of conduct are necessary to maintain communal life, just as they are necessary to maintain a united married life'.[74] Coming from a confirmed bachelor, this analogy is interesting. These 'suitable lines of conduct' he found in the Torah. 'Torah is the foundation; undermine it, and your edifice of Jewish life must fall', he wrote to Ben Yehuda, the well-known Zionist.[75] From community-consciousness, the scientist had moved miles further.

Like a social-anthropologist, he gave the example of Sikhs in India—bearded, turbaned, and distinctive. 'Living as they do in a land of many races, who vary in blood, sentiment, morals and culture, this powerful people have come to know that, for a group of human beings to preserve their cohesion, *well-defined and continual manifestations* are necessary, acquiescence in which is a declaration of *allegiance* to the group, and neglect of which is a *betrayal*, since it endangers the groups bonds and existence'.[76] His reference to 'allegiance' and 'betrayal' is understandable; as a professional he longed for group-cohesiveness but could never achieve it. He noticed how the Scots formed a majority in IMS by helping each other through a 'nearly pried-up gravitation'.[77] Haffkine wanted the Jews to gravitate round the Torah and its language.

For this he had a biological explanation as well. 'Just as an organism is differentiated into separate organs, functioning differently, but coordinated and promoting the welfare of the whole body, so the association of men into intimate groups, bound by ties of blood, religion, locality, or other material or ideal bonds, tends to that spirit of mutual help which is at the base of all biological progress'.[78] With his impeccable scientific credentials (based on reason and rationality), he was not always sure on how to encapsulate faith and science together. On one occasion he would say, 'there is no conflict between the Jewish faith and science', as all advances in science point to the Jewish conception of one power with no beginning and no end (this is what the ancient Hindus also thought!). On another he would reflect, 'we need again masterminds equipped with the instruments of modern science and philosophy, but filled with deep and sympathetic knowledge of the law to bridge the gap between faith and reason, to reinterpret the Torah in terms of modern philosophy and science'.[79] This age-old civilizational dilemma he could not have resolved. But a year before his death in 1930 he did donate all his savings to promote, paradoxically, traditional Jewish learning.[80]

An Evaluation

By the time Haffkine took to research, two distinct schools had clearly emerged. The German school, led by Koch, concentrated on the isolation and exhaustive study of individual bacteria and thus laid the foundations of several highly specialized branches of bacteriology. The French school, led by Pasteur, concentrated on the problems of the prevention of infective diseases by calibrated inoculation and thus developed the science of immunology.[81] Haffkine chose to follow Pasteur in letter and spirit. Germany at that time had no large colonial stakes. But France and Britain had enormous imperial interests and both recognized the importance of Pasteur's methods and programmes. Bruno Latour has made a critical study of the role of Pasteurians and *Institute Pasteur* in the colonial process.[82] The 'new doctor' worked in the laboratory and at the same time prescribed or at least influenced administrative regulations. They acted like 'Solon' and without them the 'Colonial Leviathan' could not have been built, much less sustained. The biologists themselves were pretty aware of their self-importance. To Rudolph Virchow (a pioneer in cellular pathology), politics was 'nothing but medicine on a grand scale'. Similarly, was medicine nothing but politics on a mass scale?[83] The story of Haffkine would confirm a political reading of the laboratory. But unlike Latour's 'heroes', Haffkine could not tame the Leviathan. He petitioned, beseeched, and fell. Again, unlike Yersin, here is a Pasteurian with little difference; he treats the patients, advises the government, and also reflects on the social questions. Haffkine does not fit in the Latourian mould.[84]

It is, however, not difficult to see the close relationship between the microparasites and the macroparasites (i.e. the colonizers). Control over one was crucial to the success of the other.[85] Yet some scholars argue that its role in the 'stabilization of colonial rule was far more limited'. This role was conditioned and constricted by the values, opinions (and opposition) of the indigenous society, and the ground realities of a colonial economy.[86] This is a valid argument but only to a limited extent. Parasitology had given many colonizers (especially those with lofty utilitarian views) a sense of purpose and a practical programme. The microscope had supplanted the sword.[87] Given the political will, it was possible to move. Haffkine could show charts of success when he had the political support, and he flopped the moment it was withdrawn.

Support, in both academic and administrative terms, was crucial. Haffkine was lucky to have the support of the top bacteriologists of the time, Metchnikoff, Roux, and Pasteur himself. Later Koch also defended his prophylaxis. In contrast, Jaime Ferran who was certainly the first to inoculate human beings against cholera in 1885, was not so lucky. Practising medicine in a peripheral town of Spain, his claims to vaccine against a number of bacterial disease were viewed with disbelief and disdain in the scientific metropolis.[88] Haffkine had better guidance. He moved with greater diligence, more accuracy, and had the benefit of a close peer-scrutiny so long as he was in Paris. Pasteur's recommendation had facilitated his shift to India.[89] This also ensured him an enormous administrative support. But his direction had changed. He was now taking 'a laboratory product' to the man on the street. He was no longer a 'discoverer' but a 'deliverer' delivering to the masses what was perceived scientifically to be good. This process of 'deliverance' was no less challenging nor devoid of innovations: the 'stalactite' growth in plague bacilli, for example, or the way he conducted human testing of his vaccine. He was perhaps the first to define the principles of controlled field-trials.[90] Yet of all the medical men in India a microscopic few like Ross and Donovan were obsessed with and inching towards a fundamental discovery.[91] Ross and Haffkine shared certain traits. Both were acutely aware of their self-importance, both disdained bureaucracy, and both put a premium on 'men', not institutions. While on the verge of his malaria-vector discovery, Ross wrote, 'we do not want laboratories, we want men'.[92] Haffkine would say, 'the worker is the chief item, not bricks and mortar, etc'.[93] Both believed in taking laboratory results to the common man; they believed more in prevention than in cure and sought active state intervention. As their expectations could not be fully met, both suffered exhaustion and frustration. However, unlike Haffkine, Ross had higher literary and argumentative skills which he used with deadly effect.[94] In addition, Ross had a British origin, a medical degree, a rank in IMS, and a fundamental discovery to his credit. Haffkine had none of these.[95] Naturally he would often withdraw, sulk, and look for support when opposed. But, unlike Ross, Haffkine did not seek pecuniary rewards. Ross had even petitioned the Parliament for remuneration.[96] Haffkine could petition only his peers for restoration of his honour. Recognition was enough for him which he did receive in ample measure atleast in the first half of his career. Not every one in the IMS was opposed to him. Simpson, Ross, Thornhill supported always.[97] But Ross and Haffkine were natural dissenters and they exercised their right to differ a little more freely.

Right from the beginning of the plague out-break Haffkine differed from the schemes of disinfection, segregation, and forced hospitalization which the government medical officials had launched.[98] This was apparently not liked. To him the only plausible method to combat the epidemic was individual preventive treatment. The government would rather put the blame on the ignorance and insanitary conditions of the natives.[99] The government had its own reasons to panic, and so had the people. They could hardly come to terms with each other. Certain measures evoked sharp opposition and even riots.[100] But there were many who came forward with little or some persuasion to accept Haffkine's prophylaxis. So there was no single, homogenous response from the Indian society. It varied from place to place, time to time.[101] Haffkine himself had a fine understanding of Indian society. In a letter to a senior official (which for obvious reasons remained unanswered), he wrote:

> The natives here are, of course, not the prodigies of imbecility, superstition and ingratitude which some good papers occasionally amuse themselves in representing them to be. Every civil surgeon or practitioner who has had an occasion of extracting a cataract or stone, or rendering any other good to a native, will say that such a description does not accurately represent him. Stories of superstitious fabrications attributed to the people are sometimes manufactured, sometimes only favoured and exaggerated, by an unwilling or incapable executive.[102]

Thus, unlike Yersin in Hong Kong, Haffkine took a keen interest in Indian affairs. To make matters worse for himself, he criticized the official agencies, especially the IMS. The Americans had nothing like the IMS in the Philippines; 'Yet look at the doctors in Philippines, is India superior to them?'[103] On the eve of his departure from India, he wrote, 'In Rogers' and Lister's places no non-IMS man will ever have a chance. By plotting, giving false evidence, lying, false representation, spying, the gentlemen now in possession will keep out any man not of their set'.[104] Convinced of his special position as a scientific researcher, he proved to be a difficult person. No wonder, even before Mulkowal, he had received subtle snubs.[105] Living in a difficult world and plagued by a deep sense of insecurity, he demanded loyalty but could never command it. He had no professional medical training or degree, yet he personified what a doctor should be:

> The doctor should have faith in the remedy; he should be interested in the success of his mission; he should have at heart exclusively the interest of the people he is dealing with; no thought of reporting a success or fear of being blamed for failure should preoccupy him.[106]

A century later when medical attention is gradually shifting from the etiology of AIDS virus to the possibility of a vaccine against it,[107] the life and work of Haffkine could well be instructive.

Acknowledgement: This work was made possible by the grants from the Edelstein Centre for History of Science, Technology and Medicine (Jerusalem), The Wellcome Trust (London) and the International Institute of Asian Studies (Leiden). I am greatful to Ella Andriesse, Ilana Lowy, Wim Stokhof, Tony Travis and Shaul Katz for their care and interest. Shaul made my visit to Jerusalem a trip into culture and history.

A slightly different version of this paper was published in *Science, Technology and Society*, 4, 2, 1999, pp. 240-271.

References

1. W. Haffkine to H. Thornhill (Medical Officer in Jaffna, Ceylon), Feb. 28, 1896; Haffkine Papers (hereafter HP), Ms. Var 325, file 332, preserved at the archive of the Hebrew University Library, Jerusalem.
2. Haffkine's Memorandum to Lord Curzon, Dec. 22, 1900, HP, file (hereafter f.) 367.
3. M. Worboys, 'The Emergence of Tropical Medicine: A Study in the Establishment of a Scientific Speciality', in G. Lemaine *et al.,* (eds.), *Perspectives on the Emergence of Scientific Disciplines,* Paris, Mouton, 1976, pp. 76–97; Bruno Latour, *The Pasteurisation of France*, Massachusetts, Harvard University Press, 1988; D. M. Haynes, 'From the Periphery to the Centre: Patrick Manson and the Development of Tropical Medicine as a Medical Speciality in Britain 1870–1900, Ph.D. Thesis, University of California, Berkeley, 1992; David Arnold, *Colonizing the Body,* Delhi, Oxford University Press, 1993, Deepak Kumar, *Science and the Raj,* Delhi, Oxford University Press, 1995.
4. George H. Bornside, 'Waldemar Haffkine's Cholera Vaccines and the Ferran-Haffkine Priority Dispute', *Journal of History of Medicine*, 37, 1983, pp. 399–422; Ilana Lowy, 'From Guinea Pigs to Man: The Development of Haffkine's Anticholera Vaccine', *Journal of History of Medicine and Allied Sciences*, 47, 1992, pp. 270-309.
5. Note dt. April 4, 1899, HP, f. 79.
6. E. Lutzker and C. Jochnowitz, 'Waldemar Haffkine's School Day's', *Jewish Currents*, October, 1980, pp. 26–32; see also Selman A. Waksman, *The Brilliant and Tragic Life of W. M. W. Haffkine*, New Brunswick, Rutgers Univ. Press, 1964.
7. Ilana Lowy, *op.cit.*, p. 276, Note 4.
8. *Ibid*, p. 274.
9. *Ibid*, p. 277, also HP, f. 339.
10. *Ibid*, p. 279.
11. W. J. Simpson, 'Waldemar Haffkine', *The British Medical Journal*, Nov. 8, 1930, pp. 801-2.

12. E. H. Hankin, 'Remarks on Haffkine's Method of Protective Inoculation Against Cholera', *The British Medical Journal*, II, Sept. 19, 1892, pp. 569–71; also HP, f. 397.5.
13. *Ibid.*
14. W. H. Haffkine, 'A Lecture on Vaccination against Cholera', *The British Medical Journal*, II, Dec. 21, 1895, pp. 1541-44.
15. *Ibid.*
16. HP, f. 327.
17. W. J. Simpson, 'Two Years of Anti-cholera Inoculations in Calcutta', Calcutta, 1896; HP, f. 336.3.
18. Circulation no. Medical 266/272 dt. March 26, 1896, HP, f. 327.
19. G. C. Mukherjee, Medical Officer, Purulia, to the Sanitary Commissioner, Bengal, April 11, 1898, HP, f. 387.2.
20. Haffkine to Secretary to GOI, July 31, 1908, HP, f. 408.
21. W. M. Haffkine, 'Epidemiological Notes', Calcutta, 1911 (printed for private circulation), HP, f. 387.12.
22. *Indian Medical Gazette*, Feb. 1897, p. 44.
23. *Ceylon Independent*, Jan. 17, 1896; Clipping in HP., f. 332.
24. The vaccine-enthusiasts expected an effective anti-malaria vaccine much before Ross could pin down its real cause. Now, even after a century, around 40 per cent of the world's population is still at risk from malaria, and yearning for cheap effective vaccine. In recent years a vaccine called Spf 66 seemed to reduce infection rates by 31–55 per cent in early tests. The findings now have been controverted and a new study considers this vaccine useless. *The Statesman*, Delhi, Sept. 29, 1996.
25. Haffkine to Owen, Dec. 17, 1897, HP, f. 443.3.
26. W. B. Bannerman, 'The Plague Research Laboratory of the Government of India', *Proceeding of the Royal Society of Edinburgh*, XXIV, 1902, pp. 113-44.
27. E. H. Hankin, *The Bubonic Plague*, Pioneer Press, Allahabad, 1899, III; one of the reasons Hankin wrote this tract was to combat such rumours. This had a forward from Haffkine.
28. K. L. C. Raja, 'Vasoorikerivekkal', *Mangalodayam* (in Malyalam), II, Trichur, 1910.
29. W. M. Haffkine, 'On Preventive Inoculation', *Proceedings of the Royal Society*, 65, 1899, pp. 252–71.
30. W. M. Haffkine, 'What to do Against the Plague in India', (a hand-written note), HP, 344.12.
31. W. B. Bannerman, *op.cit.*, Note 26.
32. Curzon to Hamilton (Secy. of State for India), Nov. 27, 1902, Curzon Papers, Mss. Eur.F.111/161, p. 380, India Office Library and Records (IOLR), London.
33. Elgin to Hamilton, Feb. 24, 1898, Elgin Papers, Mss. Eur.F.84/16, IOLR. p. 36.

34. *Ibid.*
35. HP, f. 369.
36. *Report of the Indian Plague Commission*, London, 1900, ch. iv; also HP, f. 345.1.
37. Elgin to Hamilton, August 25, 1898, Elgin Papers, p. 136, Note 33.
38. A. Godley (Under-Secretary of State) to Curzon, May 3, 1899; Curzon sent a reply quite characteristic of him: 'Haffkine is a Russian, and that it might seem a little strange to place one of his nationality at the head of an Indian Institute. I should hardly find an English Professor in a corresponding position at Tashkent'. Curzon to A. Godley, May 24, 1899, Curzon Papers, Eur. F111/158, pp. 58c, 92d.
39. HP, f. 334, quoted in Ilana Lowy, *op.cit.*, p. 301, Note 4.
40. As Haffkine recalled in a talk with Gibson (on March 7, 1910), 'Bannerman himself had been pulled out by the ears by me from Madras where he was serving as a deputy sanitary commissioner and was engaged in supervising drains and sewers and vaccination duties; had there been no laboratory of mine and no plague prophylactic, Gibson would have continued to visit the *qalis* and lanes under the then Plague Commission'. HP, f. 444.111.
41. A. Godley to Curzon, Nov. 10, 1899, and Curzon to Hamilton, Nov. 16, 1899, Curzon Papers, pp. 197, 241.
42. Haffkine to Surgeon-General Harvey, Dec. 14, 1899, and Harvey to Haffkine, Jan. 18, 1900. HP, f. 87.
43. Home, Medical, nos. 103–16, March 1902, Pt.A, National Archive of India.
44. 'Knowing as we do the unselfish devotion and labour you have bestowed on the work of endeavouring to prevent the ravages of cholera, plague and typhoid fever, etc. with much success, we feel convinced that you will if possible accept this post, which we trust will enable you to continue your grand work in this country and will also, we are sure, add many more laurels to your already world-wide reputation.' Nehal Singh (Maharaj Rana of Dholpur) to Haffkine, May 9, 1897; HP, f. 443.3. In addition, the Dholpur and Patiala chiefs were willing to provide money for Ronald Ross also to do malaria research. Ross was then working under difficult conditions. But he was stopped by the government to accept any 'native' offer. Ross Archive, 301/072 and 01/110, School of Tropical Medicine, London.
45. *Parliamentary Debates on Indian Affairs*, 1896, p. 351; 1898, p. 820, IOLR, v/3/1599 and 1601.
46. G. Hamilton to Curzon, Feb. 16, 1899, Curzon Papers, Eur.F.111/158, p. 20.
47. The Bishop of Calcutta to Curzon, June 22, 1900; Curzon Papers, Mss. Eur.F.111/201, pp. 114, 248.
48. Haffkine to the Secretary to Govt. of India, Jan. 8, 1901, HP, f. 368.
49. HP, f. 444.9.

50. Curzon to Hamilton, Nov. 27, 1902, Curzon Papers, Mss. Eur.F111/161, p. 380.
51. Curzon to Hamilton, Nov. 13, 1902, *Ibid*, p. 403.
52. Curzon to Hamilton, Nov. 5, 1902, *Ibid*, p. 401.
53. The Bombay Government did not pass this information to the Punjab Government or the Government of India. As Curzon noted, 'I do not feel at all clear that the Bombay Government is not equally, or nearly equally, to blame'. Curzon to Hamilton, Dec. 18, 1902, *Ibid*, p. 444
54. Report of the Punjab Plague Inoculation Commissioner, HP, f. 364.1.
55. Haffkine's Note on Mulkowal, Aug. 10, 1907, HP, f. 326.
56. *Summarised Report of the Plague Research Laboratory for 1902–1904*, Bombay, 1904, p. 8.
57. Haffkine to the Government of Bombay, Nov. 8, 1902, HP, f. 347.
58. Mamorandum dt. May 7, 1903, HP, 49.9.
59. Soon after the incident, Ibbetson (an influential member of the Viceroy's Council) had concluded that 'it would very probably be necessary to dismiss him'. Curzon Papers, Mss. Eur F.111/206, p. 1989.
60. Home Dept. to Viceroy, Nov. 15, 1903, *Ibid*, 111/208, p. 212.
61. Eli Chernin, 'Ross Defends Haffkine: The Aftermath of the Vaccine-Association Mulkowal Disaster of 1902', *Journal of the History of Medicine and Allied Sciences*, 46, 1911, pp 201–18.
62. Ross Archive, Mss.02/159 for details, see Deepak Kumar, *op.cit.*, pp. 168-71, Note 3.
63. *The Journal of Tropical Medicine and Hygiene*, X, 3, 1907, pp. 33-45.
64. *The Times*, July 29, 1907, HP, f. 364.9.
65. HP, f. 326.
66. A. Godley to Haffkine, Dec. 5, 1906, HP, f. 364.9.
67. Hamilton to Curzon, Dec. 4, 1902, Curzon Papers, p. 384.
68. HP, f. 408.
69. This collection called Calcutta Books of General Notes (1908-15) is preserved with Haffkine Papers in Jerusalem. HP, f. 411.1.
70. HP, f. 415.1, 421 and 422.
71. Letter to the Editor, *Pall Mall Gazette*, June 4, 1913; *The Indian Medical Gazette*, July 19, 1914, p. 291.
72. I could not see any reference in the Haffkine Papers on his religious views or Zionism till 1911.
73. HP, f. 251.
74. W. M. Haffkine, 'On Jewish Endurance', *The Jewish World*, Nov. 29, 1916, pp. 15-18.
75. Haffkine to Eliazor Ben Yehuda, April 21, 1922, HP, f. 228.
76. W. M. Haffkine, 'A Plea for Orthodoxy', *The Menorah Journal*, April 1916, pp. 3-13.
77. 'In my laboratory in India, I, at one time, suddenly became aware of being surrounded by assistants taken from the ranks of the official Indian

Medical Service, all of whom were Scots—not one Englishman, Irish or Welsh. Unnoticeably to myself, they had induced me, whenever I needed additional help, to apply to the government for a man of their own. In that they manifested, In believe, less dislike of others than well understood and neatly pried-up, gravitation with regard to each other...'; Haffkine to D. I. Macht, July 23, 1929, HP, f. 85.9.

78. Address at a Jewish meeting in New York (not dated, probably 1916), HP, f. 56.

79. HP, f. 228. Such efforts had been made from time to time. Centuries ago, Shem Tov Ibn Falgura (1223–1291), a medieval Jewish rationalist, sought to synthesize the fidelity to Torah with a commitment to western philosophic and scientific wisdom. Raphael Jospe, *Torah and Sophia: The Life and Thought of Shem Tov Ibn Falagura*, Cincinati, Jewish Union College Press, 1988, p. 12.

80. HP, f. 247.

81. William Bulloch, *The History of Bacteriology*, London, Oxford Univ. Press, 1983, p. 255; George Newman, *The Rise of Preventive Medicine*, London, Oxford Univ. Press, 1932, for 'controversial' details see, G. L. Geison, *The Private Science of Louis Pasteur,* Princeton, Princeton Univ. Press, 1994, Thomas D. Brock, *Robert Koch: A Life in Medicine and Bacteriology*, Madison; Science Tech. Publications, 1988.

82. Bruno Latour, *op.cit.*, pp. 1-145, Note 3.

83. David Arnold (ed.), *Imperial Medicine and Indigenous Societies*, Delhi, 1989, p. 18.

84. Latour's major example is Yersin in Hong Kong. He portrays Yersin as 'interested in nothing, or almost nothing, for in each agent he took only what might link it along an obligatory passage that led him, by forced stages, to vaccination'. At one point, Latour asks scholars 'to allow the actors to define themselves', yet he is unable to do so in his own otherwise brilliant analysis because he bases his account only on printed sources, predominantly the three French medical journals.

    Variety of sources would perhaps allow one a more eclectic perspective. But as Latour himself admits, 'I use history as a brain scientist uses a rat, cutting through it in order to follow the mechanisms that may allow me to understand at once the *content* of a science and its *context*'. Obviously a promise not fulfilled because of a selective use of historical data. Bruno Latour, *op.cit.*, pp. 12, 51, 95-10, Note 3 (emphasis as in original).

85. In 1898, Patrick Manson (who later founded the London School of Tropical Medicine) wrote, 'I now firmly believe in the possibility of tropical colonisation by the white races. Heat and moisture are not in themselves the direct causes to any important tropical disease. The direct causes of 99 per cent of these diseases are germs... To kill them is simply a matter of knowledge and the application of this knowledge'. M. Worboys, 'The Emergence', p. 85, Note 3.

86. Mark Harrison, *Public Health in British India*, Cambridge, Cambridge Univ. Press, 1944, pp. 228-34.

87. Warwick Anderson, 'Laboratory Medicine as a Colonial Discourse', *Critical Inquiry*, 18, 1992, pp. 506-529.

88. For this Ferran was perhaps himself responsible. His ego, 'secretative' methods, tall claims, and adverse publicity deprived him of an early and due scientific recognition. E. O. Shakespeare (who was deputed by the U. S. Senate in March 1885 to report on cholera in Europe and India) was advised by his medical friends in London and Berlin that 'a personal investigation of the Ferran question was now beneath the dignity of serious scientific consideration'. Still when he visited Ferran, he was struck by his skill and 'beautifully stained microscopic preparations'. For details see, E.O. Shakespeare, *Report on Cholera in Europe and India*, Washington, Government Press, 1890, pp. 711-714; George H. Bornside, 'Jaime Ferran and Preventive Inoculation against Cholera', *Bulletin of the History of Medicine*, 55, IV, 1981, pp. 51-532.

89. To quote a despatch from the then Secretary of State for India to the Viceroy, 'One is naturally sceptical about remedies but Pasteur's eminence is such that any suggestion of his is worthy of attention', Kimbereley to Lansdowne, Nov. 18, 1892, Lansdowne Papers, National Archive of India, Micro. 1050–1661, Reel 2, p. 82.

90. George H. Bornside, 'Waldemar Haffkine's', pp. 414–415, Note 4.

91. For details see, Ronald Ross, *Memoirs*, London, John Murray, 1923, and Marry Gibson, 'The Identification of Kala Azar and the Discovery of Leishmania Donovani', *Medical History*, 27, 1983, pp. 203-213.

92. Ross to Manson, May 10, 1898, Ross Archive, Mss. 02/155, Note 62.

93. Commenting on Tata Institute of Research (opened at Bangalore in 1909), 'If I had say a 50 lakhs to dispose off and wished to secure a discovery which to benefit the whole of mankind, I would try ('buy') a worker... On the other hand you may provide the worker with anything you like but surround him with thieves and swines... or else build palatial institutes and put there not the worker but a set of thieves and liars'. Note dt. 10.07.1913, HP, 443.5.

94. Ross once threatened to sue even his mentor, Patrick Manson for an 'indirect' criticism of his work at Liverpool. Manson had to apologize and pay £ 5 as charge for the legal notice! Royal Society of Tropical Medicine and Hygiene Papers, WTI/RST/F56-65, CMAC, Wellcome Trust, London.

95. Leonard Rogers (1868–1962), an IMS who founded the Calcutta School of Tropical Medicine in 1914, considered Haffkine 'a foreign bacteriologist without registrable medical qualifications'. This is how he was viewed by probably majority of the IMS. Rogers Papers, PP/ROG/A.55/106, CMAC, Wellcome Trust, London.

96. Ross argued, 'Science has become ... the premier industry of the world', and that 'there should be *payment for results* in addition to the present system ... *of payment for expectations*'.

    Quoted in Eli Chernin, 'Sir Ronald Ross, Malaria, and the Rewards of Research', *Medical History*, 32, 1988, pp. 119–141 (emphasis as in original).

97. When the Secretary of State refused to exonerate Haffkine publicly of the Mulkowal affair, Simpson wrote to Ross (June 9, 1907): 'Poor Haffkine, I fear the Government are determined to stand by the position

they have taken up... it is however a bad day for science when truth is dominated by passions and expediency'. Quoted in R. A. Baker and R. A. Bayliss, 'William J. R. Simpson: Public Health and Tropical Medicine', *Medical History*, 31, 1987, pp. 450-465.

98. HP, f. 364.9.

99. To this Haffkine's reply was, 'would it be practical and helpful if, upon a visit to the poor of London, in connection with some misfortune, one suggested to them, as a remedy, to lift their lot from the condition they were in?' Haffkine to the Secretary of State, Sept. 19, 1911, HP, f. 388.2.

100. For details see I. J. Catanach, 'Plague Policy and Popular Unrest in British India, *Modern Asian Studies*, 22, 1988, pp. 723-755; *idem*, 'Plague and the Tensions of Empire 1896–1918', in D. Arnold (ed.) *op.cit.*, pp. 149-171, Note 83.

101. R. Chandavarkar, 'Plague Panic and Epidemic Politics in India 1896-1914', in T. Ranger and P. Slack (eds.), *Epidemic and Ideas,* Cambridge, Cambridge Univ. Press, 1992, pp. 203-240.

102. Haffkine to H. Butler, April 21, 1911, HP, f. 407.2.

103. 'The present Director General of the IMS is a good bed-side manner man... the present Sanitary Commissioner with the Government of India, can he be quoted as a demonstration of the superior results of the IMS system?' HP, f. 444.11, Note 40.

104. Note dt. 10.07.1913, HP. f. 443.5 Little did Haffkine realize that Rogers himself suffered much. The IMS set up was such. In 1898 Rogers in spite of his strong credentials, could not get a pathologist's position at Lahore, because a senior IMS lobbied for his nephew! Even in 1913, Rogers was denied few beds on a regular basis at Calcutta Medical College Hospital for work on *kala-azar*. This Rogers considered 'the last and saddest of my experience'. L. Rogers, 'Note on the difficulties encountered by IMS officer in research' (TS), Rogers Papers, PP/ROG/ A.55/100–110, Note 95. for more details, Helen J. Power, 'Sir Leonard Rogers: Tropical Medicine in the Indian Service', unpublised Ph.D. thesis, University College, London, 1993.

105. When Haffkine was honoured with CIE, the same decoration was given also to a Lieut. Colonel 'whose sole work was to check the groins and arm-pits of the passengers in Bombay dock'. Haffkine was reminded of 'when we were youths in the Gymnasium of Berdiansk, Liova Tzyboulevsky (a Jew) was to be given a gold medal; a fairly dumb-headed Russian was given the gold medal also as an off-set to the success of the Jewish youth... The English as represented by the Lords Curzon and Sandhurst, the trumpeters of English *fair play*, are every bit as fine sportsmen as were those Ukrainian pedagogues of Berdiansk'. HP, f. 167 (emphasis as in origianl).

106. HP, f. 344.12.

107. In early September 1996, Professor Thomas Lehner of Guy's and St. Thomas Hospital in London reported to the British Association for the Advancement of Science a new vaccine against SIV (the monkey eqivalent of HIV). But the question of the suitability of the animal model remains. As a critic puts it, 'however good the animal model is, there isn't one that mimics human disease well'. Reported in *The Statesman*, Delhi, Sept. 12, 1996.

Indigenous Medicine

12
Evolution of Ayurveda Through The Ages

—*Brahmananda Gupta*

Pre-vedic

Health-care system was prevalent even in pre-vedic period. We hear of the Indus valley civilization, pre-Harappan cultures of Mohenjodaro, Harappa, and Kalibangan which were considered to be highly developed. Excavations of Mohenjodaro exhibiting underground sewerage system, public bath, private bathrooms, and wells evidently reveal the knowledge of public health and hygiene. From the archaeological findings of bones and skulls in the skeletal remains, we get enough evidence of diseases, method of cranial surgery for brain disorders, use of knives and other instruments, metallic rings around the teeth, use of metals such as gold, copper, silver etc., for medicinal purpose, and use of 'Silajit', the antimony-preparation as medicinal remedies, which suggest the highly developed technology and scientific mind of Harappan culture.

Vedic Period

There are some discussions on health related topics in all the Vedas. Diseases and their treatment, medicinal herbs and their efficiency for removing the ailments, have been described here and there. But in comparison to the Rig Veda, *Sama* and *Yajur*, *Atharvaveda* appears to be more elaborate in dealing with the mode of treatment. That is why perhaps in later days both *Carakasamhita* and *Susrutasamhita* claim Ayurveda to belong to *Atharvaveda*. But we also find references where Ayurveda has been claimed as a separate veda i.e., *Pancamaveda*, in addition to the four existing ones. Others, however, would like to ascribe Ayurveda, an ancillary status to the veda i.e., *Upaveda* and finally *Carana-Vyuha* would like to call it an annex of *Rgveda*. Whatever may be the fact, that Ayurveda is a system introducing a scientific mode of treatment, has been accepted by all.

In the *Rgveda* itself many diseases, medicinal, herbs and fundamental principles of Ayurveda have been discussed. Reference to diseases such as jaundice (RV1.9.7.11–13), heart disease (RV1.50.11.12), etc. can be found. *Rgveda* tells us stories about the vedic physicians Asvins, who rejuvenated Cyavana (RV1.116.10), provided an artificial limb to Vispata, wife of Khela (RV1.116.16), and cured blindness (RV1.116.16) and leprosy (RV1.88). The basic principles of Ayurvedic treatment based on *tridosa* viz. *vata*, *pitta,* and *kapha* and the seven basic elements of the body viz. *rasa* (nourishing fluid of plasma), *rakta* (blood), *mamsa* (flesh), *meda* (fat), *asthi* (bone), *majja* (bone-marrow), and *sukra* (semen) can be traced.

Medicinal plants (RV.X.97.1) possessed the potential power to overcome the diseases and pain of the body. Proper food and diet have also been given a predominant place in the *Rgveda.*

With regard to the date of RV, scholars are of different opinions ranging from 7500 BC to 1000 BC.

Although the RV mentioned the occurrence of the diseases due to the imbalance of the three factors of the body called the '*tri-dhatu*', popularly known as *tridosa*, *Atharvaveda* discusses the same 'tridosa-theory' in a slightly different way. According to AV, the ailments can be caused by three elements viz. *abhraja* (i.e., due to moisture-ladden cloud), indicating excess of *kapha* element, *vataja* (due to wind), and *susmaja*, indicating *pitta* or fiery element (AV.XVII.3.5) in the body.

Atharvaveda also mentions the division of the *vayu* in the body as *prana*, *apana*, *udana*, *vyana,* and *samana* (AV1.2.12) and refers to the *ojas asthi* vital fluid (AV.II.18). Elementary human anatomy has been described in the *Atharvaveda* (AV.X.2) and important organs of the body have not been missed (AV.II.33). It may be interesting to note that *Atharvaveda* asserts that 'In the beginning (of creation) water brought an embryo into being' (AV.IV.2.8).

Atharvaveda also mentions blood circulation in the vessels (AV.X.2.11.). Among the diseases of head and neck, diseases of liver, skin diseases, genito urinary diseases (*prameha*), gynaecological and obstetrical diseases, the use of many medicinal herbs have also been mentioned.

Asrva (bleeding) was treated by Pippali and munja grass application. The vedic people primarily considered treatment through application of the sun-rays, water, wind, and medicinal herbs.

Four types of treatment have been mentioned in the *Atharvaveda.* They are:

(a) *atharvana cikitsa* (b) *angirasa cikitsa*
(c) *daivi cikitsa* (d) *ausadhi cikitsa.*

(a) In the *Atharvanic* type, the chanting of mantras was primarily considered. This type can be considered as faith-healing by way of psychotherapy or psychiatry or psychological type of treatment.

(b) The *Angirasa* type was mainly the medical treatment based on application of medicinal herbs and products of animals and birds.

(c) Under *Daivi* type of treatment, cure with the help of natural elements such as sunrays, water, earth, etc., was applied for healing purpose. It may be regarded as some forms of naturopathy treatment where phenomenon of nature plays the role of a healing agent.

(d) The *Ausadhi* type of treatment is undertaken as the curative treatment by the application of finished products of medicines.

Atharvaveda, which according to some scholars, belongs to circa 1500–1000 BC, contains huge materials of Indian medical science, known as Ayurveda and denotes the knowledge of how to maintain a prolonged healthy life. But the *Atharvaveda*, like other Vedas as a whole, being by-and-large socio-religious and ritualistic, was mostly regarded as magico-religious by foreign scholars.[2]

Viewed from a different angle it may appear that prayer to god may appeal to the common mass as a method of faith-healing which stimulates the will power of an affected person to fight out his ailment. The spiritual-cum-mental therapy, if I am permitted to say, is gaining popularity even in modern times. The enthusiastic acceptance of *yoga*, meditation, etc., even in the western world, reveals that the control of mind and peace of mind contribute much to the well-being of an individual as well as that of the society. In this world of competition, hectic life full of stress and anxiety, the psychosomatic approach of the *Atharvaveda*, reflected in Ayurveda, goes a long way to make life more happy. Moreover, the charms and incantations, used for healing purpose, were assigned to the duty of a priest and not to the duty of a physician. But apart from a few such religious-bias, the *Atharvaveda* contains a large amount of materials dealing with human anatomy, classification of diseases, herbal medicine (*bhaisajya*) applicable to these diseases, etc. Mention has also been made of practitioners, fully trained in medical science (*vaidya*), and also some wandering medical practitioners (*carana-vaidya*) in the then set up of the society.

From the earlier times, on account of the division of work, different duties were allotted to different sections of people. A hymn in the *Rgveda* contains the idea by pointing out that there was a threefold list of skilled professions, namely carpenters (*taksan*), medical healers or physicians (*bhisaj*), and priests (Brahmin) (RV.9.112.1.). This reveals that in the early Indian society the physicians had a separate and almost an equal status other than that of the priests. In almost all the ancient civilizations priests have enjoyed a privileged status other than the common people all over the world. But the service of the physicians was no less important. They had to combine the expertise, craftsmanship, and the intellect of a wise man. The common people respected the physicians for the skill and knowledge they possessed. At the time of battle or fight, the physicians were asked to accompany the king to the battle field to save the lives of kings and those of the soldiers. But the enhanced position and indispensability of a physician was envied by other high-ranking privileged castes, advisers of kings and law givers, who ultimately lodged a campaign to cut down the importance and status of a physician in society. That is why in the early Brahmanas viz., the *Satapatha Brahmana* of the later Vedic period (c.900–500 BC), we notice that physicians and medicines were denigrated by the priestly hierarchy, who rebuked the physicians for their impurity and their associations with all sorts of common people.[3] Some passage from *Taittiriya Samhita* also hints at some such priestly contempt for physicians narrated through a symbolic mention of a celestial physician, called *Asvinikumaras*. In course of time after the Vedic period even the Smriti-text writers like Manu took up the fight against the physicians to denigrate their status in society.

The Brahmana literature gives us detailed information also on medical science viz., the basic constituents or elements of the body, known as '*dhatus*', the visible external body parts (such as head, ear, nose, mouth, etc.), the unseen inner-body-parts, (such as heart, spleen, lung, liver, kidney, vein or artery, foetus, the inner membrane of the embryo, food habits and drinks etc. Various medicinal plants like *apamarga, aswagandha, udumbara, khadira, bilva, bibhitaka* etc., have also been described in the text.

The Sutra literature and the Upanisads also contain a lot of information regarding body parts, their ailments, cause of ailments, treatments, and food-habits. *Kausika-sutra* is very important from this point of view. It contains a lot of medical imformations of that time. This particular text may be considered as a go-between the *Atharvaveda*, on the one hand, and Ayurvedic texts, on the other. It is so, because it for the first time categorically puts, both the faith-therapy and the medicinal-therapy side by side, thus bringing some credibility to the system.

Later Vedic Period

The knowledge accumulated in the entire Vedas, Brahmanas, Aranyakas, Upanisads, and Sutra literature perhaps took a concrete shape in the later Vedic period, when specialized attempts were probably made by the *Rsis* to compose, one after another, specialized medical texts in all the eight branches of Ayurveda. For the information of those earlier texts, however, we have to rely on the statements and anecdotes of the *samhita granthas* of Caraka, Susruta, Vagbhata and other later commentaries as well, for the simple reason that many of the earlier evidences and texts are no longer or not yet available to us. We hear that Ayurvedic science dealt with eight branches:[4]

1.	*Salyatantra*	General Surgery
2.	*Salakya*	ENT, including eye and head diseases
3.	*Kayacikitsa*	Internal medicine
4.	*Bhutavidya*	Psychiatry
5.	*Kaumarabhrtya*	Paediatrics
6.	*Agadatantra*	Toxicology
7.	*Rasayana*	Geriatrics
8.	*Vajikarana*	Aphrodisiac

Many medical texts were also compared in these branches. But unfortunately most of these texts are either lost altogether or not yet traced. Only the texts of Harita and Bhela have been retained in a bad torm. *Ayurvedasastra* was not contined to the treatment ot human beings only, but it also included the treatment of diseases of animals and even plants. Texts on *Asvayurveda*, *Hastyayurveda*, *Gavayurveda* relating to the treatment of horses, elephants, cattle and trees (*vrksayusveda*) were written by Nakula, Salihotra, Parasara and others. Ayurveda suggests not only the cure of diseases but its importance lies primarily on the prevention of diseases. That is why, it recommends code of general ethics and good conduct and diets to be followed during the day-time, night-time, and in different seasons. It may be interesting to note that the term 'Ayurveda' could not be traced to the Vedic texts. Although it can be said that it must have gained importance before the time of Sanskrit grammarian Panini, who mentioned it twice, and the term Ayurveda occurs also in the Mahabharata.[5] Of the eight schools mentioned earlier, the Agnivesa cum Caraka School was known as 'School of Medicine' and Susruta School as the 'School of Surgery'.

One of the classical texts of the ancient Ayurvedic literature is called *Carakasamhita*. The *Carakasamhita* is in reality a compilation of ancient Indian medical-art based on the discourse of Atreya Punarvasu on diseases, method of diagnosis based on some careful observations of the clinical symptoms, the etiology, the pathology, and also the personal nature of the patient, his constitution, and disposition. It contains a systematic description. The text appears in the form of a dialogue between the teacher and the taught, an Upanisadic tradition of *Guru-sisya* discourse. *Carakasamhita* is mainly a treatise on Ayurvedic therapeutics.

The other classical text of Ayurveda known as *Susrutasamhita*, may appear to some scholars a little modern in its approach and may appeal to some physicians of today, as it contains valuable information regarding the objective and scientific approach of the ancient physicians, the knowledge of the diseases, dieteties, pharmacological and surgical therapies. Strangely enough, the older *Susrutasamhita* has described in the text many instruments that appear susprisingly similar to modern ones and some of them may be used even today.

The modern acupuncture system owes its origin to the *Susrutasamhita*. Susruta has dealt with the idea of needing a type of therapy in connection with *Marmas* i.e., 'vital points'. That is why the sensitive parts or the 'vital points' have been regarded as '*marmasthanas*'. In Ayurvedic concept these *marma*-points are connected through bio-energy channels known as *Nadis*. Through these underlying channels the bio-energy or body-force termed as prana is carried from one point to other points of the body. These '*marmasthanas*' can be highly sensitive when touched or pressed by needles, finger tips etc. When these *marmasthanas* or pranic-energy channels are pressed by needle or massaged or applied with hot compress, some sort of relief can be obtained. Thus the *marma* treatment was used for therapeutic purpose in the old tradition of Susruta.

Susruta was translated into Arabic language and Rhazes, an Arab physician of repute, quoted very often from Susruta calling him 'Husrut' or 'Sarad' as an authority of surgery. The speciality of *Susrutasamhita* lies in the fact that it deals elaborately and systematically with the surgical operations of ancient India. It describes how to remove stones from ureter or blooder, how to undertake a plastic surgery of the nose, cataract couching, cauterization, application of leaches in high blood-pressure, treatment of *Ksara* (Alkali), etc.

Prof. P. C. Roy placed *Carakasamhita* before 500 BC, in the pre-Buddhist period. The entire philosophical bias of a medical text like Caraka, its affinity to Atman-Brahman unity, discourse on rebirth (*punarjanma*), salvation (*moksa*), chapters on ominous signs (*aristalaksana*) and many others show that the text of Caraka stands closer to the Upanisadic doctrines, prevalent in the early Indian post-Vedic society, than the much developed texts of later origin. Moreover, a serious and systematic study of the philosophical doctrines of *Carakasamhita* may give an impression that some of the philosophical schools, organized from the Upanisadic doctrines, might have received impetus from *Carakasamhita* in later period. Investigation of the philological style and coining of words also arrive at the same conclusion ascribing an earlier date to Caraka. At the end of the later-vedic-period *Carakasamhita* and *Susrutasamhita* might have been composed in their original form.

The last of the three classical authors (Vrddhatrayi) is Vagbhata or Vagbhatta or Vahata,who is known as the author of *Astangasamgraha* and *Astangahrdaya*. The author might have lived in the 6th century. The Chinese traveller I-sing, who came to India between AD 671–695, disclosed his acquaintance with an Ayurvedic text called *Astangahrdaya*. This book, with the other two earlier medical texts of Caraka and Susruta, was translated into Arabic and Persian language in the 8th century in the court of Persian emperor Harun-Al-Rashid. In the medical treatise *Astangasamgraha* the author discloses his family identity, birth place, and his education career. This book is composed in both prose and poetry. The other book *Astangahrdaya* appears to be a more mature product of old age, which is more popular, authentic, and largely known outside of India, and it has been translated in many foreign languages. Jejjata, an Ayurvedic commentator of 9th century and Cakrapanidatta of 11th century have very often quoted from *Astangahrdaya* naming its author as Vagbhata.

Buddhist Period (600 BC–200 BC)

Now we come to the Buddhist period, the beginning of which can be considered to belong to a high order and nurtured in the elderly tradition of the later Vedic texts. This period in which, centres for Indian medical studies were opened and Ayurvedic medicine was taught at the universities of Kasi, Taksasila, Nalanda can be considered as the golden era of Ayurvedic treatment. In the earlier Buddhish literature, in opposition to Brahmanic literature, the name 'Ayurveda' was, however, replaced by the term '*tigiccha-satta*' (*cikitsa sastra*). At the time of Buddha, Agadatantra and Salyatantra (Sallakatthakam) perhaps got an upper hand.

Buddha has been depicted in the text as calling himself the incomparable physician, and surgeon as well (*anuttaro bhisako sallakattho*, (Milinda p. 215). In the early Buddhist period medical treatment and surgery developed to a greater extent. Buddhist texts, particularly the *Mahavagga*, supply a lot of information. Jivaka, who was a physician and a renowned surgeon, belongs to this period. He was a contemporary of Buddha and there are a lot of anecdotes with regard to his expertise knowledge. The *Sivi Jataka* refers to the marvellous treatment of Jivaka who had taken out the right and left eyes from the sockets of King Sivi. Jivaka completed seven years of medical training under Bhiksu Atreya at Taksasila University and became a famous surgeon.

With the propagation of Buddhism outside India, Ayurvedic medicine spread over to Tibet, Central Asia, Sri Lanka, Indonesia, Java, Sumatra and to many other countries. In the later Buddhist period, the doctrine of '*ahimsa*' (non-injury) and compassion towards all fellow-beings became very popular and as a result of it, surgical operations were looked upon as causing injury (*himsa*) and pain to patients. Probably for this reason surgery was discouraged in the later society. Thus, the study and practise of surgery being utterly neglected, extensive study of the eight branches (*astanga*) of Ayurveda suffered a lot and only the branch of *Kayacikitsa* (inner medicine) and *Rasayana* survived.

Muslim Period

With the advent of Muslim rule in India from 10th century onwards, the Unani system of medicine was introduced in India and it enjoyed the royal patronage of the Muslim rulers. During the Khilji and Tughlak rule, the Unani system of medicine was endorsed with official recognition of the Delhi Sultanate. Thereafter the Mughal rulers invited Muslim physicians and surgeons from Persia. Abul Fazl reports that in the court of Emperor Akbar twenty-nine eminent physicians came from Arab countries to pay homage to the king. The Mughal emperor Akbar being tolerant and liberal in attitude also invited some Ayurvedic scholars. Throughout Muslim rule in India, Unani medicine enjoyed royal patronage and acquired the status of a state-recognized medicine system. This new introduction hampered the growth of traditional Ayurvedic medicine. But it somehow maintained its popularity being backed by the common people of India, traditionally nurtured through the ages. The violence of the Muslim conquest and its anti-Hindu and anti-Buddhist warfare weakened the older cultures as a whole to such an extent that they could not maintain the ancient Indian art and science at their highest levels.

British Period

Ayurveda was being taught and practised in the old traditional way in the first two decades of the 19th century in Bengal. The British rulers did not bother about it as the East India Company employed its own English doctors and did not take care of the Indian health system. At best the Indians were employed as 'subordinate health-workers' in the British hospitals. Those Indians who had a certain skill in medical service were attached to regiments and civil stations under the name of 'Native doctors'. As the demand for the medical service increased, the 'Calcutta Native Medical Institution' was founded in 1822 under superintendants Jamison, Breton, and Tytler. Here a second class native doctor was brought up. In this way, the British rules tried to familiarize the indigenous population with western medical science out of personal utilitarian considerations. But till then they also tolerated the indigenous system of medicine. In the newly built Sanskrit College, which was opened in the year 1824, the introduction of Ayurvedic classes in 1827, took place so that from that time onwards for a shorter period both western medicine and Ayurveda were taught side by side in the same institution. Dr. Tytler was lecturing on European medicine while Indian professors were interpereting the classical texts of Ayurveda. But this friendly co-existence of European and Indian medicine did not last for a long time.

In 1935, under the advice of Lord Macaulay the Ayurvedic classes in the Sanskrit College were closed and a new medical college in Bengal was established with a view to declare the European medicine as the only acknowledged system of medical study. Two European professors of the Sanskrit College, Dr. Tytler and Dr. Jamison, tried in vain to prevent the government from undertaking this step by sending their famous Memorandum to the Educational Secretary of India. 'In the confrontation between the British orientalists, supporting the old Indian culture, and the Anglicists, who wished to supplant the indigenous tradition by the English culture, the Anglicist had been victorious'.

The British policy fortified this trend by granting free studentship and scholarship and by distributing free of cost medical training materials, such as books, charts, and models etc. Moreover, the students, who had chosen the European system of medicine were supported by the government. They could rejoice at the idea of having much better chances of getting a job and a good position in life. The students who passed successfully the final examination of the Medical College obtained certificates enrolled as 'Native Doctor'. They constituted the first class of 'Native Doctors', the second class having been the Indian students who passed through the Calcutta Native Medical Institution, and the third class were those who had got their training in the British Hospitals. In these decades, it seemed as if the allopathic medicine would be on the point of replacing fully the traditional Indian medicine. But in this crisis a much renowned Indian personality elevated the prestige of Ayurvedic medicine in Bengal.

It was Kaviraj Gangadhara Roy who exercised a great influence in the propagation of Ayurveda throughout the 19th century and also in the first two decades of the 20th century. He started medical practice as an Ayurvedic physician and opened a '*tol*' (medical school) for educating a great number of brilliant students coming from different parts of India. As a physician, Gangadhara acquired a legendary fame based specially upon his skill in the therapeutic use of medicine in diagnosis and in prognosis. In the field of Ayurvedic scholarship his commentary on *Carakasamhita*, named *Jalpakalpatar* was a unique contribution. Gangadhar Roy drew the attention of the common mass of India to the old traditional Indian medical system called Ayurveda and upheld its old prestige. In his 'Kaviraji tol' he nurtured the brilliant students of Ayurveda and sent them to different parts of Bengal and India.

A junior contemporary of Gangadhara Roy was Ganga Prasad Sen of Kumartulle, Calcutta. While Gangadhara Roy fought for the cause of Ayurveda outside Calcutta avoiding any direct confrontation with the allopathic medicine, Ganga Prasad Sen tried to compete with western medicines in the market. Kaviraj Sen edited Ayurvedic journals, produced Ayurvedic medicines at home, and sold them in the open market for public awareness.

From 1920 onwards, India passed through a phase of national awakening when the national movement against the foreign rule was set in motion and a tendency to be self sufficient in every field of national life came to the forefront. Keeping pace with this idea of national upliftment, many new schools, colleges and universities were opened and a galaxy of Ayurvedic scholars and practitioners came forward and brought a new spirit to usher in a Bengal Renaissance. Many committees such as Chopra Committee, Osman Committee etc., were formed to suggest ways and means for national improvement.

After independence in 1947, Government of India and state governments allotted funds for research in Ayurvedic medicine. State dispensaries and hospitals were opened in the districts to serve the poverty stricken ailing people. But inspite of this planning to boost the national health-care in India, nothing concrete came out of it.

In recent years a new trend is being noticed in different parts of the globe. In order to get rid of the dangerous maladies and to avoid the injurious side-effects of modern medicines, people in different parts of the globe are graduating towards 'herbal medicine' which is the new name of Ayurvedic herbal treatment.

Yogic postures (*asanas*) and breathing exercises in the form of *pranayama* are being taught in the schools of UK and in other parts of the globe. Chinese accupuncture, a modern developed version of the Sirabedha of Susruta, is giving relief to patients all over the world. But it is a pity that no concerted efforts are being noticed to reorganize the traditional medicine of Ayurveda in our country for thc time being.

References

1. *Atharvanir angirasor daivir manusyaja...........uta/ausadhyah prajayante yada tvam Prana jinvasi.* AV.XI.4.16
2. Why Ayurvedic medicine, originating from Veda, was called magico-religious is explained in the text of a young scholar: 'Much in Hinduism ultimately based on the ideas of the vedic period, the time of long migrations of Aryans (as the Indo-Iranians called themselves) to India and their settlement (in this country). The world attitude of this time seems to be, at least to a great extent, the so called magical one, in which the distiction between the religious and non-religious holy and unholy is meaningless'. Rahul Peter Das in 'Heilvorstellungen in der alt-indischen Medizin'.
3. Gods said, 'We will not invite you Ye(=Asvins) have wondered and mixed and mixed much among men, performing course'. SB.IV.5.14.
4. C.S.I.30,28; S.S.1.1.6; A.H.1.1.5; *Mahabharata* II. 5.16., II.25 and *Harivamsa*, Chap. 29.
5. *Kratukathadi-sutrant* at-thak/IV.2.60;
Kathadibhyasthak/IV.4.102.

13
Travails of Traditional Medicine

—*Subrata Pahari*

Before taking the plunge, two points should be cleared (i) what is traditional medicine? and (ii) what is the actual thrust of this paper?

According to some leading scholars (F. Kennett, R. Jalota, O. P. Jaggi *et. al.*) traditional medicine is a sort of antique treatment based on both supernatural and natural cure. It is deeply related to the culture, convictions, and the climate of a particular country and its creed. The ingredients of this system can easily be procured from that particular region where it emerged. The rudiments of this system have been handed over from generation to generation through both written and oral tradition.

Out of some growing needs, several systems of antique medicine originated in some ancient civilization i.e., Greek medicine, Chinese medicine, Egyptian medicine, and more certainly Indian traditional medicine. Amongst these, Indian traditional medicine is considered one of the oldest and compact systems of treatment. It is also believed that almost all of the said systems to some extent are highly indebted to Indian traditional medicine.[1]

Unlike other traditional systems, Indian traditional medicine does not mean any single system of cure. It consists of different types of supernatural, natural, empirical, and therapeutic system of cure i.e., ayurveda, unani, siddha, yoga, tantric and folk medicine, of which ayurveda is a more complete, compact, and multifarious system of scientific treatment. In this regard, a certain section of people like to consider that ayurveda (*astanga ayurveda*) is the genesis of all indigenous systems but as research progressed, its eight folds were transformed into eight separate systems of cure. But this view is not generally accepted. However, some western scholars like F.L. Dunn and D.C. Jarvis have classified these systems into some other stratum. According to their opinion, allopathy and homeopathy are entitled to 'cosmopolitan medicine', ayurveda, unani and yoga to 'regional medicine', and tantric and folk medicine to 'local medicine'.[2]

In this context, we have to remember that unani is basically a foreign system of treatment. It originated in Greece (Unan) and developed in the soil of Arab. So how is it included in Indian traditional medicine? In response, it may be said that basically unani is a combined system of treatment; it is a synthesis of almost all the frontline systems of antique medicine. But the fact is that, towards its origin and development, the contribution of traditional medicine (especially ayurveda) is immense. Since its introduction in India, it was assimilated with Indian indigenous medicines so deeply that it is very difficult to differentiate it from Indian medicine.[3] That is why, what has been practised in India as unani is now being called *unani tibb*. This interaction was made at least in four different ways:

1. Direct interaction between unani and traditional medicine in the soil of India.
2. Interaction between *kabirajas* and *hakeems* in the royal courts of Arabian rulers.
3. Interaction through the immigrant students who used to come to India for medical education.
4. Indirect interaction of Greek medicine and Egyptian medicine to which unani is highly indebted of which are also highly indebted to Indian traditional medicine.

For example, the use of cubeb, rocksalt, plantago ovator, aniseed, and, sparmint is what Indian physicians learnt from the *hakeems* and the *hakeems* learnt the use of ginger, camphor, cinnamon and lac from Indian *vaidc* and *kavirajas* Besides these, some Arabic and Persian medical texts like *Samrud*, *Sarak* and *Badan* were translated from the Indian texts of Susrut, Charak and Nidan respectively. That is why, certain sections of people prefer to consider unani as the facsimile of ayurveda.[4]

Regarding the thrust of this paper, it can be said that Indian traditional medicine has a hoary antiquity. It assumes a chequered character through the vicissitudes of history. Since its inception in remote past, it has remained an indispensable part of the Indian system of cure. Even today, it is being practised with great persistence and zeal. But its prolonged journey was not so easy and comfortable. It had to go through various ups and downs. Some internal and external hurdles made its journey very tedious and troublesome. Finally, it succeeded in crossing over the hurdles. Here, at first, we would like to know, what were the travails of this system and then, under such adverse condition, while most of the antique medicines of the world became obsolete, how Indian indigenous medicine is able to retain its glory.

In this paper, the travails of traditional medicine are examined in three separate sections (a) pre-British period: 3500 BC–AD 1757 (b) British period: AD 1757–AD 1947 and (c) post British period: 1947 onwards and the mystery of its success is disclosed in the last phase of this paper.

(A) Pre-British Period: 3500 BC–AD 1757

There is no doubt that traditional medicine is one of the oldest and most compact medical systems in the world. It has had different branches i.e., ayurveda, yoga, siddha, tantric, and folk medicine. At the very outset, there was no compact medical system in our country. People used to administer various herbals, metals, and animals as medicine in order to cure their diseases. As the time progressed, they indulged themselves into deep medical research. As a result various superficial and empirical systems emerged. The unearthed Indus plates, the remains (neem, sea fish and the bone dust of deers and rhinos) of Harappa, and the bored skulls discovered from Bhurjaham (in Kashmir) can help a lot to assume the nature and feature of the primitive system of Indian medicine.[5]

The superficial concepts of pre-Vedic medicine developed some rudimentary forms towards the end of the Vedic period and by then, it was divided into four separate disciplines (supernatural, natural, empirical, and therapeutic). However, concerned experiments and researches were going on. The scholars and the rulers of that time extended their support to the same. As a result of the joint venture, the *astanga ayurveda* (eight fold ayurveda) emerged during the classical period (1000–800 BC) of Indian history. The followers of ayurveda tended to believe that ayurveda (science of life) is the mother of all prevailing Indian systems. But the unearthed Indus plates and the Vedic literature (*Rig Veda* and *Atharva Veda*) strongly indicate that at least yoga and folk medicine are older than ayurveda. But it is quite right that siddha or *rasatantra* is an indispensable part of ayurveda whereas tantric medicine is the synthesis of ayurveda, yoga, and folk medicine.[6] The practitioners of this system prefer to use minerals and metals, or in other words, alchemy rather than herbals. At present, these systems are very popular in south India.

Travails came first just after the inception of ayurveda or more accurately, after the innovation of *Rasayana* or alchemy (chemical, minerals and metals). The discrimination of its users and practitioners made the situation very grim and complicated. Anyway, the travails which it had to face during the pre-British period, may be classified into the following:

(a) Discrimination of its users and practitioners,

(b) Unequal development of its different branches,

(c) Effects of the Buddhist injunction and customs,

(d) Influence of the Muslim invasions,

(e) Advent of some foreign medicines (unani, allopathy, and homoeopathy.

Usually, the men of high profile preferred ayurveda and siddha; those from the religious and spiritual world were very much fond of yoga and tantra, while the commoners used to favour folk medicine. So, each section had tried to develop its respective systems. But in this process, only ayurveda developed considerably. This uneven progress upset its practitioners so immensely that they began to look down upon other indigenous systems. Not only so, this incident also created an unprecedented interdisciplinary conflict among the practitioners of ayurveda. Since the days of the *Atharvaveda* and *Kaushikasutra*, the alchemy section of ayurvedic medicine made immense progress, especially the discovery of *parada kajjali* (sulphurate of mercury) by the great Nagarjuna which ushered in a new era in the history of Indian alchemy. This epoch making discovery influenced the alchemists so strongly that they started claiming *rasatantra* or siddha as an independent system of treatment. Consequently the practitioners of ayurveda were divided into two separate groups *Banausadhi Sampradaya* (herbalist) and *Rasausadhi Sampradaya* (alchemists). This unhealthy competition lasted till the sixteenth century. It ended with the publication of the *Rasajalnidhi* (an ayurvedic text) by Kaviraj Gopal Krishna Bhattacharya. In Bengal it lasted till the end of the end of the nineteenth century.[7] In this context, we must say, if the rhythm of combined research continued, Indian alchemy as well as Indian ayurvedic pharmacology would have reached dizzy heights. Unfortunately, it did not happen.

The influence of the Hindu and the Buddhist injunctions and customs over traditional medicine was immense. It had highly affected the origin and development of Hindu surgery. This pernicious symptom was first traced at the time of the *Yajurveda*, because it declared '*visaka apabitra*' i.e., physicians are impure.[8] Then Lord Buddha's cult of non-violence added to it a new dimension. By this process, Manu, the famous orator of the Hindu Sastra, proclaimed, *chikitsakan debalakan barjashu habyakabbyayo* i.e., physicians and washermen have no right to participate in any auspicious occasion of the Hindus.[9] As a matter of fact, the *vaids* and *kabirajas* who used to enjoy the most respectable place in our society (as second god), with this injunction, gradually descended from their earlier positions. For this reason, Dhundhukanath (famous Buddhist Sahajia) was forced to pray for a panacea (chemicals), which could be used as an alternative form of surgery.[10] So the surgery section of the traditional medicine was gradually undermined and this also created a big gulf between Indian and western surgery in near future.

The travails of traditional medicine were intensified with the invasion of the Muslims. Their rampant attacks on the citadels of the Hindus and Buddhist academic institutions caused an irrecoverable loss to the legacy of traditional medicine. Moreover, they brought unani with them. Naturally, their patrons promoted unani in place of traditional medicine. It was no doubt a direct blow to indigenous medicine. But this indiscrimination did not last long, because within a short while they came to know that unani was not sufficient enough to serve their purpose, and even their subjects were also very fond of traditional medicine. So they willy-nilly extended their support for the promotion of traditional medicine.

There has been some controversy regarding the attitude of Muslim rulers towards traditional medicine. R. N. Chopra expressed the view that with the advent of Muslim conquerors, the decline was more rapid.[11] But A. L. Basham is of the opinion that there is no record of such animosity in the field of medicine.[12] However, the history of Indian medicine stands witness to how traditional medicine became the victim of passive negligence of Muslim rulers[13] during the reign of the sultans, especially during the time of Firoz Tughlaq (1351–1388). In contrast, the Mughal rulers were quite cordial in this matter.[14] Most of the translations of Indian medical texts were possible during this period. Some Hindu *vaids* and *kavirajas* were appointed as court physician in the Mughal court. However, some regional or local rulers had already started this tradition long before the Mughals. In this regard, Nawab Hussain Shah of Bengal (1493–1519) deserves special mention. Kabiraj Mukunda Das was his court physician.[15]

The pangs of traditional medicine was to reach its zenith with the advent of western medicine. Since the days of Akbar (1556–1605), some European doctors got appointments in the Mughal as well as some local courts. They succeeded in winning the faith and conviction of some Indian kings and chiefs by curing some complicated cases. For example, Dr. Gabriel Boughton cured successfully the third degree burns case of the daughter of Shajahan.[16] Thenceforth, they were easily appointed in almost all Indian royal and local courts. Not only so, some well-to-do families at that time also appointed European doctors to act as their house physician. So Indian traditional medicine as well as unani were to face another period of acute crisis.

In this connection, it may be cited that though the larger section of Indian people were fond of *ayurveda* and *yoga*, they did not hesitate to take the help of other prevailing systems when their first choice failed. For example, Great Ashoka (273–232 BC), Sasanka (AD–606 637), Lakshman Sena (AD–1179 1205), Nawab Hussian Shah (AD–1493 1519) and Mirjafar (AD–1757 60)[17] were notable among the recipients of folk and tantric medicine. But they did nothing for the cause of these systems. If they did so, we would have these systems in some other advanced and sophisticated form. Anyway, according to the chronology of Indian history, the pre-British period is divided into two sections ancient and medieval. If it is justified, it may be said that the real development of traditional medicine was made during the first half of the modern period and the second half remained almost barren in respect of medical experiment and research.[18]

(B) British Period: AD 1757–AD 1947

Another mighty blow came upon this system during the days of the Company's rule. The trouble of traditional medicine reached its zenith in this period. These can be classified into four separate sections:

1. The hostility of the colonial government as well as the patrons of allopathy,
2. The impact of some epoch-making discoveries on traditional medicine,
3. Interdisciplinary conflict between the practitioners of ayurveda,
4. The monopoly drug trade of the Company.

The famous Portuguese ruler Garcia-de-Orta was the harbinger of such repression. He was the first ever European who directly issued an ordinance declaring that the Christians of his kingdom would no longer be able to consult any indigenous or local physician for their treatment.[19] But this ordinance was not very effective because his subjects could not confine themselves only to western medicine during the epidemic and endemic-stricken days.[20]

In Bengal, the situation was quite different because, from the very beginning, the Company had no such reservations. They were totally indifferent to matters of health, disease, and medicine. They used to suggest to their officials to consult with the local medicine men, if needed.[21] But within a decade, the whole situation changed dramatically. In fact, three vital factors were responsible for this changing scenario—

(a) the devastating outbreak of cholera, malaria, *kala-azar,* and small-pox, (b) the growing demand for western medicine and (c) failure of traditional medicine in curing some lethal diseases.

The main constraint which lay behind the Company's confusion in taking any clear-cut decision in this respect, was the age-old conflict between the Anglicists and the Orientalists. It confused the Company so much that they were forced to promote both western and Indian medicine.[22]

Surprisingly, this situation changed rapidly. Since 1820, the Company assumed the paramount power of this country. Allopathy became very sophisticated by virtue of some epoch-making discoveries, and above all the age-old Anglicist and Orientalist controversy was solved in favour of the Anglicans. Considering the whole situation, Lord Bentinck (AD–1829 35), a staunch follower of utilitarianism, declared in 1835, 'medical class of the Sanskrit college and the medical class of the Calcutta Madrassa would be abolished from 1st February and a new institution (Calcutta Medical College) would be formed under the supervision of the GCPI (General Committee of Public Instruction)'.[23] It was undoubtedly a tremendous blow to the legacy and the prospect of traditional medicine. The glaring possibility of the development of traditional medicine with the help of state patronage which had peeped since 1813, was nipped in the bud. This comprehension became true with the motivated firing by the Company from Fort William to encourage Pandit Mudhusudan Gupta who dissected a human corpse in the laboratory of Calcutta Medical College in 1836.[24] Since then, the Company and the followers of allopathy joined hands to abolish the practice of traditional medicine. In this regard, they adopted four measures:

(a) They appointed some scholars (both Indian and European) to collect the name of indigenous herbs for the British Pharmacopoeia,

(b) Policy of not offering any registration and recommendation to any indigenous medical institutions,

(c) Establishment of the Company's absolute monopoly over the Indian drugs and trade,

(d) Enactment of Poison Act (1914) to perish its practice.

Though the Company abolished the medical classes in the Calcutta Madrassa and the Sanskrit College in 1835, they could not ignore the merits of the indigenous medicinal plants. So they appointed some poor scholars and *kavirajas* to rob the same for the British Pharmacopoeia. They also started some sort of double profitable trade of indigenous herbs and plants. At first, they used to purchase some indigenous herbs

(*Kuchila*) at a very nominal rate (50,000 maund *Kuchila* for Rs. 3,200 only) for the European factories, and those (Strychnine) used to be sold in Indian market at a very high (Rs. 1,12,000) market price.[25] In order to establish their absolute monopoly over Indian drug market, the Company enacted the Poison Act, in 1914. Some *vaids* and *kavirajas* were arrested on the charge of preparing poisonous drugs until the outbreak of the First World War in 1914, which obstructed much in the fulfilment of their purpose.

Besides these measures, the Company decided not to spend a single penny for the cause of traditional medicine. Whenever they were requested for the same, they either made some lame excuse of the paucity of fund or they intentionally criticized the system as 'unscientific'[26] to avoid their responsibility. Even, the frequent requests for offering registration and affiliation for some ayurvedic and unani medical institutions, schools, and colleges were also drastically turned down in a very abrupt manner.

Apart from these, some epoch-making developments and discoveries like the anatomy (1316), chemotherapy (1493–1541), blood transfusion theory (1625), blood circulation theory (1628), germ theory (1683), physiology (1757–1766), vaccination (1796), penicillin (1928) were sufficient enough to drive traditional medicine back to the rat race. By these discoveries, it was proved that the age-long humoral theory of ayurveda and unani and the supernatural and natural causes of folk and tantric medicine are not all behind the sufferings of human beings. Moreover, the discovery that some contagious diseases like cholera, malaria, small-pox, and *kala-azar* are caused by some infection of various malignant microbes, like *Vibrio cholerae* for cholera, *Plasmodium falciparum* for malaria, *Variola virus* for small-pox, *Leishmania donovani* for *kala-azar*, cast doubt over the practice of traditional medicine during the second half of the nineteenth century.

But it is a matter of great pleasure that, in spite of all hostilities, they could not uproot this system permanently. In fact, their hostilities turned into a blessing in disguise. Because, it charged the followers of ayurveda and unani so much that, soon after the declaration of 1835, they became very active and worked towards regaining their glory. Acharya Gangadhar Roy and Kaviraj Gangaprasad Sen *et.al.* on behalf of ayurveda and Hakim Ajmal Khan, Abdul Majid Khan and Rahim Khan on behalf of unani took the charge of survival and revival of traditional medicine. By virtue of their organized campaign, each and every sphere (education, practice, publication, and research) of traditional medicine was highly enriched. This remarkable chapter of development has been demarcated as 'the renaissance of traditional medicine' in the medical history of India.

Contextually, it must be said that the revivalist trend that we easily notice in case of ayurveda and unani, is not visible in case of yoga and folk medicine. Because nobody bothered about these systems till the end of the nineteenth century. At least, the historical census of 1872 opened up a new vista for folk medicine. The Calcutta University opened a separate department on Anthropology in the year 1920 under the aegis of Sir Asutosh Mukhopadhyay, the then Vice-Chancellor. The Anthropological Survey of India was established in 1945 in order to conduct deep research on the life and culture of Indian aborigines. The Asiatic Society, the then one and only citadel of oriental learning, also extended its support for the same. Apart from these, some freelance European researchers took the initiatives in this discipline. Amongst them, E.T. Dalton's *Tribal History for Eastern India* (1872), Rev. P.O. Bodding's *Santhal Medicine* (1925), and M. Mc. Alpin's *Conditions of the Santhals* (1909) deserve special mention. However, the worldwide interest can be traced from 1970s; since then, it has been cultivated by the name of 'folk medicine', 'tribal medicine', and 'ethno-medicine' with great persistence and zeal.

Similarly, very little initiative had been taken in favour of the yogic medicine till the end of the nineteenth century. Only some *sahajias* and sufis showed their personal interest in this natural system of cure before the establishment of the Company's rule. Due to their initiatives, *Amrita Kunda* (a famous yogic medical text) was translated into Arabic and Persian. Swami Dayananda Saraswati in Punjab and Swami Bijoy Krishna Goswami in Bengal made some nominal experiment in this discipline. But as the virulent side effects of some western drugs caused major harm to Indian public health, the people of this country turned towards it. Since then, they started to concentrate on this system. As a result, several yoga clubs and clinics were established. The Council of Secondary and Higher Secondary Education also included it in their syllabus on school education. Several western countries have also shown huge interest in this respect. At present, they are conducting some experiment and research on the same in outer space. In a word, yoga has become the focal point of todays' doctor's and scientists' interest.

(C) Post-British Period (1947 onwards)

It was hoped that the travails of traditional medicine would reduce after the assumption of independence, because the fellow Indians would put proper emphasis on this indigenous system. But it did not happen expectedly. So troubles are going on. The troubles of this period may be categorized into four special groups:

(a) Inter disciplinary conflict of the indigenous medicine men,

(b) Influence of state faculty of Bengal (1937) on the practice of this system

(c) Piracy of western druggists,

(d) Apathy of our present generation.

The heyday of ayurveda was very short-lived. It suffered a serious set back in the first half of the twentieth century. The patrons of this system were divided into two separate groups—*shuddhapanthi* and *mishrapanthi*. The *mishrapanthi* were in favour of taking help of modern medical technology but their opponent (*shuddhapanthi*) did not think so. Kaviraj Bijoy Ratna Sen, Gananath Sen, and Jamini Bhusan Roy belonged to the *mishrapanthi* group and Kaviraj Shyamadas Tarkachuramani, Kj. Pravakar Chottopadhyay, and Kj. Bimalananda Tarakatirta were very much in favour of traditional Vedic line.[27]

This difference of opinion was gradually transformed into a professional and institutional controversy. The institutional generally belonged to some non-medical families and learnt medicine from any registered medical institution. On the other hand, the professionals have had purely hereditary medical tradition. So they do not like to disclose the unwritten rudimentaries before any institution. According to them, it is god gifted. So it is not for general practitioners.[28] Similarly, the institutions very often underestimate the professionals for not having any proper education in physiology, germ theory, and highly sophisticated modern medical technology. This unhealthy competition is still going on. There is no sign of mutual understanding. For this reason, R. C. Majumdar (veteran historian) lamented, 'It was an intriguing problem of which no easy or immediate solution seems to be at hand'.[29]

The establishment of the state faculty of Ayurveda and Unani (1937) also gave it a new dimension. According to its declaration, any body who intended to practise these systems would be able to get registration only by producing a letter of recommendation from any registered practitioner and by paying Rs. 10/- only. This relaxation opened up a golden chance before the opportunist quacks. Veteran Kaviraj Prabhakar Chattopadhyay and many others strongly criticized this regulation. They maintained that the Faculty indirectly helped produce thousands of upstart quacks.[30] The Government of Independent India was also carefully apprised about the future of traditional medicine. They very often sanctioned more grant for the cultivation of western medicine in comparison to indigenous medicine. Their apathy stands as a serious constraint to the development of traditional medicine. For example, on one occasion, on being requested, one of our cabinet ministers said, '*taka kari kharach na kare kichu kara jay kina dekhchhi*' i.e., he will do something for this purpose without spending a penny.[31] But, even young children know very well that mere fair words cannot fill the pocket. This apathy is still very much in action, though the present government is very vocal morally but does nothing in practical. Along with our government, our present generation also is very cynical about this system. They consider this system as antique and empirical, so in their opinion, it may be used as an alternative but not as a frontline system of medicine. Naturally, this apathy offers a golden chance to the drug pirates of the west. Earlier, they unjustly included the names and the merits of different Indian herbs and medical plants in the British Pharmacopoeia, then they started their double profitable monopoly drug trade. At present, they are directly claiming the patents of some important drugs and herbs like neem (*Azadirachta indica*), ginger (*Zingiber officinale*), turmeric (*Curcumalonga*), aniseed (*Pimpinella Anisum*) and even the *bastusastra* (Ancient Indian Sculpture) of India as their own. If the Government of India does not become careful at the right time, we will lose the patents of other important herbs and drugs in near future. We are also afraid that if this process goes on, they even can claim the *astanga ayurveda* as their own.

(D) Innate Limitations

Despite some external hazards, traditional medicine has some innate limitations, which have remained partly responsible for its ongoing travails;

(a) The studies of surgery and physiology is not still up to the mark; these areas are to be developed,

(b) It has no provision of emergent cure, so the patients who require the same are forced to consult western medicine,

(c) Germ theory and pathology still remain very neglected areas in this system,

(d) Some important medical texts on these systems are yet to be recovered and still to be interpreted,

(e) The patrons of this system still believe that it is god gifted, it needs no rectification. This obstinacy must be given up.

Mystery of Success

In spite of all these limitations, it has had some inherent merits which remain ever helpful in overcoming its ongoing hurdles.

(i) It is very cheap and easily procurable. So it can give better security than others in the days of acute medicinal crisis.

(ii) It is highly suitable for the culture, climate, conviction, and the food habits of this country. As western medicine is suitable for the non-vegetarians of the cold countries, similarly it is suitable for the vegetarians of tropical countries like India.

(iii) It has no harmful side effects. It is an accomplished fact that the WHO (World Health Organization) has been banning regularly some western drugs for their dangerous side effects, but traditional medicine is free from such evils.

(iv) Its medicinal merits are immense. It is curative not preventive. Several chronic diseases like asthma, dysentery, rheumatism, and some haematological problems which at present are being considered almost incurable, can easily be cured by the indigenous medicines.

(v) Not only so, at present, some indigenous medicine men are claiming that some deadly diseases like tuberculosis, cancer, and AIDS can be cured by indigenous drugs. So it should be examined seriously.

Conclusion

In conclusion, we may say that since the remote past, traditional medicine, by virtue of its inherent merits succeeded in retaining its age-long glory and popularity. About 70 per cent of Indian people are still dependent on this system. So the time has come for putting adequate emphasis on this system especially on the efficacy of folk medicine. Because of our cynical attitude, it still remains an uncharted terrain. As the inclemency rate of virulent diseases over the aborigines is very low, we should take more initiative to verify the knowledge of the *Atharvaveda*, *Palakapya*, *Garurapurana* as well as the rudimentaries of folk medicine which have been handed over from generation to generation.

Another ominous symptom which can at present be noticed is that, influenced by the present western media, a section of Indian people prefers to call it 'alternative medicine' and in their opinion, it should not be included in the realm of frontline modern medicine. But the concerned statistics shows that about 70 per cent of Indian people are still dependent on traditional medicine and about 60 per cent area of this country is yet to be charted by modern medicine. Under such conditions if traditional medicine is considered 'alternative' then, barring English language, Christian religion, and allopathy, each and every thing in the world should be regarded as an alternative. In this context, it can be said that if it is done, then not only our traditional medicine but our traditional culture also will lose its self-identity in the near future. So it would be better to keep open all the prevailing avenues, so that one can try another, if their first choice fails.

Lastly, it is an accomplished truth that despite high techno-medical progress, modern medicine is still helpless before some deadly and so-called incurable diseases. By virtue of its highly sophisticated technology, it can only detect the nature and feature of the diseases but is still not capable of curing them. So the time has come for conducting exclusive research on these traditional systems. The panacea may be found out in this way. The proper slogan of the day should be please revive, rectify and restore it, do not try to abolish.

References

1. H. E. Sigerist, *A History of Medicine*, vol. II, New York, 1961. passim, R. C. Majumdar, 'Medicine' in *A Concise History of Science*, New Delhi, 1971, pp. 262-264.
2. D. C. Jarvis, *Folk Medicine*, London, 1960, p. 11; F.L. Dunn in *Asian Medical Systems* (ed.) by Charles Leslie, 1977, see relevant portion.
3. M. Z. Siddiqi, 'The Unani Tibb' in *A Concise History of Science*, *op. cit.*; Rudrendra Kr. Paul, 'Unani', vide *Bharat Kosh*, (in Bengali), vol. I, 1371 BS, Calcutta, pp. 443-35.
4. M. S. Siddiqi, *Studies in Arabic and Persian Literature*, Calcutta, 1956, p. 19; A. Wahid and H. H. Siddiqi, *Survey of Drugs*, Delhi, 1961, p. 10; Panchanan Neogi, *Ayurveda O Nabyarasayana* (in Bengali), Calcutta, 1314 BS, pp. 31-32.
5. *Report of the Drug Inquiry Commission,* Government of India 1964, p. 20; Asoke Kr. Bagchi, *Snayu Slayasastrer Bibartan O Snayumandaler Arbud Rog* (in Bengali), Calcutta, 1986, picture 2(a). The Vedic Age see Bharatiya Vidya Bhavan Series, Bombay, 1988, p. 181.
6. R. C. Majumdar, *op. cit.*, p. 233; B. C. Jana, 'Indigenous Systems and Indian System of Medicine', vide Annual Magazine of J. B. Roy Ayurveda Medical College and Hospital, 1991–1992, p. 4.
7. Prabhakar Chattopadhyay, *Hindu Rasayan Sastrer Itihas* (in Bengali), 1958, Calcutta, p. 188; P. C. Ray, *History of Hindu Chemistry*, vol. II, Calcutta, 1925, pp. 8-27.
8. Bijan Bihari Goswami (translated), *Yajurveda Samhita*, Calcutta, 1975.
9. Gopal Batabyal (translated), *Manusamhita*, Calcutta, 1384 BS, pp. 225-440.
10. Dhundhuknath, Rasendra Chintamani, vide *Ayurbeda Bharati*, vol. 2-4, 1370 BS, p. 57.
11. R. N. Chopra, *Indigenous Drugs in India*, Calcutta, 1933, p. 5.
12. A. L. Basham, 'Practice of Medicine in Ancient and Medieval India', vide *Asian Medical Systems*, *op. cit.*, p. 40.
13. R. C. Majumdar, *op. cit.*, pp. 266–64.

14. M. Z. Siddiqi, *op. cit.*, pp. 266 - 273; Asoke Kr. Bagchi, *op. cit.*, pp. 40- 43.
15. Abdul Karim, *Banglar Itihas* (Sultanate Period in Bengal), Dacca, 1977, p. 517.
16. William Irvine, *Later Mughals*, New Delhi, 1971, pp. 305-306.
17. Subrata Pahari, *Unish Shataker Banglay Sanatani Chikitsar Swarup* (in Bengali), Calcutta, 1997, pp. 31-32.
18. *Ibid.*
19. P. D. Gaitonde, *Portuguese Pioneers in India*, Bombay, 1983, p. 151.
20. David Arnold, 'Cholera and Colonialism in British India' in *Past and Present*, November 1986, p. 127; P. Hehir, *The Medical Profession in India*, London, 1923, pp. 2, 9.
21. O. P. Jaggi, *Public Health and Its Administration*, vol. 14, Delhi, p. 71.
22. Brajendranath Bandyopadhyay, *Kolkata Sanskrita Kaleger Itihas*, Calcutta, 1824–1858, p. 35.
23. H. Sharp, *Selection from Educational Records, 1781–1839*, part I, Calcutta, 1920, p. 24.
24. Debiprasad Chattopadhyay, 'Prachin Bharate Shalya Chikitsa O Vijnan' vide *Maulabad O Vijnan* (in Bengali), Calcutta, 1993, p. 2; W. C. B. Eatwell, *Rise and Progress of Rational Medical Education*, Calcutta, 1860, p. 21.
25. Asima Chattopadhayay, *Bharater Banausadhi* (in Bengali), 1353 BS, Calcutta, pp. 43-44.
26. *Ayurveda Sanjibani* (a medical journal in Bengali), vol. I, pp. 42, 43, *Anubikshan* (a medical journal in Bengali), vol. VI, p. 384.
27. *Ayurveda Bharati* (in Bengali), no. 2–4, 1270, Calcutta, pp. 60-70.
28. R. C. Majumdar, *op. cit.*
29. Prabhakar Chattopadhayay, *Adhunik Roger Ayurveda Chikitsa* (in Bengali), Calcutta, p. 13.
30. *Ayurveda Bijnan Sammilani* (a medical journal in Bengali), vol. VI, 1328 BS, p. 222.
31. UNI, New Delhi, 25th July 1999, vide *Bartaman* (a Bengali Daily News Paper). 25.6.1999.

Gender and Health

14

Indigenous Approach to Delivery Deaths in Colonial Bengal

—*Mousumi Bandyopadhyay*

Infantile and maternal mortality were something to which we were quite habituated for a very long time. Under the British empire, there was a conscious effort on its behalf to solve this problem. But this backfired and the results were quite counterproductive. Several discussions and seminars have been organized and there have also been a number of publications on western intervention and its impact. But seldom has there been a thought on how the indigenous approach could challenge the faulty imperial policy. My analysis would be a humble step in that direction.

I

There was an advancement in medical science in nineteenth century England, and as a British colony, in India they adopted a number of steps to introduce modern advanced medical technology, the immediate result of which was the creation of a class of native doctors trained in western scientific education. Inspite of this advancement, the early British critics of Hindu and Muslim treatment of women paid no attention to the issue of medical care for women for a long time. The doors of the medical colleges in India were closed to the women who wanted to study medicine also for a long time. As the male doctors were strictly forbidden to enter into the *antahpur*, the women were entirely dependent on the *dhais* for childbirth. In most cases they died due to improper or wrong treatment. The mortality rate of both child and mother was very high. In many cases, the absence of basic scientific knowledge, cleanliness, and the sense of hygiene led to the death of the mother and the child. The blame for high infant and maternal mortality was mainly laid on incompetent *dhais* and poor hygienic condition in the *aturghars*, where the birth took place. It was the smallest, darkest room in the house where the mother was left in the care of the *dhai*. Following delivery the midwife placed the mother on a strict diet, denying her cold water or cooling drinks even in the hottest months. Contemporary newspapers, journals and periodicals vividly depicted the picture of such condition. From the Census of India we also get a more or less similar picture:

> The character of the room depends on the means and the enlightenment of the family, but generally it is one of the worst rooms in the house, or a shed is erected outside the compound. Among the poorer classes, the woman's accomodation is wretched. A portion of one of the living rooms may be screened off, or she may have to use the *verandah*; some doctors even state that the cowshed or kitchen is occassionally used. As a rule, when a separate room is assigned, it is small, dark and ill-ventilated.[1]

A midwife, usually a woman of the Dom or Bagdi caste, attended the mother during and after childbirth. During delivery those midwives sometimes interfered with natural labour in a way that could jeopardize the health of both mother and child. The clever ones among the *dhais* accumulated certain amount of expertise either from their predecessors or from their own experience. But they had no idea of the mechanism of labour, nor of the in-built forces which delivered the child. She used crude, artificial force to induce delivery often with disastrous results. Available data suggests that the infantile and maternal mortality rate was considerably higher in Bengal than in England. During the decade ending 1885, the infant mortality rate in England was 142 per 1000.[2] During the first two decades of the 20th century in Bengal, one in five babies died before their first birthday.[3] In 1921, infant mortality rates were still on the increase and were, even among the *bhadralok*, double the corresponding proportions in European countries.[4] British critics focused on the prevalent practice of child marriage and consummation immediately after puberty as other reasons behind the high maternal and infant mortality in Bengal.[5]

Western observers in the early 20th century focused on the poor standards of traditional Indian midwifery. In 1901, the editors of the census commissioned a special enquiry into the methods adopted by indigenous midwives. Inspite of that, the introduction of the training programme for midwives was not undertaken on a large scale, until the establishment of the Victoria Memorial Scholarship Fund in 1903 which was an attempt to combine practical experience and scientific knowledge of the midwives. The general object of improving the treatment of childbirth in India could be approached on two lines:[6] (1) to train up midwives of a superior class and (2) to endeavour to impart a certain amount of practical knowledge to the indigenous midwives. The work of the fund bore results. The resistance of the *dhais* gradually broke down. They became accustomed to western methods to some extent and did not hesitate to call in the trained medical women if the case was complicated. However, taking the country as a whole, the response to the effort to train the *dhais* was rather meagre. It is true that some centres reported good and successful work, but the others had to admit failure because the experimens were tried chiefly in towns, large or small, where there were medical women willing to give them a trial and do the teaching work. The villages were left practically untouched. This was quite natural because women doctors were not found in the villages and *dhais* could not travel to the town for a lesson that involved time and money. The second difficulty was that only a very small percentage of Indian women were then able to read and write and all the reports state that the general ignorance of the women who attended the classes in various parts of the country was the main stumbling block. Finally, the most important factor was that courses of instruction were offered only in English and they were presented in a regular classroom format. This indeed made it nearly impossible for an adult woman with a midwifery practice to attend all the lectures and complete the assignments. It was for these reasons, where traditional *dhais* were enticed to begin training schemes, their dropout rate was close to hundred per cent.

Under such critical circumstances it became necessary to inculcate a sense of awareness among women, so that they could realize and identify their own problems. As the institutional efforts turned out to be quite futile, the role of society assumed greater significance.

II

We find that as early as in 1875, the first of a continuing stream of mother and childcare manuals like *Sishupalan* by Shib Chunder Deb, claimed that the 'ignorance on the part of Hindu families of the proper management of infants, and the great mortality that arises from the cause' compelled him to write the book.[7] This work and those that followed it, recommended reforms and imparted knowledge of the need and means for improvement known to the *bhadramahila*. Progressive *bhadralok* husbands also started taking a keen interest in the well-being of their wives. The *bhadramahilas* were encouraged to take up midwifery themselves. In 1867, the *Bamabodhini Patrika* published a series of detailed and informative articles on midwifery, covering pregnancy — its symptoms and treatment and delivery.[8] *Bamabodhini Patrika* had articles on childcare. In it was published numerous articles on the divinity of motherhood and on the essentials of bringing up a child. As a prelude to the upbringing of a child, stress was laid on care during childbirth.

Bamabodhini Patrika had published many exhaustive articles on the norms to be followed during pregnancy and the safety precautions during childbirth. There were also separate discussions on what a pregnant woman should wear, what food habits she should develop, permissible working limits, and what state of mind she should remain. It was stated that pregnant women should wear loose-fitting clothes and should have light but nutritious food. Regarding permissible work limits, an example was cited stating that rich and poor women suffered during childbirth, not the middle class women. That means, sitting totally idle is not correct and overworking is also not advisable. It was stated that a cheerful disposition and reading of holy scripts and moral sciences was advisable.[9]

In this connection the different symptoms of pregnancy were also described. Among them nausea, salivation, lactation, enlargement of belly, growth of the foetus, and changes in the uterus were vividly dealt upon.[10] From the time of conception to delivery, detailed discussion was made for all the stages. Labour pain,[11] general symptoms for delivery, and at each stage the role of the *dhai* and the parturient women were all discussed. How the oilcloth is to be placed under the abdomen of the mother, how the uterus is to be tested[12] were all the subjects of the *dhai*. From the second half of the 19th century it was felt that all women should know about this subject so that before calling the *dhai* they can take necessary precaution.

During childbirth, the *dhais* took recourse to age-old traditions and even if complications cropped up, their actions and steps were not always in line with th advancement of science in the 19th century. The aspects on which the *dhais* had no know-how were sometimes brought up in scientific discussion like, for instance, caesarian delivery or unnatural delivery, removal of placenta[13] and so on. On perusal of this article, one can actually see how the scientific thought started entering the educated Bengali society. In *Bamabodhini,* the *dhais* were instructed to carry a surgical knife, a pair of scissors, female catheter, stethoscope, and a silk thread on going for a call.[14]

From this we get a panoramic view of the changing attitudes during the last half of the 19th century. That these subjects are suitable for the reading of women and that there should not be any inhibitions during the discussion of them were by and large realized by most of the people, barring a few exceptions. *Bamabodhini* clearly stated that during pregnancy a lot of harm and mishaps of the mother were caused by superstitions and ignorance, hence the mother had to be conscious of her norms during pregnancy.[15] This sort of an outlook would not have been possible without some scientific thought. Mothers took notice of new information in so far as they could. The changes reflected desire on the part of educated Bengalis to derive benefit from modern scientific knowledge and a growing humanitarian concern for the welfare of both the mother and the child. The quackery of the untrained midwives gradually brought awareness to the enlightened section of the Bengali society and everyone admitted that some sort of education and training should have been imparted to the *dhais*. A very well-known journal of the time, *The Calcutta Journal of Medicine* edited by Mahendralal Sarkar, noted:

> Females, especially widows, when they unfortunately become the victims of disease, hardly meet with any sympathy and attention unless or until the disease reaches a height when indifference is culpable in the extreme. The greatest cruelty is shown during confinement. At time when the utmost possible care and attention is necessary, the parturient female is confined to a place in the house having no hygienic recommendations whatever, and hardly better than a dungeon.[16]

The same periodical further states,

> It is most lamentable to think how many parturient females, for want of timely and proper aid, are, with children in their wombs, falling into the grasp of death; how many children die before seeing the light or are born only to die, and how many mothers, escaping for the time being from the effects of avoidable accidents or diseases become afterwards bedridden for life.[17]

The housewives no doubt had a responsibility to look after the management of the *sutikagriha* and to monitor the working of the *dhais*. Unfortunately, due to lack of proper education, especially scientific education, they were as ignorant as the untrained midwives. But what is noteworthy is that gradually the women themselves were becoming conscious on this subject, and very often a few articles were published in the contemporary periodicals where the women themselves wrote about their role in case of childbirth. They wrote, 'The facilities of the *aturghar* should be supervised by the other ladies of the house. The *dhai* attends the mother and the child but not with sufficient care and attention. On superstitious grouds other family members stay away from the *aturghar*. They should be reminded that the mother and the child are at considerable risk while under the supervision of an illiterate *dhai*. Particularly during this time it is the duty of other members of the households to stay with the mother and the child and take proper care of them.'[18]

As a matter of fact, our country had a significant process of curing patients that is the process of community healing. The watch word of imperial medicine was segregation. It was concerned with the etiology of diseases and the human body as a machine of many parts to be sectionally repaired. But traditional medicine and medical care depended on community healing and family care. The patient and, in case of childbirth, the mother was treated in body and mind in her presonalized circumstances. No doubt, the total perception of the patient as a human being, a member of the family and community, and having an interactive mind is important in effecting a cure.[19] It was for this reason that the *aturghars* were made at the side of the dwelling houses and the mothers were not sent to the hospitals for delivery and subsequent nursing. So when due to the observances of unnecessary and superstitious rituals and customs, the mother was segragated for a long period, a number of indigenous newspapers and periodicals raised their voice against the custom. A number of them stated that housewives would be of much help for the parturient women. The *Calcutta Journal of Medicine* wrote,

> ... In diseases peculiar to women, specially those of the lying in-room the services of a good housewife were of incalculable value. Her importance might be imagined from the extent of the demand for women doctors which is now felt in every civilized country, and her necessity determined by the apprehension so justly entertained that most of the organic disease of women are attributable to a bashful evasion of the doctor in the first stages of disease and to defective disclosure of symptoms after diseases have been fully developed.[20]

A number of doctors who were serving in different parts of rural Bengal also realized the grave situation. One of them, Ram Lall Dey, LMS, Medical Officer, EB Railway wrote a letter to the *Medical Gazettee* as early as in 1866 stating the miserable condition of the women of the district of Koosthea, where he was engaged in his practice. He wrote,

> ... Most painfully aware of the many instances of suffering and danger to the lives of mothers and their unborn children which not unfrequently fall under the sad experience of medical men, practising either among the natives of the metropolis or the rural inhabitants of the Mofussil, owing to the heedlessness and natural tendency of the general public to put too blind a faith and confidence in native midwives or dhyes who go around in this country with no erudite head or experienced finger, obstructing or subverting, but not aiding and facilitating nature in her process of parturition, I beg, Mr Editor, to draw your kind attention to this

> fact, hoping that the evils arising from the systems may be properly laid before the public...and some remedy devised to put a thorough check to this most barbarous and pernicious practice....[21]

Thus almost every sector of society became anxious to improve the standard of skill of the traditional midwives because they would be more experienced than doctors and, as women who had children themselves, had more empathy with their patients. However, faced with the problem of India's high infant and maternal morality rate, poverty and poor living conditions did not become central issues for discussion for the British Government. To them the sole problem was the *dhai* and its solution was to provide them modern scientific training schemes. Yet, none of the schemes was really designed to train the *dhai*, but rather to replace her completely. But this sort of replacement constituted a major problem in the way of success of the *dhai* training scheme, because the workings of the indigenous *dhais* and the trained midwives were different. The trained midwives visited homes and like doctors delivered babies and left. Cleansing up the afterbirth and nursing the mother during the days of confinement were not part of their duties.

The colonial authority considered the *dhais* an incurable social pathology. They were hell bent on the termination of the *dhai* class as they felt that there was no way by which those illiterate and unsophisticated *dhais* could be trained up to the levels of western methods. But the people of our country started to believe that if the traditional *dhais* could learn the basic principles of hygiene, grasp the notion that excessive bleeding was a danger signal rather than beneficial cleansing, and learn to call for assistance in difficult cases, then a great many lives could be saved. But how to make the *dhais* do that was the big question. A number of books written by the eminent doctors of the time on midwifery in the vernacular language proved to be effective in this matter. One such book was *Dhatrishiksha and Prasutishiksha* written by Dr. Jadunath Mukhopahyay in 1891. In the preface he wrote about the significance of the book. He wrote,

> Midwifery is practised by many native females who are either quite ignorant of the art or have gained but a slight experience in it which can avail them nothing in the management of intricate cases. Serious and fatal results have, in too many instances, been known to have ensued from the ignorance, and yet they are seldom deterred from plying their vocation. It is therefore of the utmost importance that they should be taught practical midwifery, a profession which they at presence take to without any previous training. It is true that native midwives seldom know to read or to write, but if there were in existence a work in their

> vernacular giving practical lessons in the art they follow, they would no doubt avail themselves of the earliest opportunity of getting at those lessons either by trying to read the book themselves or by getting it read to them by others. It appeared to me that such a book can only be adopted to their comprehension by being written in the form of a dialogue, dialogue which is the most impressive of all methods of conveying knowledge to simple and unsophisticated minds. The aid of the teacher is dispensed with and the widest scope given for entering into explanation for which a serious treatise is not at all fitted. I have accordingly ventured to publish a guide to practical midwifery in Bengali in two parts. The first part treats of management of pregnancy, management of natural labour, management of parturient females and the proper nursing of the child till it is two years old. The second part treats of preternatural labour and of abdominal presentations with their treatment, puerperal haemorrhage, management of twin cases, of dismenorrhoea and menorrnagia, signs of pregnancy, abortion and consequent effects.[22]

The author had the confidence that apart from being of use to native midwives, who had indeed a very large practice in this country, this might be read with profit by educated Hindu females who would no longer place themselves in the hands of ignorant women in one of the most critical periods of their life.[23] A number of leading newspapers of the time admitted the significance and necessity of such books and expressed their views in their papers. *Abalabandhab* wrote, 'Jadubabu has correctly stated that by learning midwifery men have not been of much help to women. Many women have died in the hands of midwives after acute suffering but yet no one had mentioned in the house that a doctor should come for the delivery. In this situation, there is no other alternative to women becoming self-reliant in matters related to midwifery.'[24]

Apart from Jadunath Mukhopadhyay, a few others also wrote books on this subject in vernacular namely, *Dhatrividya* by Khirodaprasad Chattopadhyay in two volumes (1886), *Dhatrividya* by Alokchandra Dasgupta (1887), *Dhatrividya* by Rajendranath Mitra (1888), *Dhatrividya O Naari Chikitsa* by Sekhar Kumar Basu (1888), and *Dhatri Sahachar* by R. G. Kar and S. C. Basu (1893). What was necessary was the publication of such books, as many as possible, so that the indigenous *dhais*, not only in towns but mostly in rural areas, would have access to such books and could acquire knowledge for their practical work in day to day life. Classroom training in a foreign language could not train the indigenous *dhai* in the required number. Smt. Hemanta Kumari Chaudhurani very aptly commented on this subject in a contemporary

Bengali journal *Antahpur.* She wrote that for teaching these subjects small books in simple language circulated among women could be of great help. For educating married women on this subject, conducting weekend lectures by trained female doctors or discussions in every village along with reading of books can be of immense utility. With the help of her husband, a woman could learn a lot from various books. The magazines for women could also play a pivotal role by publishing articles on these topics and imparting education in the story-telling mode.[25] The journal also stated that they would always welcome suitable articles on these subjects and would gratefully publish them.[26] The same journal also wrote that although at that time in large cities qualified *dhai* and medical practitioners were saving the lives of many and were helping the Indian women to come out from the shackles of superstition, but even then India had not reached a satisfactory level, as qualified *dhais* were still not available at all places . Even in some towns there was no provision for qualified *dhais,* not to mention the villages. As most of the people in our country were poor they could not afford qualified *dhais.* Even with the help of the Lady Dufferin Fund there was a great dearth of books for our women. So that section of society on whom the life of the future generations are totally dependent had to be educated first. It is a matter of great shame that the amount of compassion we show while having children is not all to be seen while bringing up the child. The would be mothers are never taught regarding childbirth, child bearing, and rearing of the newborn.[27]

All these articles, discussions, and treatises and many others were intended to inject awareness among the womenfolk as well as the professional birth attendants for generations. Although this effort was not sufficient due to the enormity of our population, but pitted against the erroneous imperial policy, this was the only effective measure which produced some meaningful result.

However, these measures ultimately failed to suffice the need. Women required medical assistance not only at the time of delivery but throughout their life as a human being. Contemporary women magazines started to focus on the health and hygiene of women in different articles and started to apprise the society of the need for having female doctors. In an issue of the *Antahpur*, Smt. Hemanta Kumari Chaudhurani described the health condition of Bengali women under the head '*Bharatmahilar Swasthya*' in this way:

> ... The majority of Indian women do not enjoy a good health. The health of the mother or the wife if is on the decline, it has a far reaching influence

> on the children. It also results in a general disorder of the family life. When the wife falls ill, both she and her husband have to suffer. Sickness dampens all the other charms of life ... on gauging their health we get a very dismal picture, some are with impaired vision, some are with chronic headaches or with some other ailments. We are becoming conscious about the cleanliness of the roads, but what about the state of affair at our *antahpur* where childbirth actually occurs, and we have a very strongly bonded relationship during our entire lifespan, have we every spared a thought! ... The dwelleres of the *antahpur* on whom the country, society and the family is dependent for its peace and tranquility, are really in a sorry state! The country that boasts of Jana, Laxmibai, Padmini and Karmadevi and other brave women who sided with their menfolk even in battlefields is now producing women who faint at the sight of a drop of blood! They are neither physically strong, nor mentally and tears are their only possessions.[28]

Thus, this article is a testimony of the fact that lack of health among Bengali household women could be a major cause of disharmony both in the family and in conjugal life. In another issue of the *Antahpur,* Smt. Sarojini Devi wrote under the title '*Mahilar Swasthya Sambandhe Koekti Katha*' that,

> Women in Bengal, particularly Hindus, were in a pathetic state of health. Headaches and colic pains were a regular feature and ailments of the uterus were a constant source of agony of a very large member of women. Quite a few of them deprived of being a mother. It is what is called as the progress of modern women? Is this conducive to having healthy, gritty, hardworking and enthusiastic Bengalee children for tomorrow?[29]

Thus there arose a genuine demand for lady doctors.

III

The first organized work of teaching women in western medicine was taken up in India in the Madras Presidency. This was initiated by the efforts of Dr. Balfour, Surgeon General and Mrs. Mary Scharlieb, an English woman. Gradually Punjab and Bombay followed the footsteps of Madras. Surprisingly enough, Bengal, which has always prided itself on its advancement and intellectuality, was way behind in receiving women as medical students in medical college and schools. The question of admitting women to the medical college was raised in 1875, 1879 and 1881 but with no practical results. It was around this time that various indigenous periodicals, women's magazines, and newspapers again became vocal in advocating the cause of medical education for women.

They lamented Bengal's backwardness in this matter and urged the Government of Bengal to allow women to pursue medical studies. The *Brahmo Public Opinion* said,

> ... if there be any one country where, more than at another, the want of lady doctors is most keenly felt, it is no doubt India. The system of *Zenana* seclusion makes it nearly impossible for male doctors to be very useful in treating female patients, consequently, a very large number of our women come to premature death from want of proper medical attendance. We know of instances, where, with the utmost difficulty female patients could be induced to allow the doctor to feel their pulse only. Besides, there are diseases peculiar to them, which it is simply impossible for male doctors properly to diagnose or treat. The establishment of medical institution for the tution of lady students is an urgent necessity in these days in India [30]

The *Bamabodhini Patrika* also whote that,

> Everyone with prudence will admit that as for men, medical education is equally necessary for women. There are certain types of female diseases which can only be appreciated by women and even if those are understood by men, their treatment by males cannot be as effective as by females. Its necessity is more felt in India than in other countries. How is it possible to have proper medical treatment of females of our country where we believe that it is against our religion to come out before any unknown male person who does not belong to her family? Amongst the doctors there are many who have such character that it requires to be carefully considered whether respectable ladies can at all be presented before them. Even many ladies hesitate to appear before those doctors, who have carved the reputation of having good moral character and behaviours. Under such situation, it is no wonder that many Indian women prefer to face death rather than to undergo treatment under such doctors. Women in thousands thus suffer from the diseases and embrace premature death ... As the necessity of female doctors is being perceived, so does the instances of good performance of females in the field of medical education come in. The door of medical education is open to females in America and England and in those countries their membership is increasing every year, and those female doctors are competing with their male counterparts not only in their countries but also outside. In this country too a few *bibi* doctors have already made their graceful appearance. With a blend of religious sentiment and modesty along with education they proved themselves quite worthy of treating the females of the *antahpur*.[31]

Finally, in 1883, Kadambini Ganguly got admitted at the medical college and her success story is now history. A number of indigenous newspapers namely, *Charuvarta*, *Samsad Prabhakar*, *Sanjivani*, *Bamabodhini Patrika*, *Hanneman* and many others expressed their strong support for the opening of the medical college for women. Kadambini completed her certificate course in 1886. Subsequently, she acquired some medical qualification after going to England. She was destined to remove the misery of our sisters. In the meantime, in 1885, 'The National Association for Supplying Female Medical Aid to the Women of India' commonly known as the Lady Dufferine Fund was established. It encouraged the establishment of maternity hospitals as well as baby clinics. But there was opposition to the Dufferin Fund. The Dufferin women doctors were compared with female missionaries who had come to India with the aim of destroying the indigenous cultural system. The newly founded *Zenana* hospitals were denounced as an insult to the art of Indian childbearing. The Hindu revivalist newspaper *Bangabasi*, which fostered cultural indentity in the form of protests against colonial domination, blamed the Dufferin Fund for a singular lack of knowledge: 'The *Zenana* hospital is an outcome of a movement which was started duly, gauging the conditions of native life'.[32] In 1923, a Calcutta newspaper *Hitabadi* alleged that Indian women including middle-class women, were treated worse than dogs in the Lady Dufferin Hospital, whereas European and Eurasian patients were treated well.[33] The Dufferin Fund failed to satisfy the native women doctors in general as it did not provide suitable opportunity to them for proving their worth in their jobs. Kadambini Ganguly (nee Bose) was no exception to this. She was one of the unfortuate victims who had to suffer from the discriminatory policy and professional employment gave her direct experience of frustration. The vernacular press voiced strong objections to the amount of public revenue spent in hiring European lady doctors, who did not speak vernacular languages, when qualified Bengali lady doctors were available in increasing numbers. European lady doctors also charged high fees thereby putting their services above the means of those most in need.[34] In a broad sense, initial sexual discrimination in England was being turned into racial discrimination in India. Discrimination against women doctors in England forced them to look to the colonies for employment. In India, English women doctors were able to take advantage of the racial discrimination of the colonial power to monopolize all available positions. This seriously hindered the advancement of Indian women doctors who were left to labour under the oppressive effects of dual discrimination on grounds of both sex and race. A number of native newspapers decided not to remain as mere spectators to this injustice. For example, *Bengalee* reported,

> ...the standard of qualifications proposed by the Central Association for determining the different grades of lady doctors for employment under it, is in it itself so arbitrary and calculated to act so injuriously to the interests of female medical students of this country that we fear many of our young ladies will be deterred from persuing their medical studies or accepting employment under the Association. It has been distinctly laid down that for the highest grade of appointments 'at present the registered medical women must come from Europe or America'. This decision of the Central Association seems to be so ill-advised and objectionable that we shall not all be surprised, if it will strengthen the apprehension so generally entertained by the people that one of the objects of the National Association is to provide a living to a member of English medical women who are struggling for existence. We are quite willing to encourage real merit, but wherever it may be found. But the proposed classification is not likely to encourage merit, but will maintain a distinction which is by no means desirable and based upon considerations of race....[35]

Kadambini took charge of the Calcutta Zenana hospital three times successively but had to continue as an 'officiating doctor' throughout the period. She was never entrusted with the responsibility of a full department. Kadambini was offended and wrote an open latter to the newspaper condemning the attitude and acts of the colonial government. She wrote,

> ... By the present arrangement, English medical women, though they may not at first possess higher qualifications than their Indian sisters, will soon acquire much better skills by performing hospital duties for It is a recognised fact that hospitals exist for two purposes— the treatment of the sick poor and the education of the medical profession and that the performance of hospital duties quietly improve the qualifications of a doctor. The Indian medical women will miss all the advantages of such professional duties by their exclusion from the medical charge of important hospitals or by being placed in an inferior position there, for in the inferior class of hospitals, few cases of importance will ever come for treatment and in the large and important hospitals, major operation and other important duties will always be performed by the senior position in charge. No opportunity has yet been offered to Indian medical women to show whether they are capable of taking responsible charge of large and important hospitals. It must not be forgotten that it is the opportunity and surroundings which makes the individual. Now without giving Indian medical women opportunities to prove their capabilities, it is not fair to them to pronounce that they are not competent to hold first class

> appointments and to be placed in responsible charge of large and important hospitals....[36]

Ultimately with severe disappointment she resigned from her government service and took to private practice which she continued till the end of her life. She carved fame and popularity by her service of women and children and this made her a legendary figure in the history of medicine as well as of women in our country. Kadambini was the trend setter. It was in 1885 that two women were allowed to join the full fledged MB course of the Calcutta Medical College. They were Bidhumikhi Bose and Virginia Mary Mitra—both Bengali and native Christians. Bidhumukhi was a famous social worker and a reputed medical practitioner. Her younger sister Bindubasini Bose was also a meritorious medical student having passed MB in 1891 from the Calcutta Medical College. Like her elder sister she was also engaged in private practice and became successful. Virginia Mary Mitra also excelled in her results. She stood first in first MB examination. Though she did not get a rank in the final MB examination, she did pass with high grades. She started her professional career with government service—with the Bhagalpore Zenana Hospital, but in 1893 she left her job and returned to Calcutta for private practice. In 1894, she got married to Dr. Purnachandra Nandi, after which she gave up independent private practice though she did look after her husband's patients and at times gave them medicine.

Jamini Sen is a very leading Bengali name in the history of medicine in India involving women. She passed the LMS in 1896 from the Calcutta Medical College after which she started private practice. During her entire career, most of the time she gave service as a government service holder and being an Indian, she had to face various types of discrimination although she acquired foreign qualification from England. Her sister Kamini Roy wrote on one such instance:

> Even with higher qualifications and ability Indians were never held at par with the British or Eurasians and were denied equal status, opportunities and respect. Hence in 1914 when all the three European lady doctors had to be transferred from women's hospital at Agra on disciplinary grounds, Jamini was handed over the baton. She was substituting for them, and that too at such a gruelling summer time at Agra. However, after six months when the dispute was settled and the European doctors were called back, Jamini was sent to Simla where there was a biting cold.[37]

However, she served in many places and tried to reach out to the patients for treatment in every possible area. She also started to write books on medical practice like *Prasutittva*. She died in 1932 and with her death ended the illustrious career of a highly acclaimed lady doctor of the early 20th century. These women and after them many others came to the forefront with the same mission. Unfortunately, in most cases, these endeavours have not been formally put on record. Quite a considerable number of lady students also passed from different medical schools. Among them Haimavati Sen from Campbell Medical School, who served at Chinsura for a long time, deserves a special mention. Most of these students served as hospital assistants under the imperial government. Within their limits they tried to reach out to the masses and particularly to those who were in distress. In such a small spell it is not possible to touch up all their efforts and contributions. I would love to elaborate on them at some other opportune moment.

At the end, it would be most pertinent to spare a thought for the present scenario at the dawn of the 21st century. It is true that there is a declining trend of the mortality rate in India, but even today the maternal mortality rate here is alarmingly high. Sepsis, abortions, haemorrhage, toxaemia, and anaemia account for the large majority of all maternal deaths over the decades of the 1980s.[38] India's maternal mortality ratio is estimated at 400–500 per 1,00,000 live births– about fifty times higher than that of many industrialized nations.[39] This appears to be an underestimate and a more realistic estimate is probably 555 though higher estimates in the range of 700–900 have also been made.[40] However, a large number of maternal deaths are preventable, if attention is paid to three principal underlying conditions among women in India viz., (1) poor health care (2) poor nutrition and (3) high and closely spaced fertility starting from adoloscence.[41] But the most important factor to which attention should be given even in the present day is antenatal care (ANC) and care during birth. The concept of special care during the antenatal period is not unknown traditionally in India. Pregnancy is associated with a number of cultural practices, ranging from the concerning diet to special rites. By and large, however, existing traditional practices concerning diet, combined with traditional omissions, notably the reluctance to seek antenatal care, do little to enhance reproductive health. The maternal and child health programme seeks to address this period of neglect. Under the maternal and child health programme, all pregnant women are to be routinely followed up either in the health centres or at home, and provided immunization, iron supplementation, and regular check ups to monitor the pregnancy. But the available data suggests that this service reaches only a few pregnant women. On the national level, it is estimated that no more than 40–50 per cent of all pregnant women in India receive any antenatal care at all.[42]

Contact with the health care network at the intranatal stage is even poorer than at the antenatal stage. At the time of delivery no more than twenty per cent of all women have some contact with medical or paramedical personnel. In 1984, no more than 15 per cent of all rural births were performed in an institution, and as many as two-third were delivered by untrained workers and others. There are also rural areas of the country where nine out of ten births are delivered by an untrained attendant. In these circumstances, the role of the estimated 5,00,000 traditional birth attendants in India— about one per 1000 population— becomes specially important.[43] Collaboration between the health sector and the traditional birth attendant is an important way of bridging two very different cultures concerning reproductive health but this link has not yet been effectively exploited.

RCH (Reproductive and Child Health progamme) is a package which includes services for both mothers and children. In West Bengal the actual implementation stage for RCH is yet to begin. In keeping with the objectives of the RCH scheme NGOs have been given special responsibility. In this new approach NGOs are to play a very important role. As the Swaminathan Committee recommends, a new climate of partnership between government and voluntary and non-governmental organisations will be created to encourage the extensive participation of such organizations at all stages and levels in the national programme for population stabilization and social development.[44] The Government. of West Bengal has indentified four major NGOs in the field — (1) CINI (2) GANA UNNAYAN PARISHAD (3) W. B. VOLUNTARY HEALTH ASSOCIATION and (4) TAGORE SOCIETY FOR RURAL DEVELOPMENT. In almost all the districts of West Bengal a Government–NGO combined effort is being planned.

Thus, even after independence, for the mass of rural women the problem associated with childbirth has remained almost the same as it was during the colonial period. During the colonial regime, due to the partisan attitude of the government the other factors behind maternal and infantile mortality were suppressed. Under the Raj the responsibility of the *dhais* became all important. At present, due to the so-called proper documentation, the other reasons have come into limelight no doubt. But even in that context the responsibility of the *dhais* cannot be overlooked. Although in the urban sector the problem is not so acute, in rural sector the biggest support comes from the indigenous *dhais*. Hence the need for training the *dhais* properly is the need of the hour. We have to bear in mind that there are some villages in West Bengal where unless real complications arise, deliveries take place at home as pregnant women have to be taken across the river to avail institutional delivery. It thus involves a much bigger question of transport and infrastructure development throughout the state which the RCH programme cannot tackle. The state of the government hospitals also need improvement. But the first and foremost thing which is to be taken care of is the reorientation of the *dhai* class. In a country of huge population there is a tremendous shortage of man power or I would prefer to say woman power. So what is necessary is not brushing them aside as quacks but to regenerate their skill, recycle their knowledge, and update their wisdom so that they can solve at least a part of the pressing problem. It is obvious that the colonial government could not or rather did not understand our problems but the question is whether we ourselves have recovered from the clutches of colonial hangover and have realized our problem or not.

References

1. *Census of India*, 1911, v. 1, p. 328.
2. *Ibid*, 1921, v. 1, p. 209.
3. *Ibid*, pp. 209, 230
4. *Ibid*,
5. Dagmar Engels, *Beyond Purdah? Women in Bengal 1890–1936*, Delhi, 1999, p. 130
6. *Nineteenth Annual Report of the Bengal Branch of the National Association for Supplying Female Medical Aid to the Women of India for the year 1904*, Calcutta, 1904, p. 59.
7. Meredith Borthwick, *Changing Role of Women in Bengal 1849–1905*, NJ, 1984, p. 159
8. *Ibid.*
9. *The Bamabodhini Patrika*, Kartik, BS 1284, pp 616-619.
10. *The Bamabodhini Patrika*, Aswin, BS 1274, p. 59.
11. *The Bamabodhini Patrika*, Agrahayan, BS 1274, p. 637.
12. *The Bamabodhini Patrika*, Chaitra, BS 1274, p. 710.
13. *The Bamabodhini Patrika*, Jaisthya, BS 1275, pp. 32-33.
14. *The Bamabodhini Patrika*, Poush, BS 1274, p. 676.
15. *The Bamabodhini Patrika*, Aswin BS 1274, p. 597.
16. 'Midwifery in India', in *The Calcutta Journal of Medicine*; April 1869, vol. II, no. 4, p. 136.

17. *Ibid*, p. 137.
18. Nanibala Dasi, 'Sutikagare Prasutir Susrusa' in *Antahpur*, September 1903, p. 108.
19. Chittabrata Palit, 'Epidemics and Empire: A Critique of Public Health Policy in Colonial India', in *History*, vol. II, no. 1, 1999, The University of Burdwan, 1999, pp. 59-67.
20. 'Treatment of Diseases in Rural Bengal' in *The Calcutta Journal of Medicine*, Oct. to Dec. 1874, vol. VII, nos. 10 to 12, p. 378.
21. Correspondence on 'Dhyes or Native Midwives' in the *Indian Medical Gazette*, Oct. 1, 1866, p. 311.
22. Jadhunath Mukhopadhyay, *Dhatrishiksha and Prasuti Shiksha* vol. 1, Chinsura, 1871, pp. 1-2.
23. *Ibid.*
24. *Ibid.*
25. Hemanta Kumari Choudhury, 'Sutikagriha' in *Antahpur*, November 1902, pp. 133-138.
26. *Ibid.*
27. *Ibid.*
28. 'Bharat Mahilar Swasthya' in *Antahpur*, July 1901.
29. Sri Sarojini Devi, 'Mahilar Swasthya Sambandhe Koekti Katha' in *Antahpur*, December 191, p. 269.
30. *Brahmo Public Opinion*, June 18, 1883.
31. *Bamabodhini Patrika*, Shraban B.S. 1290.
32. *Confidential Report on the Native Newspapers*, January 28, 1893.
33. *Ibid*, Sept. 23, 1923.
34. Meredith Borthwick, *op. cit.*, pp. 325–26.
35. *Bengalee*, October 6, 1888.
36. Narayan Dutta, 'Abalabandhab Dwarakanath O Kadambini' in *Amrita*, January 18, 1980.
37. Chitra Deb, *Mahila Dactar Bhin Groher Basinda*, Calcutta 1994, p. 132.
38. Shireen J. Tejeebhoy and Saumya Roma Rao 'Unsafe Motherhood: A Review of Reproductive Health' in *Women's Health in India: Risk and Vulnerability* ed. by Monica Dasgupta, Lincoln C. Chem and T. N. Krishnan, Delhi 1998, p. 129.
39. *Ibid,* p. 125.
40. *Ibid.*
41. *Ibid,* p. 129.
42. *Ibid,* p. 135.
43. *Ibid,* p. 141.

44. Mausumi Manna, *A Report on Reproductive and Child Health: A Perspective on the New Policy. The Case of West Bengal*, Sachetana Information Centre, Kolkata, January 2001.

15

Western Approach to Infantile Mortality and Delivery Deaths

- *Aparajita Dhar*

The late nineteenth and early twentieth century Bengal under the aegis of colonial rule witnessed an upswing in the curve of infantile mortality and delivery deaths. Available data suggested that in European countries great strides had been made to improve the condition under which children of all classes were born. In England, the rate of infantile mortality for the ten years from 1876 and 1885 was 142 per mile. It was also stated that improvement had been most rapid since the beginning of the twentieth century, and the rate in 1920 was as low as 80 per mile. How far India was from realizing the importance of the due care of mother and child at the time of birth, and how great was the waste of life which resulted from the failure to realize this and to acquire the necessary knowledge to set matters right, was shown by the fact that the rate of infantile mortality was nearly three times as great in Bengal as in England, and there was so far no sign of improvement. During the first two decades of the twentieth century, in Bengal, one in five babies died before their first birthday.[1] The rate reported by the Commissioner for Public Health with the Government of India for 1927 was 167 per 1,000 births and of these 49.54 per cent took place during the first month of life.[2]

I

The causes of infant mortality were stated to be several. Of direct causes, the principal were unskillful midwifery and disregard of the rules of hygiene, the lying-in-room being generally dark, damp, ill-ventilated outhouses. The practice of cutting the umbilical cord with dirty instruments (e.g., a piece of split bamboo or a conch shell) and of applying cowdung ashes to the freshly cut end commonly resulted in tetanus-neonatarum and caused a very large number of deaths among healthy infants every year. Cleanliness was very often conspicious by it's absence, and the application of anti-septic dressing was very rare. Other dangers that threatened the young child were caused by insufficient clothing combined with exposure as well as the ignorance of the proper treatment of infantile diseases. The census reports also pointed out that the figures given by Dr. Pearse, the Health Officer of Calcutta, for 1909 pointed to the fact that out of 2,700 children that died within the first month, 1,000 children died of tetanus and occasioned by ignorance in matters of hygiene relating to childbirth on the part of mother and those attending to her.[3]

The colonial masters thus castigated the indigenous midwives that it was their incompetency, lack of obstetric expertise, and poor hygiene in the lying-in-room that were responsible for the escalation in the number of deaths.

According to British critics of Bengali sexual practices, high infant mortality was decisively caused by the early consummation of marriage. Criticisms of early consummation was, from the British point of view, a better stick with which to browbeat the Bengalis in the case of dirty *aturghars* and untrained *dais,* men here at best negligent observers.[4] In 1909, Major W. W. Clemensha, Sanitary Commissioner of Bengal claimed that 'out of 2,700 children that die within the first month (in Calcutta) more than 1,200 or nearly 50 percent, come under the heads of premature birth and debility at birth ..... probably early marriage is the preponderant factor'.[5] High maternal mortality was also due, according to British critics, to child marriage and consummation immediately after puberty.[6]

As far as maternal mortality and delivery deaths were concerned Dr. Kedarnath Das, the eminent gynaecologist and P. C. Mahalanobis, had collected the primary statistics from the original records of the Eden Hospital Calcutta. The statistical analysis of the rates of maternal deaths at delivery and the proportion of still births in males and females among Bengali Hindus was carried out systematically for the period 1850s to 1901. Out of 6481 recorded cases, there were 431 deaths which gives an average death rate of 66.5 per cent.[7]

It was noted in the Bengal census in 1921 that there was a phenomenal excess of female mortality in Bengal during the first part of a woman's reproductive age period.[8] Even in the early thirties the maternal mortality rate was believed to be very high in our country. An investigation carried out by the All India Institute of Hygiene and Public Health showed that it was as high as twenty-four per thousand live births. A further study investigated every female death associated with pregnancy, child bearing, and peurperium over a period of one year. It was found that sepsis caused the largest number of deaths in the child bearing group. Anaemias and toxaemias of pregnancy were also the major causes of maternal deaths. To provide a rational basis for a campaign against the high mortality due to anaemia, a study was carried out on 467 pregnant women clinically chosen as anaemic. Evidence of iron deficiency was found in the whole series of cases.[9]

The Age of Consent Committee Report stated that the maternal mortality was at its maximum in the earliest ages. In relation to the order of confinement the maternal mortality rates was highest in the first confinement. Also in the first birth order, the earlier the age of the mother the greater was the risk of maternal deaths. The incidence of neo-natal mortality was greatest in the first birth order when the mother was under twenty years of age. According to the Age of Consent Committee Report there were 3½ times as many still-births and neo-natal deaths in the case of girls below 16 as there were in the case of women between 20 to 30. Some witnesses stated that various causes conspired to engender the evil results of high maternal and infantile mortality. No one would deny that poverty, ignorance, tuberculosis, bad midwifery conditions, and insanitation all contributed to the appalling maternal and infantile mortality in India.[10]

The role of the *dai* or the indigenous midwife who acted as the sole gynaecological consultant before and after childbirth has been ascribed to as a factor responsible for the escalating delivery deaths. Therefore, one colonial response to the horrors perpetrated by the *dai* was to seek to oust the traditional specialists and replace them with 'modern' agents and specialists. Women were encouraged to give birth not in their own homes, darkened rooms and squalid out-houses but in lying-in or maternity hospitals. Attempts were also made to recruit a new kind of midwife from among women who were not from the same lowly background as the traditional *dai*, and who had some educational and medical training. Infact, the moves to replace traditional Indian midwives or *dais* could be seen as one of the most striking examples of the growing attempts to incorporate women into a colonizing medical discourse. Attention began to be drawn towards them from the 1860s and 1870s as European doctors and missionaries learnt more about their crude and often dangerous techniques, and as the scale of infant mortality in India began to be recognized. The activities of the *dais* were freely labelled 'barbaric'. In the course of an appeal for funds to provide medical aid for the women of India in 1890, Lady Dufferin referred to 'the condition of those women who debarred from all skilled medical relief, are subjected to the barbarous practices of ignorant midwives'.[11]

II

The colonial government at this time was thus motivated by the desire to impart training to the native *dais*. In a letter dated 25th March 1873, the Under Secretary to the Government of India (Home Department) T. J. Chichele Plowden wrote to the Secretary to the Government of Bengal, (Judicial Department), relative to the working of the scheme imparting training to the native women in practical midwifery. He wrote that 'the results of the experiment, are certainly not encouraging, but the Governor-General-in-Council hopes that so important a measure will not be abandoned until all that is possible has been done to make it succeed. A similar attempt to improve the obstetrics of the country has not failed in the North Western provinces'. His Excellency in Council also observed that

> the scope of the experiment should not be confined solely to cases of actual childbirth, in the bulk of which very little professional knowledge is wanted, but that it should extend also to the diagnosis and treatment of special female diseases. Most of them are known to be of obscure character, often simulating other diseases and frequently of a very distressing nature, yet usually curable if taken up early. Native women, especially of the upper classes, from their confined and secluded lives are liable to attacks of this class of disease, and in which they absolutely refuse to place themselves under the treatment of medical men, though they would gladly resort to trained midwives.[12]

The *Indian Medical Gazette* also wrote that such a desideratum had long been felt by the European as well as native medical practitioners in Calcutta, particularly by those who have had many opportunities of treating diseases among the inhabitants of the Calcutta *Zenanas*. Henry Goodeve, Duncan Steuart and their successors—the professors of midwifery in Calcutta, having each in turn made more or less endeavours to supply such a want to their effect—left the grand want of educated native midwives quite unprovided for, and so far as practical results were concerned, the western science of obstetrics had as yet done nothing in aiding the native *dais* to bring timely aid to her country woman in her hour of sorrow and travail.[13]

Imparting training to the indigenous midwives was no doubt an attempt to combine practical experience and scientific knowledge. However, despite her experience, a midwife was often ignorant of basic, sanitary principles. The Calcutta Medical College Hospital and the Mitford Hospital in Dacca first opened courses for midwives in 1870. A European midwife attended the delivery of R. C. Dutt's third daughter in 1873—an instance of compromise between a traditional midwife and a doctor, as well as a status symbol.[14]

The General Report of Public Instruction in Bengal reported that, in the 1890s, Eden Hospital trained an average of 10 students a year. While the numbers are not insignificant, it is clear that Eden's programme was incapable of educating enough midwives to replace traditional birth attendants.[15]

Reformers agreed that if *dais* could learn the basic principles of hygiene and grasp the notion that excessive bleeding was a danger signal, and learn to call for assistance in difficult cases, then lives could be saved. Enticing *dais* to the training classes was however difficult enough. Convincing them of the superiority of western medicine and the importance of deferring to the western medical practitioners was close to impossible. At any rate, western trained doctors were not willing to share 'all'. The 'kits' given to retrained *dais* contained soap and scissors but not forceps, speculums or chloroform.[16]

The lack of serious attention to retraining *dais* is especially interesting given the virulence of the rhetoric denouncing them. The attack began as early as the 1840s when British doctors decried the torture inflicted on Indian women by *dais*. When half-hearted schemes to retrain *dais* failed to work and professional midwifery courses turned out dozens rather than hundreds of graduates, there was little soul-searching as to why. Instead, the *dais* became the symbol of superstition and dogged resistance to change, often described as a pathology that needed to be rooted out.[17]

III

In the 1880s, one of the most important Victorain responses to the conditions of female health and childbirth in India was the foundation of The National Association for Supplying Female Medical Aid to the Women in India.[18] Begun in 1885, the Countess of Dufferin Fund as it was popularly known, became the first programme with official support to focus on medical care for Indian women.[19] It encouraged the establishment of maternity hospitals as well as baby clinics.[20]

The main object of the fund was to train Indian women in medicine at both licentiate and degree level, so that they might treat female patients. It was deemed essential to penetrate the 'veil of the zenana', if any lasting cultural impact were to be made upon the Indian people. Medicine, as we see clearly in case of the Dufferin Fund, was intended as a bearer of western cultural values that would bind Indians more to their colonial masters.[21] The government had decided that training Indian women in western medicine boosted their claim to benevolent rule and promised to bring the Raj into direct contact with the zenana.[22]

The Dufferin Fund was, however, not designed to provide medical care to the entire gamut of women. The Fund maintained that the medical care for women had to be provided by women in 'Women-only' hospitals. It was common knowledge that poor women who worked alongside men did not observe purdan but this strata did not concern the Fund's founders. The women of most interest to the British were the upper classes and castes who observed female seclusion. British officials wanted to win the hearts and minds of the elite, zenana hospitals were to be staffed and run by women and outfitted with the necessary curtains, partitions, and separate entrances to allow the '*purdahnashin*' to observe all rules of sex segregation. This was the ideal, an ideal outfitted by British men on women whose definition of purdah was rigid and idealized.[23]

This ideal became evident in the Annual Reports of the Fund which stated that

> the difficulty of pursuading purdah women to avail themselves of the advantage of Dufferin Hospitals is one which the committee has continually before it, and the question of making fresh efforts to gain the confidence of purdah-nashins has again been seriously considered, in communication with Lady Dufferin... The fact that "purdah" women have not yet commenced to make use of existing buildings, in such numbers as those working in the interests of the Fund could wish, cannot be denied....it also appears that buildings if they are to attract "purdah nashins" must be absolutely detached from the main hospital where non-purdah women are admitted and must be strictly closed to males, whether for inspection or other purposes.[24]

Although Dufferin hospitals and dispensaries, opened after 1885 with private donations and government support, provided employment for many women, some labelled the organization exploitative and discriminatory. The fund favoured foreign women over Indian women. Infact, India provided jobs for British women graduates who found it difficult to practice at home. The circle was a comfortable one; tales of *zenana* provided the raison d'etre for British women's medical training, many of those trained pursued lucrative careers in the empire, and feminism was removed from 'home' where it might turn against British men and given free expression in India where it legitimized British rule. By sponsoring British medical women for women only hospitals, the Raj posed as both humanitarian and sensitive to the needs of the *zenana*.[25]

At the level of imperial rhetoric, the work of the Dufferin Fund was proudly acclaimed for bringing the benefits of western civilization to Indian women. And yet for all the viceregal rhetoric, it is indicative of the secondary importance which was actually attached to medical work for women that it was left to wives of viceroy and governors, that the Fund operated through a series of volunteer branch committees with only a weak central structure rather than being taken up as official business. The government offered its goodwill but would not take up the work itself. It believed that if it did so, private subscriptions would dry up, the burden of administration would fall upon its already overworked officials, and it would be obliged to carry the additional burden of pay and positions for women doctors. And yet without that communication the activities of the Dufferin Fund were difficult to sustain and unable to command public support.[26]

IV

In the 1920s, discourses on childbirth and female health took place against a changed political background. Motherhood and fertility were no longer condescendingly regarded as predominantly moral issues, but as social problems linked with women's health and living conditions. Hospitals for women were opened all over the country. Although only a few women were affected by these activities, the initiatives were a sign of the times. During the early 1920s, so-called 'female issues' had gained predominance because middle-class women's campaigns for female enfranchisement had gained attention in Bengal as in other Indian provinces.[27]

One of the conseqences of establishment of childbearing as a central concern of medicine was the development of the view of pregnancy as a pathological condition. Ante-natal care had acquired importance in England mainly after World War I, when the monitoring of the health of the unborn child and the mother became a key element in health policies. Oakley argues that this acted towards placing women's bodies and their reproductive function firmly in the control of the medical establishment.[28]

In India also the need for ante-natal supervision was becoming the order of the day. Dr. N.A. Purandare M.D.F.C.PS. honorary obstetrician Wadia Maternity Hospital, honorary gynaecologist King Edward Memorial Hospital, and honorary lecturer in G.S. Medical College Parel, Bombay, wrote an article in the *Journal of the Indian Medical Association*. This was entitled 'How to Avoid Maternal and Foetal Dangers'. According to Dr. Purandare, one of the greatest advances that had been made in the sphere of obstetrics in the recent years was the establishment of anti-natal supervision with a view to adopting 'prophylactic measures' to secure the safety of the mother and the child during labour. To attain this aim, he wrote that the expectant mother would have to be guided in respect of her food and hygiene and examined in general to exclude complication and, from an obstetrical point of view, to determine the presentation and position and to judge of the relative size of the head and the pelvis. In giving instructions regarding food and hygiene the object was that she should keep such good health during pregnancy as to prepare her to pass through the process of childbirth and lying-in-period without trouble. She should have good nourishing diet composed of milk, fruit, green vegatables, carbohydrates, the element supplying sufficient vitamins especially vitamins A and D, the former for raising her defensive forces in the organism against infection, and the latter for encouraging calcium metabolism so needed during pregnancy, not only for her economy, but for the proper development of the foetus.[29]

Emphasis was also laid on the examination of the expectant mother in general systematically to discover any complications arising from pregnancy, such as anemias, and toxaemias of pregnancy or any morbid condition in connection with other parts of the body such as lungs, heart, alimentary canal, urinary, and nervous systems.[30]

In the early decades of the twentieth century, the medical pracitioners were expressing concern over the problems in gynaecological diagnosis and treatment of the patients. Bhibuti Bhusan Bhattacharya, MB wrote and article in the *Calcutta Medical Journal* entitled 'The Gynaecological Diagnosis and Treatment in General Practice', in which the author meant to bring to attention certain discrepancies generally noticed in gyneacological practice. He pointed out that it was a common knowledge that in every household of Bengal there were some women suffering from gynaecological ailments. As a rule, the mothers did not like to express anything about their diseases, if by chance their ailments were known, there was no proper way of treating them. Due to this neglect they were ever sickly and one could well imagine the result— headache, pain in lower abdomen, colic, acidity constipation, palpitation, hysteria, leucorrhoes, and bleeding, urinary trouble or some such trouble were always noticed among them. No treatment or maltreatment gradually led the mother to chronic invalidism.[31]

Having suggested that 'Routine Method of Examination' was essential for proper gynaecological diagnosis, the author wrote, 'History of not only present illness but also of past health, puberty, and menstruation, pregnancy (etc.) are taken one by one. Next from head to foot she is thoroughly examined — no parts of her body are neglected in a hurry. A special care is taken of her mental and neurotic conditions ...

After such a routine general examination if required, her blood, urine, stool etc. should be examined and even the aid of X-rays, cystoscope etc. should be taken to come to a definite diagnosis of the case. Instead, to give off hand diagnosis in haste without proper examination is extremely bad'.[32] The author also urged upon the fact that the 'cervix uterus' of the patient was to be dealt with as a definitive organ with a distinctive function.

The author concluded his essay by saying that

> want of proper examination may produce great many dangers. Therefore, it is essential to make the proper diagnosis by a routine examination before proceeding to treat any gynaecological case. At the same time it should be our look out to induce our women folk by all means to allow examination. To allow the dumb weaker sex to die or lead a life of invalid only for proper medical examination to observe social customs would be suicidal to the policy of national and economical welfare. The social reformers as well as the medical profession at large shoud take of the matter in right earnest to mend or end this deplorable custom.[33]

Infantile mortality and delivery deaths had reached epidemic proportion under colonial rule. Although western approach to the entire problem had been lackadaisical, yet attention was drawn to women's health in the early decades of the twentieth century. Western trained Indian doctors laid emphasis on ante-natal and post-natal care to reduce the rates of death among mothers and children.

References

1. *Census of India, 1921*; VI.I p. 209.
2. *The Indian Medical Gazette*, Nov. 1930.
3. *Census of India, 1911*; VI. I p. 30-31.
4. Dagmar Engels, *Beyond Purdah? Women in Bengal 1890–1930,* Delhi, 1999, p. 129.
5. *Census of India, 1911*; VI. I p. 479.
6. Dagmar Engels, *op.cit.*, p. 130.
7. *Sankhya*, 1933–34, Calcutta, vol. I.
8. *Census of India, 1921*; VI. I p. 255.
9. All India Institute of Hygiene and Public Health, Silver Jubilee publication.
10. *The Age of Consent Committee Report, 1926-27.*
11. David Arnold, *Colonizing the Body: State Medicine and Epidemic Diseases in Nineteenth Century India*, Delhi, OUP, 1993, p. 257.
12. Government of India Proceeding, Judicial Department (Medical Branch), File No. 63, No. 7, April 1873.

13. *The Indian Medical Gazette*. 1866, Oct. p. 311.
14. Meredith Borthwick, *The Changing Role of Women in Bengal* (*1849–1905*) New Jersey, 1984, p. 159.
15. Quoted in Gerldine Forbes, 'Colonial Imperative and Women's Emancipation: Western Medical Education for Indian Women in Nineteenth century Bengal', *Modern Historical Studies*, vol. 2 pp. 188-204.
16. *Ibid.*
17. *Ibid.*
18. Dagmar Engels, *op.cit.*, p. 138.
19. Geraldine Forbes, *op.cit.*
20. Dagmar Engels, *op.cit.*
21. Mark Harrison and Biswamoy Pati (ed.), *Health, Medicine and Empire: Perspectives on Colonial India*, New Delhi, 2001, p. 74.
22. Geraldine Forbes, *op.cit.*
23. Geraldine Forbes and Tapan Roy Chaudhuri (eds.), *The Memoirs of Dr. Haimabati Sen: From Child Widow to Lady Doctor*; Delhi, 2000, pp. 30-31.
24. *Tenth Annual Report of the National Association for Supplying Female Medical Aid to the Women of India for the year 1894*, Calcutta, 1895, p. 17.
25. Geraldine Forbes, *op.cit.*
26. David Arnold, *op.cit.*, pp. 263–64.
27. Dagmar Engels, *op.cit.*, p. 141.
28. Supriya Guha, 'The Nature of Woman: Medical Ideas in Colonial Bengal in India' *Journal of Gender Studies,* 3, 1 (1996), pp. 23-28.
29. *Journal of the Indian Medical Association*, 1932, pp. 316-317.
30. *Ibid.*
31. *Calcutta Medical Journal*, vol. 19, 1924, pp. 152-153.
32. *Ibid.*
33. *Ibid.*

16

Patronage, Philanthropy, Western Medicine: Gender and Health in Nineteenth Century India

—Sujata Mukherjee

I

In nineteenth century India, western medical activities were sought to be carried out in institutional locales such as hospitals, dispensaries as well as asylums. These apparatuses formed the most obvious and concentrated zones for the practice of modes of diagnosis and intervention conducted in medical terms. The technology of the curative clinic permitted that 'exact superposition of the "body" of the disease and the body of the sick man' which Foucault describes at the opening of *The Birth of the Clinic.*[1] The modern clinical hospital became the hub of a web of medical activities. Dispensaries were to extend consultation and medication to patients without the need to intern them. It has been suggested that the medicalization of social space and the hygienic transformation of the family (over the nineteenth century), can serve as two exemplars of the technical enactment of medicine's liberal vocation. Medicine sought to construct public space through sanitary legislation, health regulations etc. On the other hand, it also sought to construct private space, in particular the domestic environment of home and family, in a form conducive to the promotion of health of the family members. 'Over the 19th century, the government of conduct in the name of health was to assume a more liberal form, that is to say, it operated according to a division between a "public" domain to be rendered pure, clean, healthy and sanitized by authoritative action, and private spaces to be governed not by reducing freedom but by regulating.'

The hospitals,[2] dispensaries,[3] asylums opened in colonial India formed the nucleus from which western medicine sought to establish its superiority over indigenous forms of medicine. In this enterprise, the patronage and philanthropy of Indian elite also played a very positive and collaborative role. Richer sections of the Indian population provided funds for running dispensaries, hospitals, and colleges. Historians have point out that medical philanthropy and patronage in India sprang from a variety of motives.[4] It was seen by the Indians as a means of extending leadership over one's own community and society. It must be remembered that India had a strong cultural tradition of philanthropic and charitable works, which found fresh outlets in the colonial era. Medical philanthropy was also partly a political strategy. The Indian elite wanted to utilize it as a means of gaining prestige, influence, and recognition from the colonial regime.

It seems that the Calcutta elite's (which included the English educated Indian intellectuals) patronage and philanthropy for western science as well as medicine sprang from the belief that western science which was integral to western culture, was an important modernizing force.[5] People like Ramkamal Sen,[6] Dwarakanath Tagore,[7] Motilal Seal,[8] were great patrons of western science and philanthropists who generously contributed towards promoting western medicine.

In general the Bengali intelligentsia welcomed the institutionalization of western science. The Hindu College established through the efforts of the *bhadralok* or the new elite in Calcutta in 1817, had to teach apart from the humanities, subjects like 'geography, chronology, astronomy, chemistry and other sciences'.[9] The college received a donation of scientific equipment from the British India Society of London for teaching astronomy, optics, mechanics, and chemistry in 1823.[10] In 1823, when the General Committee of Public Instruction decided to spend government fund to set up a Sanskrit College in Calcutta, Rammohan Roy strongly protested against the move. In a letter to Lord Amherst he wrote:[11]

> If it had been intended to keep the British nation in ignorance of real knowledge, the Baconian philosophy would not have been allowed to displace the system of schoolmen, which was the best calculated to perpetuate ignorance. In the same manner the Sanskrit system of education would be the best calculated to keep this country in darkness, if such had been the policy of the British Legislature.

He urged the government to employ European gentlemen of talent and education to interest the natives of India in mathematics, natural philosophy, chemistry, anatomy, and other useful sciences, which the natives of Europe have carried to a degree of perfection that has raised them above the inhabitants of other parts of the world.

Towards the end of 1831, a small hospital was established in Calcutta for the treatment of patients as well as for imparting clinical instructions to the students of the Native Medical Institution.[12] The moving spirit behind the establishment of the hospital was Ramkamal Sen, who made a liberal donation and took a very keen interest in the development of medical education from the very beginning. The hospital was planned on a small scale and accommodated thirty patients in the indoor department. It had an outdoor department as well. Naba Krishna Gupta, the senior and most advanced student of the medical class was appointed apothecary. He was assisted by other students by rotation each month.

The Calcutta Medical College[13] (CMC) from its very inception, was enthusiastically supported by the Calcutta elite. Many luminaries of Calcutta including Dwarakanath Tagore, Ramkamal Sen enthusiastically supported medical education given at the CMC by instituting scholarships and prizes for brilliant students. Dwarakanath's special concern for medical philanthropy was evident from the fact that he instituted scholarships of Rs. 2,000 per year for three years.[14] Already in 1833, he was elected a member of the committee of the Leprosy Society.[15] In 1835, he joined with Motilal Seal and Rajah Protab Chandra Singh to plan the establishment of a fever hospital for the poor.[16] Four students of the college were sent to England through financial help of Dwarakanath Tagore, Professor Goodeve, and partly of the government.[17] Three of them including Dwaraka Nath Bose, Bhola Nath Bose, and Gopal Chunder Seal passed the examination for the Member of the Royal College of Surgeons (MRCS) in 1846 and returned to India to join the uncovenanted Medical Service. Surjee Coomar Chukerbutty remained there, obtained the MD degree of the University College of London and became the first Indian to pass the examination for the Indian Medical Service and join the covenanted Medical Service. He also became a distinguished professor of the Medical College holding the Chair of Materia Medica from 1864 till his death in 1874.

In 1837, Madhusudan Gupta[18] suggested that Calcutta Medical College start a programme to train midwives and also build a lying-in hospital for poor women. In 1840, a large female (lying-in) hospital was constructed in the Calcutta Medical College grounds by a liberal public subscription. It contained 100 beds and afforded instructions in midwifery.[19] In 1841, Dr. H. Goodeve, who had been appointed in 1837 to the chair of anatomy and medicine, took charge of anatomy and midwifery.[20] It seems that from the middle of the 19th century the *bhadralok* in Bengal showed eagerness to adopt new medical skills in case of childbirth though it was accessible to few who could afford high cost. The report of the midwifery hospital stated in 1848 that all of their college graduates — six or more in number practicing in Calcutta were 'habitually called to take charge of the women of the families they attend during their confinements'.[21]

II

In the case of health care for women, while the colonial state showed initial apathy,[22] piecemeal and sporadic efforts spearheaded by individuals (both Indians and Europeans) bore important results. Both the Indians and Europeans came forward as patrons to provide female medical aid. The main activities broadly aimed at providing maternal care by opening training centres for midwives and also at broadcasting facilities of health care to women by bringing trained female doctors from abroad and opening the doors of medical education for aspirant female doctors in India. For the white elite, apparently the basic initial stimulus for this interventionist role came from writings of people like James Mill who articulated a version of gender relations as being prevalent in India, which would justify British presence. He wrote in his *The History of British India:*

> The condition of women is one of the most remarkable circumstances in the manners of nations ... The history of uncultivated nations uniformly represents the women as in a state of abject slavery, from which they slowly emerge as civilisation advances ... As society refines upon its enjoyments ... the condition of the weaker sex is gradually improved till they associate on equal terms with the men and occupy the place of voluntary and useful coadjutors. A state of dependence more strict and humiliating than that which is ordained for the weaker sex among the Hindus cannot easily be conceived.[23]

As the 19th century progressed, the traditional practices of childbirth and maternal care were discredited. One important target was the unhygienic condition under which birthing was taking place in India. Childbirth took place in a special room called the *aturghar* or *sutikagriha.* Dr. Stewart, a Professor of the Calcutta Medical College was horror-stricken to see the 'filthy, smoky and crowded hovels, to the straw of which the unfortunate Bengallee females are condemned by native usage in the hour of suffering'.[24] Meredith Borthwick has shown that early medical literature on the horrors of childbirth in India emphasized the place of birth as being the main cause of the high rates of mortality among both mothers and infants.

It must be remembered in this connection that with increasing urbanization in 19th century India, a sanitary perspective was sought to be introduced in patterns of medical thought.[25] As early as 1835, a committee was appointed by the government to enquire into the state of health of city and suburbs of Calcutta and to collect information regarding its ventilation, drainage, and municipal arrangements. This committee was formed at the suggestion of Mr. Renald Martin, then surgeon of the Native Hospital and after 12 years published a three volume report which came to the conclusion that 'a very large amount of disease in Calcutta was caused by the absence of cleanliness, drainage and ventilation and that the hospital accommodation of the city was most inadequate for its wants'. In 1876, the health officer for Calcutta presented a detaied picture of the unhealthy and unhygienic practices of the *aturghar* and the same kind of portrayal was available in the census reports of 1911.[26]

In India (as elsewhere), childbirth was attended by aged women and *dais* or midwives who were described as 'experienced and courageous women of advanced age and with clean clothes before whom she (the birthing mother) may not feel shy, who have cut their nails and who cheer her with friendly words'.[27] The *dai* generally was a lower caste Hindu or poor Muslim. In Bengal, she could be a *hadi* or *dom,*[28] in north India she was generally a *chamar* or of the sweeper caste[29] and in the south, she was of the barber caste. There was little incentive for the *dai* to hone her skills or for the midwife to develop any professional trait as in Europe, even before the coming of medical men. It had the classic traits of a traditional occupational grouping devoid of professionalism. The recruits were a caste-based restricted hereditary group and often the calling was handed within a family from mother to daughter.

The duties of the *dai* could extend from cutting the umbilical cord, washing the puerperal garments and burying the placenta, to living in the home of the parturient mother and giving her and the infant regular massages and warm fomentations. Thus they had to perform menial tasks but received meagre pay. Many studies of medical profession have a tendency to glorify the role of midwives. It has been emphasized that the they had more empathy for their patients than the doctors. The *dai* appeared to symbolize rites exclusive to women which involved non-Sanskritic ritual performance.[30] Among the Calcutta elites we find a mixed attitude towards the midwives. People like Lal Behari Day portrayed a kindly and well intentioned village midwife.[31] On the other hand, many accounts highlighted the ignorance of the *dai* which was blamed for jeopardizing the health of both mother and child by interfering with the process of natural labour. Many accounts recorded cases of how midwives began pulling the heads of infant as soon as it appeared or of how the placenta was removed by hand immediately after the infant had fully emerged. According to Geraldine Forbes, many treatises written by the Bengalis were actually translations of English works and attacked the traditional method of birthing.[32]

Many travellers' and medical men's accounts in the 19th and early 20th centuries suggested that birthing process in India was no less hazardous than it was in England. Little was actually known about pre-natal and post-natal care.[33] In fact, in England in 1868, 26 per cent of children died before the age of five.[34] Undoubtedly, in most parts of the world in the 19th century, child delivery was a hazardous process and also painful till the discovery of chloroform in 1847. According to Meredith Borthwick, some Bengalis thought that European women had overcome the difficulties of childbirth by observing the rules of health, but as shown by P. Branca, cases of puerperal fever was actually a frequent cause of maternal mortality in England. At the same time, new medical techniques were developing in England raising the standard of midwifery.[35]

It seems that from the middle of the 19th century the *bhadralok* in Bengal showed an eagerness to adopt new medical skills in case of childbirth. It was, however, accessible to few who could afford high cost. Borthwick has pointed out that many Bengali women, in fact, shunned doctors because they were skeptical about the capacities of a doctor.[36] In many cases, there was continued dependence on the midwives while at the same time doctors were also called.

III

According to Forbes, 'the Indian way of giving birth would probably not have received attention it did had it not been for the increase in the numbers of missionary women in India in the latter half of the century'.[37] It has been pointed out by Balfour and Young that the stimulus for the first *dai* training schemes was provided by the missionaries who had gained access to the purdah as teachers and were grieved to see their young pupils dying in childbirth.[38] In the 1860s, a number of missionary societies came forward to sponsor separate women's associations which were meant to recruit and train female missionaries. These associations tried to focus on spreading education in the *zenanas*.[39] The conditions in *zenana,* in fact, became the focus of critical attention and it was considered to be a place of dirt, darkness, and disease.[40] A vast body of Anglo-Indian discursive writing was produced in the second half of the 19th century focusing on the Indian women, and one most striking thing about this was its preoccupation with the *purdah*. In the opinion of Indrani Sen, 'while "native" men evidently sought to control their women's sexuality and bodies by shutting them up inside the zenana away from the colonial gaze, the efforts of the Anglo-Indians were geared towards bringing these very women out in the open through the gradual eradication of the purdah system. In this conflict between the two groups, the "native" woman's body became, in effect, the terrain upon which the cultural contest was staked out.'[41]

The hegemonic ambitions of western medicine were represented by the activities of women missionaries from England and the United States, who came to India from the 1860s, and established hospitals, dispensaries, and training centres for midwives and nurses. Dr. Humphrey, a member of the American Methodist Episcopal Church established a medical training school for women in Nainital in 1869. The school, however, did not last for more than three years. The same mission sent Dr. Clara Swain, a graduate of the Women's Medical College of Pennsylvania, to Bareilly in 1870. She started a small class with three married women and fourteen girls from the mission's orphanage. In 1873, thirteen of them passed their final examination in the presence of three doctors and were granted certificates of practice. Before long, missions on both sides of the Atlantic began to champion the ability of women to apply the 'double cure': 'healing the body while they healed the spirit'.[42] Miss Fanny Butler, the first British medical woman came to India in 1880. Swain, Butler and other missionaries opened dispensaries, hospitals, and training centres for midwives and nurses.[43] Dr. Aitchison, a civil surgeon in Punjab launched a scheme in 1866 in Amritsar to train *dais*.[44] In 1886, the project was revived by Miss Hewlett, a medical missionary of the Church of England Zenana Missionary Society.

The role of medical missionaries is important in more ways than one. It was they who made a small but influential group of Indians desiring medical attendance in childbirth, thus creating the climate for later more widespread work. The missionary women commented on what seemed to them the horrors of childbirth and the appalling customs and beliefs surrounding the occasion of birth. It has been pointed out by a missionary author, who was not herself a doctor but who described the practices of Bengali village midwives in the mid-nineteenth century, that 'unscientific' and 'unchristian' customs seem to have been indistinguishable.[45]

In course of time, there was the growth of a strong public opinion in England as well as India that Indian women were in urgent need of female physicians. Dr. Frances Hoggan (one of the first British women to qualify as a doctor) argued that the IMS had failed to render the medical requirements of Indian women and that only women doctors could best serve the interests of Indian female patients.[46] She pointed out that the 'shrinking' of women patients from male doctors was not a 'prejudice' to be disregarded but a 'natural' attitude and it was the 'right of Indian women' to expect this sentiment to be 'respected and not outraged'. She also suggested that the government should produce two classes of women practitioners: ordinary practitioners for the country and the more accomplished section capable of teaching and practising in the bigger towns.

It seems that George A. Kittredge, an American businessman in Bombay was touched by this plea. In his view 'to be successful in this country, women must be recognised as the equals of men in the medical care of their own sex. This recognition could never be gained by those who have taken a partial medical course and an inferior degree in an Indian University'.[47] The Medical Women's Fund was set up to raise public subscription for promotion of female medical education. Kittredge started to raise funds among his Indian friends to bring female physicians from Europe or North America. He was helped in his endeavour by rich physicians from Europe or North America. He was also helped in his endeavour by a rich Parsi, Sorabji Shapurji Bengali and was able to collect Rs. 40,000 within two months. The effort gained further momentum when Pestonji Hormusji Kama came forward to offer a donation of more than 1.5 lakhs to meet the cost of establishing a hospital for women and children. The Cama hospital was opened in August 1886.

In 1847, Mary Scharlieb, the wife of an English barrister in Madras who later became a London gynaecologist persuaded authorities in Madras to allow women students to attend classes at the Madras Medical College.[48] A new chapter in the history of medical education in India opened in 1875 when four students (including Mrs. Scharlieb) were admitted to the three-year certificate course of the Madras Medical College.

In Bengal also an attempt was made during the same time for admitting female students to medical training. In 1875, Neel Kamal Mitra submitted a petition seeking admission for his granddaughter, Biraj Mohini to the Bengali course at the Calcutta Medical College. Mitra, however, insisted that Biraj Mohini should be given a separate curtained-off seat and taught dissection in the presence of her husband or himself. This proposal, however, was turned down.

In 1881–1882, Abala Das and Ellen D'Abrieu, who had passed the entrance and the F A examination respectively of the Calcutta University went to Madras with government scholarships to study medicine since they were barred from entering the Calcutta Medical College. The Council of the Medical College was opposed to the idea of admitting female students to the Medical College although the government was in favour of it. Brahmo reformers of 19th century Bengal were enthusiastic supporters of medical education for women. The admission of female students who had passed the First Arts Examination to the Calcutta Medical College was permitted by a resolution of June 23, 1883. The first beneficiary of this new rule was Kadambini Basu, one of the first female graduates in India, who later married the Brahmo reformer Dwarakanath Ganguly. In 1883, Kadambini entered the Calcutta Medical College and was awarded the GBMC degree in 1886.[49]

Rules were relaxed in 1886 by providing for admission of girls who had passed either the entrance or a special preliminary examination to a three-year course in the Medical College.[50] The Maharani of Cossimbazar made a donation of ruppees one lakh fifty thousand for the construction of a hostel for the female students.[51] The government offered scholarships of Rs. 20 per month to all female students. Bidhu Mukhi Bose and Virginia Mary Mitter received these scholarships and became the first Indian women to graduate during 1888–1889.

The first systematic and regular attempt to provide medical help to Indian women started in 1885 with the establishment of the Dufferin Fund or the National Association for Supplying Female Medical Aid to the Women of India. Mary Scharlieb and Elizabeth Bielby (missionary doctor at Lahore) personally met and informed Queen Victoria about the lack of medical care for Indian women and the Queen asked Lady Dufferin, the new Vicereine to investigate into the scope of providing medical help to Indian women. On her initiative, the Fund was established in August 1885 with three aims: to provide medical teaching and training to women, to organize medical relief, to supply female nurses and midwives in hospitals and private houses.

It has been pointed out that 'The Dufferin Fund was a distinctive example of what became a characteristic effort of the Government of India, to graft onto India the English model of philanthropy, which colonial rulers believed represented a progressive civic ideal'.[52] After the revolt of 1857, the British regarded the native rulers and aristocrats as bulwarks of empire and certain philanthropic endeavours like donation for schools, hospitals were earmarked as acts aiming at achieving progress with stability by which Indians could be rewarded with titles under a newly reorganized system of Indian royal titles. The Indian elite generously contributed to the Fund. The Central Committee of the Dufferin Fund started to collect subscription in August 1885. By January 1886 more than Rs. 70,000 was contributed by Indian maharajas and nawabs.[53]

In 1888, the Campbell Medical School at Sealdah opened its door to the first batch of 15 female trainees. The Campbell School was established in 1872 to accommodate the students of the Bengali vernacular class of the Calcutta Medical College opened in 1853. The majority of medical men were opposed to women's entry to Campbell. According to R. L. Dutt, officiating Civil Surgeon of Rungpore, there was no need for medical women of the Hospital Assistant class in the mofussil. He also pointed out that Indian women who wanted to become doctors should attend medical college and those with less education should take the midwife course.[54] Sir A. W. Croft, Director of Public Instruction, Bengal, wrote in favour of opening Campbell to women.[55] Dr. S. C. Mackenzie, the Superintendent of Campbell Medical School, received 15 applications from female candidates. He pointed out that these candidates were ladies belonging to the most respectable *brahmo* families of Bengal.

According to Forbes, the opening of medical education to women by the imperialists was prompted by the desire to the penetrate the *zenana*. 'Nevertheless, their gesture proved of benefit to Indian women seeking professional opportunities and to their clients, hundreds of thousands of women and children who now received medical attention.'[56]

It must be admitted that the new medical knowledge was not really affordable to the majority of the population and they had to depend on the services of traditional care-givers who were gradually discredited by the British civilizing discourse of science and progress. As discussed elsewhere,[57] there existed a vigorous female domain of healing in early 19th Calcutta. Medical knowledge existed both within the household and among certain recognized women specialists who had commendable skill as practitioners. Moreover, from the point of view of patients, available statistics show that benefits derived from efforts of spreading western medicine in British Bengal were not very noteworthy. In fact, in 20th century Bengal, the maternal as well as infant death rate continued to show upward trends belying any expectation that promotion of western medicine would lead to comparatively better health status for women.[58]

References

1. M. Foucault, *The Birth of the Clinic*, London, Tavistock, 1973, p. 3.
2. A General Hospital was built up in Calcutta for Europeans as early as 1707. The Presidency General Hospital started in 1768 also accommodated only Europeans. In 1787, the government built up another hospital at Dum Dum chiefly for vaccine inoculation among soldiers and their families.
3. It seems that the establishment of charitable dispensaries from the 1830s was one of the earliest attempts to provide western medical care for the Indian people. Dispensaries became local centres for vaccination against smallpox and for conveying western ideas about sanitation and hygiene.
4. David Arnold, *Colonizing the Body: State Medicine and Epidemic Disease in Nineteenth Century India*, OUP, Delhi, 1993, pp. 269-274.
5. Members of this new elite were in many cases descendants of the early indigenous collaborators of European merchant communities who ventured new opportunities and became opulent by serving the mushrooming European commercial houses in Calcutta as *banians* and *dewans* or business intermediaries. With the introduction of the permanent zamindari settlement they became powerful proprietors of landed properties in Bengal gaining further wealth and prominence. It appears that in early 18th century, the Tagore family which later rose into prominence lived in the swamps of Calcutta and acted as suppliers of goods and provisions to captains of ships and free merchants. Darpanarayan Tagore (died in 1793), son of Joyram Tagore who served as *Amin* to the East India Company was a prominent merchant and *banian* of Calcutta. See Pradip Sinha, 'Social Changes', in N. K. Sinha, (ed.), *The History of Bengal (1757–1905)*, University of Calcutta, 1996, (second edition), p. 391.
6. Ramkamal Sen (1783–1844), founder of the famous Sen family of *Kalutola*, initially worked as a compositor in a Hindustani Press on eight rupees a month. He attracted the attention of Dr. Wilson, who later became Professor of Sanskrit in the University of Oxford. He was first promoted to some 'subordinate situation' in the establishment of the Arabic Society, which introduced him to the notice of some of the most distinguished members of the European society... He became a member of the Committee of the Calcutta School Book Society and helped in the compilation and translation of several useful works ... He was placed by Dr. Wilson at the head of the Native Establishment of the Mint. Later on he accepted the office of Treasurer to the Bank of Bengal ... See P. Sinha, *op. cit.*, p. 397.
7. Dwarakanath represented a unique example of far-flung and sophisticated entrepreneurial activities. The whole range of Dwarakanath's business interests included Calcutta house properties, zamindaris, indigo factories, silk filatures, insurance and banking,

commercial houses, coal mines, tea and even shipping. For a discussion of his career and activities see Blair B. Kling, *Partner in Empire: Dwarakanath Tagore and the Age of Enterprise in Eastern India*, Calcutta, 1981.

8. Motilal Seal attained great prominence in the thirties and forties of the 19th century. He has been described a successor of Ramdulal De, the Bengali millionaire who died in 1825 and showed great talent for combining commercial activities with strong speculative skill to the Calcutta money market.
9. Kapil Raj, 'Knowledge, Power and Modern Science: The Brahmins Strike Back' in Deepak Kumar, (ed.), *Science and Empire: Essays in Indian Context (1700–1947)*, Delhi, 1991, p. 120.
10. Aparna Basu, 'The Indian Response to Scientific and Technical Education in the Colonial Era' in Deepak Kumar, (ed.), *Science and Empire*, p. 126.
11. S. N. Sen, *Scientific and Technical Education in India 1781–1900*, New Delhi, 1991, p. 162.
12. The Native Medical Institution or the School for Native Doctors was established in Calcutta in June 1822 to train native doctors. It imparted three-years' training in medicine in vernacular languages. Major English works were translated in Indian languages. The trained doctors were to serve in the army or civil department. The institution became operational in 1824 and existed till 1835.
13. The Calcutta Medical College (CMC), which was established by the order of 20 February, 1835, ushered in a new era in the history of medical education in India. The CMC was the pioneer institution of the east for a systematic education in western medicine. Its stated purpose was to train native youths aged between 14 and 20 irrespective of caste and creed in the principles and practices of medical sciences in accordance with the mode adopted in Europe.
14. B. Kling, *op. cit.*, p. 48.
15. Brajendra Nath Bandopadhyaya (ed.), *Sambadpatrey Sekaler Katha 1818–1840*, 2 vols., Calcutta, 1949–1950, II, p. 315.
16. Kissory Chand Mitra, *Memoir of Dwarakanath Tagore*, Calcutta, 1870, pp. 26–27, p. 64.
17. S. N. Sen, *op.cit.*, pp. 272–3.
18. Madhusudan Gupta was a student of the Native Medical Institution and later became a superintendent of the Hindustani class at Calcutta Medical College. In 1836 he, along with four others, performed dissection on human body.
19. *Centenary Volume of Calcutta Medical College*, Calcutta, 1935, p. 23.
20. *Ibid*, p. 24.
21. M. Borthwick, *The Changing Role of Women in Bengal, 1849–1905*, Princeton, 1984, pp. 156-7.
22. David Arnold has suggested that in the first half of the 19th century, medicine remained an essentially male-oriented and male-operated

system. He has also shown, however, that it became part of the environmental paradigm. The first direct state intervention into Indian women's health came in the 1860s, in the form of the Contagious Diseases Act (1868). It was designed to protect the health of the soldiers and regulated the treatment and quarantine of prostitutes and soldiers in lock hospitals to mitigate the evil of venereal diseases. Discussions about women's health, however, became part of the dominant environmentalist paradigm even as early as 1770s, when John Clark discussed the effects of India's climate on the European female's complexions. Within this dominant paradigm, health of white women was regarded as marker of European vulnerability to Indian climate.

23. James Mill quoted in Dipesh Chakrabarty, 'Postcoloniality and the Artifice of History: Who Speaks for the Indian Pasts?', *Representations, 37.*
24. Dr. Stewart, *Report on the Statistical History of the Female Hospital*, GRPI for 1846–47, Appendix E, no. 10, p. CLXXV.
25. *Centenary Volume of Calcutta Medical College*, pp. 31-35.
26. See Dagmar Engels, *Beyond Purdah? Women in Bengal 1890–1930*, Delhi, 1999, p. 125.
27. J. Jolly, *Indian Medicine*, trans. from German by C. G. Kushikar, New Delhi, 1977, p. 69.
28. Borthwick, *op.cit.*, p. 155.
29. G. W. Briggs, *The Chamars,* Calcutta, 1920, pp. 24–26, 53–54, quoted In Charu Gupta *Sexuality, Obscenity, Community: Women, Muslims and the Hindu Public in Colonial India*, Delhi, 2001, p. 177.
30. Janet Chawla, *Child-Bearing and Culture—Women-Centred Revisioning of the Traditional Midwife: The Dai as a Ritual Practitioner*, New Delhi, 1994, pp. 2-3, 80-2.
31. G. Forbes, 'Managing Midwifery in India', in D. Engels and Shula Marks (eds), *Contesting Colonial Hegemony: State and Society in Africa and India*, London, OUP, 1994, p. 156.
32. *Ibid*, p. 157.
33. B. Ehrenreich and D. English, *Complaints and Disorders: The Sexual Politics of Sickness*, London, 1976, p. 23.
34. P. H. Chavasse, *Counsel to a Mother*, London, 1868, p. 3.
35. P. Branca, *Women in Europe since 1750*, London, 1978.
36. M. Borthwick, *op.cit.*, p. 157.
37. G. Forbes, 'Managing Midwifery in India', pp. 157-8.
38. M. Balfour and Ruth Young, *The Work of Medical Women in India*, London, OUP, 1929, pp. 13-14.
39. G. H. Forbes, 'In Search of the "Pure Heathen": Missionary Women in Nineteenth Century India', *Economic and Political Weekly*, XXI/17 (26 April 1986), pp.WS2-WS8.
40. Janaki Nair, 'Uncovering the Zenana: Visions of Indian Womanhood in Engliswomen's Writings, 1813–1940', *Journal of Women's History,* 2, 11, spring 1990, pp. 88-94.

41. Indrani Sen, *Woman and Empire: Representation in the Writings of British India (1858–1900)*, New Delhi, 2002, p. 53.
42. G. Forbes, 'Colonial Imperatives and Women's Emancipation: Western Medical Education for Indian Women in Nineteenth Century Bengal', *Modern Historical Studies*, Journal of the Department of History, Rabindra Bharati University, vol. 2, 2001, pp. 83-102.
43. M. Balfour and Ruth Young, *op. cit.*, pp. 13, 29, 16-18.
44. G. Forbes, 'Colonial Imperatives...', p. 86.
45. Editor's introduction to excerpts from Hannah Catherine Mullens, 'Phulmani to Karunar Bibaran', in Susie Tharu and K. Lalitha (eds.) *Women Writing in India, vol. 1: 600 BC to the Present*, New York, 1991, p. 205.
46. D. Arnold, *op.cit.*, p. 261.
47. G. A. Kittredge, *A Short History of the "Medical Women for India" Fund of Bombay*, Bombay: Education Society's Press, 1889, p. 3.
48. Mary Scharlieb, *Reminiscences*, London, 1924, pp. 29–30.
49. Malavika Karlekar, 'Kadambini and the Bhadralok,' *Economic and Political Weekly*, 21, 19 (April 26, 1986), pp. WS25-WS21.
50. Sir Alfred Croft, *Review of Education in India in 1886 with Special Reference to the Report of the Education Commission*, Calcutta, 1888, p. 287, cited in S. N. Sen, *op.cit.,* p. 514.
51. S. N. Sen, *Ibid.*
52. Maneesha Lal, 'The Politics of Gender and Medicine in Colonial India: The Countess of Dufferin's Fund, 1885–1888', *Bulletin of History of Medicine*, 68, 1994, pp. 29-66.
53. *Ibid.*
54. 'Female Medical Education (Campbell Medical College)', *Proceeding of the Lieutenant Government of Bengal, General Dept., Education.* (West Bengal Archives), (November, 1887): File 21–26.
55. *Ibid.*, 2498 (April 6, 1887): File 21–7.
56. G. Forbes, 'Colonial Imperatives...', p. 97.
57. Sujata Mukherjee, 'Women, Medicine and Empire: Female Practitioners and Patterns of Health Care in Colonial Bengal', *Historical Studies*, Journal of the Department of History, Rabindra Bharati University, vol. 2, 2001, pp. 187-204.
58. Sujata Mukherjee, 'Disciplining the Body? Health Care for Women and Children in Early Twentieth Century Bengal' in Deepak Kumar (ed.) *Disease and Medicine in India: A Historical Overview*, New Delhi, 2001, pp. 198-214.

Social Work

17
Social Construction of Health: Changing Paradigms

—*Vijay Kumar Yadavendu*

The ahistorical progression of the science of health divested of its social and economic moorings reveals a commitment to a science characterized by positivism and extreme rationalism. Above all, it reveals a manifest commitment to methodological individualism which continues to dominate the understanding of epidemiology up to the present.

As the discipline of medical sociology and psychology interact with health, a similar reification of the quantitative method is seen at the expense of the development of a theory of a society which contours the occurrence of disease. This in nowhere more evident than the current marriage of behaviourism to health. Self-care, self-help, and modification in individual lifestyles are the main concerns. Such an ideology obfuscates both the cause of disease and ill health in a society and therefore, the quest for solutions. Despite the broadening, the use of social sciences is still confined in the prison of reductionism. This study tries in its different sections to expose the handiwork of such deterministic science.

Theoretical Derivation

Thomas Kuhn in his book, *The Structure of Scientific Revolution* (1962), argues that the principle characteristic of any field of scientific enquiry, during any particular epoch in its development, is the fundamental paradigm that organizes the practice of 'normal science' during that epoch. Hence, astronomy some five hundred years ago passed from the paradigm of geocentricism to that of heliocentricism and beyond.

Yet, if one were to inquire about the fundamental paradigm currently in practice, in the study of health, silence is likely to follow. At the very most, social scientists, whose primary orientation is disciplinary (e.g., economics, sociology, psychology) rather than substantive (e.g., health) would respond with paradigms from their respective disciplines; moral hazard, (sick) role, pluralism and so forth. To move closer still, pathology and medicine do have their own paradigms, but like those imposed by social science, beg the substantive issues of 'health' itself.

To first gain some intellectual distance on the subject, however, a brief look at the development of paradigm structures in the psychology of intelligence could be useful. The classical paradigm in the study of intelligence by Binet was that of a universal, genetically fixed endowment of cognitive capacity—specifically, the innate ability to solve extrinsically defined problems. That is, 'intelligence' (according to this paradigm) was (and is) assumed to be qualitatively invariant across culture and secularly invariant through societies over time. Moreover, in a particular individual, cognitive capacity was assumed to be largely fixed genetically, and the degree of its achievement was determined by the individual's social and cultural context. Intelligence testing, at its best, was aimed at measuring the endowment of such 'intelligence' whereas learning theory, and, in its more applied form, schooling are assumed to be directed at the attempt to achieve the maximum use of the differentially distributed, but qualitatively universal, cognitive capacity.

Beginning with Piaget, however, the validity of the motion of 'intelligence' as an analytical entity having a real empirical correspondent is no longer universally accepted. Instead, according to Piaget and his followers, 'intelligence is merely a continuous interaction between perception and cognition, each in its turn altering the other' [Ginsburg and Opper 1969]. Whereas Piaget's contribution lies in his apparently correct recognition that 'intelligence' is not an endowed entity, the weakness of his viewpoint and that of his followers, lies in their view of 'intelligence' as a universal process. That is, his lifetime of research has been devoted to verifying that in all societies the same stages of cognitive development are experienced. In sum, whereas the scholars of the Binet School perceive 'intelligence' as a universal entity, Piaget and his followers see it as a universal process, similar in all societies, culminating, as one psychologist has put it, in the form of a Swiss scientist [U. Neisser 1976].

Over much the same period as the development of Piaget's work, a third group of psychologists has, in effect, attempted to supplant this paradigm and pursue empirical research on the premise that 'the fundamental categories of psychological processes in man are of an historical character and that psychology must be understood as a historical science' [A. Luria 1971]. As Berry notes:

> Over the past 70 years, there have been sporadic but recurrent assertions of the notion that people raised in different cultures are different intellectually have different cognitive competencies. These assertions appear to go beyond the usually accepted notions that there are *qualitatively* differing cognitive competencies appropriate to the requirements of a particular culture. Whether all peoples have access to all dimensions, (but produce a different pattern of scores on them), or the same people have access to the some unique dimensions, is immaterial; what matters, is the assertion of more than a single universal dimension called (in the West) 'intelligence' [Berry 1972].

Continuing on this track, then, the scientific effort is directed to the identification of the 'quantitatively differing cognitive competence' and most important, to the understanding of the mechanism by which different societal forms generate and promote different 'cognitive competencies'. The present endeavour is not for the elaboration of the development of intelligence psychology, but rather the demonstration of that which is to be argued in the case of 'health'.

Individuation of Health and Medicine

The discussion of health and medicine began to emerge in early Greek society with its own theories and practitioners. Health was achieved when the four humours—blood, phlegm, yellow bile, and black bile—were in balance in the human body. Hippocrates wrote in *Airs, Waters and Places* that:

> Whoever wishes to investigate medicine properly should proceed thus: in the first place to consider the seasons of the year and what effects each of them produces. Then the winds the hot and cold, especially such as are common to all countries and then such as are peculiar to each locality ... One should consider most attentively the waters which the inhabitants use ... the mode in which the inhabitants live, and what are their pursuits, whether they are fond of drinking and eating to excess, and given to indolence, or are fond of exercise and labour.[1]

He further pointed out that human well-being is influenced by the totality of environmental factors, living habits or lifestyles, climate, topography of the land, and the quality of air, water, and food. It seems obvious that the Greeks had adopted an internal view on health and believed that medical intervention and prevention in the social and physical environment were necessary for health. Roman medicine accepted the Greek pattern. However, under the great physician Galen, the empirical content of medicine was on the rise and transition from religious to scientific orientation in the conception of health and disease began.

Medicine was integrally involved with the development of mechanistic science. Starting with Kepler and Galileo's observations of the solar system, the centuries old dialectic between the 'Platonic-Pythagorean tradition and Renaissance naturalism versus the mechanical or natural philosophy began to be resolved in favour of the latter' [R. S. Westfall 1977]. Renaissance naturalism or vitalism had upheld the union of spirit and matter in the world; it saw underlying essences reflected in all of nature. In supplanting medieval religious metaphors about disease, however, the discourses of Enlightenment provided for their secular replacement. In the case of the human body, the new metaphor was the machine. Early medical scientists such as Vesalius and Harvey saw the body merely as the homologue of machine, i.e., structured similarity. Harvey noted 'from the structure of the heart, it is clear that the blood is constantly carried through the lungs into the aorta as by two clack (valves) of water bellows to raise water' [Westfall 1977:90]. The domination of Renaissance naturalism can be seen in Harvey's view of the heart as 'the beginning of life'. He wrote:

> The mechanism of circulation was less important in understanding the body than was the vitalistic idea that the heart and blood together forming a single functioning unit which is the very seat of life [*Ibid.,* 9].

Descartes utilized Harvey's work on circulation as the basis for a truly mechanistic perception of the body. The first apparent scientific paradigm for health originated with the development of the machine model of the human body [Reiser 1978; Shylock 1969]. This new science of the Renaissance began for the first time to map out in detail the internal workings of the human body. The mechanistic view analysed living things as sets of mechanical parts such as cogs and pulleys driven by a heart-pump. People were considered machines and a sick person was compared to an ill-made clock. Empiricists like Hobbes, Bacon, and Descartes provided the philosophical and ideological groundwork behind such a model of a human being. Descrates believed that the human body worked like a machine, a machine that performs all the physiological functions of a man:

> I want you to consider (he concluded) that all these functions in this machine follow naturally from the disposition of its organs alone, just as the movement of a clock or another automate follow from the disposition of its counter weights and wheels; so that to explain its functions it is not necessary to imagine a vegetative or sensitive soul in the machine, or any other principle of movement and life other than its blood and spirits agitated by the fire which burns continually in its heart and which differs in nothing from all the fires in inanimate bodies [Westfall 1970: 93]

Descartes argued that the human body not only worked like a machine but also that the mind and the body of a given individual could be separated into two substances—one 'corporeal' or material and the other 'incorporeal' or immaterial.[2] With this conception, 'health' came to be seen as the perfect working order of human organism, likening the human organism to an automation (a self-propelling machine) [Rossdale 1965]. Moreover, the methodologies of pathology and diagnostics that developed from this view (and continues to dominate in the practice of medicine today) consider illness to be both natural (biological) and occurring on an individual basis. Treatment, therefore is pursued on an individual bio-chemo-surgical basis, relegating the recognition and implications of social causes of illness to secondary importance, though even this secondary recognition must be viewed as an 'ad hoc modification' [T. Kuhn 1962: 78]. The Aristotelian paradigm with its belief in the organic unity of living things, was gradually replaced by 'mechanistic medicine' which ultimately made possible those aspects of medicine which have been genuinely successful either in prevention or cure of disease or in providing symptomatic relief.

But the adoption of a mechanistic paradigm limits the nature and boundaries of what is conceived as the medical task. Thus, scientific medicine ultimately became curative, individualistic, and interventionist, objectifying patients and denying their status as social beings [L. Doyal 1981]. For Jewson, scientific medicine has to pass through three basic stages (which he sees as corresponding to three successive modes of production of medical knowledge), viz.: 'bedside medicine', 'hospital medicine', and 'laboratory medicine' [N. Jewson 1976]. As Doyal (1981) notes: 'these stages provide a useful means by which to understand both the development of medical thought and practice and also its relationship to broader social and economic changes'.

'Bedside medicine' which dominated western Europe from the Middle Ages until the late 18th century was available to 'minority groups' such as the wealthy and worked on a patronage system with patients choosing those particular doctors whom they believed could help them the most [N. Jewson 1974: 369–385]. Until then, the 'new science' (i.e., science after Renaissance) had little impact on medical practice and patron/doctor relationship was the very important determinant of the content of medical treatment. The patient's choice, or in Jewson's terminology, 'sickman' was the centre of medical concern, the patient being treated as a whole.

By the beginning of the 19th century, with the advent of the Industrial Revolution the concomitant process of mass urbanization and 'hospital medicine' [Jewson 1976] came into existence, and dramatic changes occurred even in medical practices. Mass urbanization led to unhealthy cities and the consequence was the establishment of big hospitals for catering to the health needs of the working population. Client-centred therapy was losing its dominance now, and even doctors excluding lay persons, midwives, etc., were becoming more organized in their profession.

Patients were no longer individuals with their own particular set of symptoms and problems, but came increasing to be seen as 'cases'—the disease became more important than the sick person [K. Figlio 1977]. It was the loss of the self in the complex social system where professionalism or individualism was on the rise. 'Hospital medicine' shifted during this period to diagnosis and classification and the Aristotelian flavour, which had characterized the theoretical base of individual centred therapy, was sidelined. Ilich has beautifully described the significance of this process:

> If 'sickness' and 'health' were to lay claim to public resources, then these concepts had to be made operational, aliments had to be turned into objective diseases. Species had to be clinically defined and verified so those officials could fit them into wards, records, budgets and museums. The object of medical treatments defined by a new, though submerged, political ideology, acquired the status of an entity that existed quite separately from both doctors and patients [Ilich 1976].

Thus, with the advent of 'hospital medicine', the emphasis shifted from a belief in disease as a disturbance of the total system to what is called 'localized pathology'. This was the period of development of new instruments and sophistication in descriptive anatomy and pathology where statistical analyses were used. The development of statistical tools substantially aided this process. The methods that developed as a consequence diminished the role even of the social, economic, and environmental factors.

With the development of the germ theory of disease, in the late 9th century, the emphasis in medical practice swung even more sharply towards the individual 'case' [Doyal 1981: 33]. The germ theory's placement of blame for most sickness and disease on micro-organisms served to effectively diminish the role of social and economic factors in the disease causation that has become the hallmark of the dominant mode of epidemiological practice to the present day. Scientific medicine or 'hospital medicine', focused on the biological problems of the individual in order to understand and treat most disease. The diagnosis of illness was made on an individual basis, and treatment or therapy was also individually prescribed [N. Coulins 1977]. Laboratory medicine was observed as the final victory of the mechanistic worldview in the latter half of the 19th century. As Doyal (1981) puts it:

> At that time, a struggle for supremacy between vitalism, (a brief in the inviolability and unity of living organism) and mechanicalism (which perceive organism merely as sets of inner-related parts) was on and finally mechanicalism got the upper hand. By the middle of the 19th century, mechanism had become dominant and experiments and vivisection had replaced comparative anatomy as the basic method for advancing medical knowledge.

At the same time, doctors became more active interventionists in the physiological processes rather than being passive observers. Medicine was on the way to gaining full recognition as a science. As Doyal (1981: 33) further notes:

> In latter half of the 19th century, both history and physiology were developed extremely rapidly and individual cell came increasingly to be seen as the central focus for understanding ill health. Cell theory and controlled clinical trials did not immediately provide any new therapy, but they did form the basis for 20th century developmonts in clinical medicine.

This biological reductionism, instrumentalism, elementalism, or positivism widened the gap between the doctor and the patient. It has been observed that this version of the natural world was a victory of the industrial bourgeoisie, which established the positivist conception of science, and of medicine [V. Navarro 1986]. Medicine has been characterized by what Jewson calls a shift from person-oriented to an object-oriented cosmology. As Doyal puts it: 'it is always individuals who become sick, rather than social, economic or environmental factors which cause them to be so' [Doyal 1981]. Stark has commented:

> Disease is understood as a failure in and of the individual, an isolatable 'thing' that attacks the physical machine more or less arbitrarily from 'outside' preventing it from fulfilling its essential 'responsibilities'. Both bourgeois epidemiology and medical ecology ... consider 'society' only as a relatively passive medium through which 'germs' pass en route to the individual [E. Stark 1977].

There are problems with this approach, which still dominate contemporary medicine. The physician deals with an individual patient (already a socially determined process) [B. Stern 1980]. The patient is not an abstract being, but of a certain age, sex, race and class and has internalized a specific historical experience from childhood to adulthood [W. Reich 1970, 1972]. The taking of purely medical history individuates the patient; however, the disease or injury from which the patient is suffering, is received as part of a collective experience in a particular historical, cultural, and social setting. These latter circumstances are as much a part of the cause, and should be part of the treatment, as purely medical facts (The medical facts themselves are social historical facts). Thus, the essence of scientific medicine's treatment of disease discourages a proper understanding of disease by excluding from consideration the most relevant internalization of the external world by the patient. As Wartofsky puts it: 'Human ontology cannot be reduced to an social or ahistorical biology without doing violence to the very specificity of human biological structure and function itself' [M. Wartofsky 1975].

By abstracting disease from its social framework and reducing it to the biological sphere, social conditions could be and were ignored. Scientific medicine became consistent with and indeed legitimated capitalist development by integrating a model of healing with the social structure; in so doing, scientific medicine has obscured the relationship between disease and the nature and form of social development. Today, heat disease, cancer, and auto accident are posited as 'diseases of civilization' [J. H. Knowles 1977]. They are conceived of as necessary consequences of economic growth and industrialism, when it is uncertain that this is so [Eyer and Sterling 1977].

The major concern of scientific medicine, consequently, is to render the body more functional in its struggle to adapt to the potentially antagonistic forces of nature. In contrast to the World Health Organization's (WHO) definition of health as 'physical, mental, and social well-being, not merely the absence of disease or infirmity', health tends to be defined in functional rather than in experimental terms, as the absence of disease. The defining of health and illness in a functional way is an important example of how a capitalist value system defines people primarily as producers. It is concerned with their 'fitness' in an instrumental sense, rather than with their hopes, fears, anxieties, pain or suffering [Doyal 1981]. In the therapeutic relationship, the task of the patient is to understand the sign and symbols of the problems as the physician reads them, and thus to accept the medical definition of both the problem and the solution. Taussing (1980) calls this process:

> The creation from a 'phantom-objectivity' with regard to disease, a process of 'denying the human relations embodied in symptoms, signs and therapy', a process by which 'we not only mystify social relations, but we also reproduce a political ideology in the guise of a science of apparently 'real things'—biological and physical thinghood'.[3]

Further Taussing concludes:

> Medical practice is a singularity important way of maintaining the denial as to the social facticity of facts. Things thereby take on a life of their own, sundered from the social nexus that really gives them life, and remain locked in their own self constitution.

From the many factors that contribute to disease—social, environmental, physical, psychological—'western' medicine tends to isolate a single physical factor and label it the 'cause'. Dubos (1959) explains that Pasteur and Koch's conceptualization of germ theory created experimental conditions that were sufficient to bring the host and parasite together to produce disease and thus minimized the influence of other factors. The focus on the doctrine of specific aetiology and germ theory facilitated the transformation of health into a commodity, amenable to sale in the market, fulfilling the basic need of the capitalist system for commodification. With this commodity fetishism, health problems become problems of the body, which require consumption of some form of technological treatment, rather than a reflection of social relations. Navarro explains this beautifully as the need for consumption, 'consumption that reflects a dependency of the individual as something that can be bought, either a pill, a drug, a prescription, a car, or the pre-packaged moon' [V. Navarro 1976].

Epidemiology and Health

This does not mean that nothing was done in the field of 'public health'. The devastation wrought by industrial and urbanization process was impossible to ignore even in the first half of the 19th century and outside hospitals, the relationship between disease and urbanization and living working conditions was becoming widely accepted. The socio-political and socio-economic events set the stage for the development of modern epidemiology, sociology, geography, psychology, and anthropology.

The development of epidemiology is rather different from other social sciences. Its 'greening period' [A. M. Lilienfeld and D. E. Lilienfeld 1980] is placed in mid-1800s, a few decades before the classics of Durkheim and Weber were published. Lilienfeld and Lilienfeld describe Louis as an important founding father of modern epidemiology. As early as 1833, he pioneered the importance of statistical methods in medicine. The construct of mortality is even older. Graunt, a London haberdasher published the *Bills of Mortality* in 1662 [K. J. Rothman 1981]. In those early days, the discovery of aetiology of infectious diseases was an important purpose of epidemiology and its development was closely connected to that of public hygiene and vaccination policy. Gradually its scope and purpose expanded beyond the area of treatment to the prevention of disease as well. After the Second World War, the emphasis on population-based epidemiological research came to be on the rise.

Traditionally, epidemiology has been associated with disease prevention and the Oxford dictionary defines epidemiology as 'that branch of medical science which treats epidemics' (The Compact Edition of the *OED* 1971). The term epidemic can be replaced with the phrase 'major public health problems'. The roots of today's epidemiology have been detected in the work of William Farr who established a tradition of careful application of vital data to problems of public health and other broad public concerns. At the time, work by sanitarians like Farr, Edwin Chadwick, and John Snow and particularly Chadwick's immense investigation published in 1842 as *The Sanitary Conditions of the Labouring Population of Great Britain,*[4] illustrated the close relationship between poverty and disease, a connection which was stressed in contemporary debates as the public health questions. Many of the major accomplishments of public health resulted from epidemiological studies in the classic tradition of John Snow's investigation of cholera, and it is at this level that the science and model of epidemiology have perhaps most clearly demonstrated their worth. Thus, serious physical hazards have been identified, legislations have restricted these hazards and demonstrable improvements in the health of the populations as a whole have been observed. Even here, however, the overriding requirement that epidemiological study examine only those factors which are conventionally regarded as objective, has effectively eclipsed many other aspects of the conditions under study. It has appeared to be enough to investigate the connections between a given illness (or range of illness) and the factors which are suspected of being associated with the conditions under consideration. Epidemiology as applied to public health at the macro level in future may thus proceed in one or two ways: either the major 'medical' issues of the day will be faced (through a recognition that events in the real world have a socio-economic setting which must be articulated and addressed via more stringent attention to underlying theoretical, contextual, as well as methodological development in epidemiology) with the corollary that political involvement is unavoidable, or epidemiology will become apparently methodologically sophisticated, but effectively irrelevant, aside in the tide of history [C. K. Cassel 1983].

In the dominant paradigm of understanding, epidemiology is regarded as 'essentially and inductive science' (*Ibid.*), and in epidemiology the casual concept is essentially a reductionistic, mechanical one (the concept of disease agent/risk factor). It is disease-centred (disease being a biomedical concept) and concerned with biological inferences. Thus epidemiology as presently constituted fails to face up to the question of how to promote health at the most basic and essential levels.

There is perhaps no more obvious illustration of medical care of basic level than that of the sort discussed by Rifkin (1985) in her text on community health initiatives in the developing world. There seems little doubt in these contexts about which conditions—both of the environment at large, and of the individual in particular—constitute the present major threats to health and well-being [M. King 1966], but there remains considerable dissension concerning priorities between those embedded, for instance, between the technologically complex and status laden medical tradition of scientific medicine, and those involved in 'low technology' health care. In this context, Rifkin (1985) cites Ross as distinguishing three types of community health development, viz, the 'external' approach, the 'multiple' approach, and the 'inner resources' approach. These approaches, as generally perceived, involve progressively more grassroots commitment and correspondingly less professional or 'expert' diagnosis and mobilization with regard to health 'needs' and 'problems' (so progressing from 'top down' to 'bottom up' approaches and planning). Of these approaches, it might at present be argued that epidemiology as usually understood, services and informs the 'top down' approach; epidemiology enable 'experts' to act (with whatever level of 'community' consultation or involvement) on 'problems' identified in professional terms. Social epidemiology, as this type of research is called, received emphasis during the war on poverty programmes of the early 1960s and, at the same time, gave some scientific justification for their inauguration and continuance [Israel 1978; I. Waldron 1977]. Studies indicated differences in occurrence, severity, and length of specific illness based upon a person's income, race, age, and especially class. While these findings became widely accepted within the discipline of epidemiology, unfortunately they had very little impact on medical education. Yet, just associating a relationship between social characteristics, disease incidence, and health status does not fully explain the totality of those relationships. To the extent that social epidemiology was content to remain on a descriptive level, it became merely a form of demography [*Ibid*].

Although the recognition of the social basis of many diseases and ill health goes far back in medical history, the greatest boost probably came with the publication of the *Chadwick Report* in England and the Shattuck Report in the US in the middle of the 19th century. Since that time, social epidemiology and environmentalist approach to health (which is considered the second paradigm in the discussion of health, for it is clearly in conflict with the biological and individual orientation of the classical school), came to be the predominant methodology. While social epidemiology allows for the use of 'multifactorial' explanation for disease occurrence, it still tends to rely upon a notion of specific aetiology and sees social and economic factors as contributive rather than causative.

The parallel between the social epidemiologist and the Piaget's school is quite striking. Both go beyond bio-individualism in recognizing that 'health' in the one case and 'intelligence' in the other, arise out of developmental process in which the individual interacts with the social environment. Both, however, generally assume the respective processes, and indeed 'health' and 'intelligence' themselves, to be universal—independent of the form of society in which they are investigated. Whereas Piaget normatively conceives of intelligence as the highest stage of universal cognitive competence, the social epidemiologists accordingly conceive health as a lack of breakdown in a universal notion of human organismic integrity. Both these assumptions are being seriously challenged in their respective disciplines.

Epidemiology is a discipline, which is concerned with health and its maintenance in a population. By definition, it is interdisciplinary in nature and calls for skills beyond disciplinary grids, which many social science approaches fall short of, whether in sociology, anthropology, or psychology. Although the social basis of epidemiology was recognized, the actual operationalization of this was in the form of discrete disciplinary inputs such as medical sociology, medical anthropology, health psychology, etc. In disease-centred epidemiology, social factors are hardly used in conceptual frameworks. In exposure-oriented epidemiology, current practice is that the factors under study are conceptualized by a specialist, e.g., nutritionists, immunologists, who are trained not to understand the phenomenon of health it its entirety, but to offer intervention and solution and not provide explanation when medicine is put into practice. The role of social sciences in health was, however, to provide explanations and offer solutions in the practice of medicine. Nevertheless, in spite of its limitations one cannot overlook the positive contribution and the changes wrought in the approach to health by areas such as medical sociology.

Medical Sociology and Health

There were works in the area of medicinal sociology in which the sociological study of illness and medicine were covered. Strauss differentiated between sociology 'of' medicine and sociology 'in' medicine. Sociology of medicine focuses on the study of medicine to illuminate some sociological concern (e.g., patient-practitioner relationship, the role of professions in society). Sociology in medicine, on the other hand, focuses primarily on a medical problem, e.g., the sociological causes of disease and illness, reasons for delay in seeking medicinal aid, patient compliance or non-compliance with medical regimens, etc. [R. Strauss 1981]. The conceptual dichotomy between these two approaches is more apparent than real. For legitimizing the cause of public health, exponents like Virchow in Germany and Chadwick in England emphasized the role of economic, social, political, psychological, and cultural factors in health and illness. Virchow, a social medicine physician, called for measures such as free public education, separation of church and state, higher wages, progressive taxation, cultural autonomy for natural minorities, agricultural collectives, and full employment [Ackerknecht 1953]. Rosen (1955) traces the term 'medical sociology' back to early 1900 Germany, related to Grotjahn's *Social Pathology* published in 1911. But it is clear that the emergence of medical sociology as an organized discipline occurred in the years after Second World War, i.e., in the late 1950s.

The 'boom' in medical sociology, the sharp increase in systematic development of the field in terms of both quality and quantity occurred during the 1970s. One thing should be made very clear and that is, medical sociology is, in a sense, synonymous with dominant American sociological paradigms. The prominent figures included Talcott Parsons, Evert Hughes, Robert Merton and August Hollingshead. Their interest in medical sociology derived from broader sociological issues. Parson's work on medicine as a social institution and illness as a deviance was an illustration of a larger theory of society; Merton used medicine as an example of a profession in the study of professions; Hughes's work was done within the framework of occupational sociology; and Hollingshead's main focus was on social class [S. W. Bloom 1979]. Parsons took a structural functionalistic perspective while the Chicago School stressed symbolic interactionism [V. L. Olesen 1975]. Parsons's functionalist orientation suffers from a particular form of ahistoricism. In capitalist society, functional health, subordinated as it is to the process of accumulation, refers only to the capacity to contribute to that process, not the capacity to perform any role or task, productive or not.

In the attempt to sketch the hopes and aspirations of medical sociology, both in the past and in the present, one is immediately confronted by an essential problem, i.e., the difficulty of finding a valid definition. Medical sociology can be described as the study of social factors in health and illness (referring to illness as the experience of becoming and being ill and its behavioural counterparts) and of the constructions of medical reality of social factors in health care. Older definitions of medical sociology as sociology of medicine and sociology in medicine [Freeman, Levine and Reeder 1979], and more recent emphasis on health and illness itself [D. L. Patrick and G. Scambler 1982] are combined in this description.

In general terms, it can be argued that the main goal of medical sociology is to improve the conditions of living for human beings. This includes analysing inequalities in the distribution and frequency of diseases as well as in the provision and utilization of health care services. It had been hoped that demonstrating inequalities would prove to be a challenge to get rid of them, and that medical sociology could provide not only the findings but also the scientific prerequisites for working and practicable solutions in health and social policy that were indicated by such findings. The analysis of medical institutions, of the providers of health care, and of their socialization, as well as of health behaviour of people, was to bring about predictive statements that would facilitate planning. Thus, many medical sociologists aimed at improving the efficacy of medicine and its institutions by analysing them, a task, which is in accordance with the humanitarian commitment of medical sociology.

This implies that medical sociology cannot be pursued without an orientation to values. This branch of knowledge, therefore, could be expected to base itself on the ethic of humanitarianism, and to be committed first of all to the social welfare of persons in time of health as well as of illness. This would inevitable lead to conflicts both with medicine and most powerful representatives, the physicians. Nor was it surprising that medical sociology, in its striving to emphasize the social dimensions of illness, turned out to be receptive to, if not even in occasions enthusiastic about psychosomatic medicine as well as the mental health movement in general. In spite of a considerable body of empirical findings, one still has a limited understanding of unequal distribution of diseases. After Parsons, it was perhaps justified to expect a 'grand theory' to be attainable also in medical sociology. But it has restricted itself to 'theories of middle range' and to even narrower hypotheses, which in the last years have tended to hide behind the pretentious concept of 'models'.

The health services system has not achieved greater efficacy and efficiency as a result of medical sociological research. The scientific parochialism that is common in this field is indeed deplorable. What are needed then, are cross-cultural surveys that would lead to such questions. There are a number of authors who recognize this to be a real dilemma, but even among the most critical, medical value scales are often accepted without question. A similar situation exists in the field of social policy. Gouldner notes:

> The state ... does not only require a social science that can facilitate planned intervention to resolve certain social problems, it also requires social science to serve as a rhetoric, to persuade resistant to undecided segments of the society that such problems do, indeed, exist and are of dangerous propositions [A. W. Gouldner 1971].

Evaluation in this case, according to Gouldner, serves to prove the inefficiency of former elites and of traditional procedures. The welfare states are using it to unmask the competitor. However, in welfare states the process does not go beyond that. It satisfies itself just by maintaining the status quo. Medical sociology then becomes a mere instrument of propaganda for the welfare state or a producer of ideologies as formalated by the German sociologist Lepsius.[5] Gouldner's insights, which he may owe to his experiences in health services research, are highly relevant for medical sociology. They reveal a vast potential, but also hidden dangers in medical sociology. Since many medical sociologists have so readily adopted medical conceptions of values, it should not be difficult to induce them to adjust to other ideologies provided only that they can be convinced—or can convince themselves—that all is done only 'for the patients' best'. In the foregoing, I have discussed some substantive aspects of medical sociology. What remains is a critical analysis of the literature itself, that is to say, a review of the publications as such. Medical sociologic writing has turned out to be a rather one-sided affair. After some tentative steps in different directions, the scientists have concentrated on a few selected areas, much like directing a wide stream into narrow channels while leaving the rest of the country, by far the larger part, untouched, a dry and unexplored waste. The torrents of publications on the topics of death and dying, health behaviour, or labelling theory, which have flooded the fields of medical sociology, are an example.

Feminist critics have viewed the medical profession as a largely patriarchal institution that used definitions of illness and disease to maintain the relative inequality of women by drawing attention to their weakness and susceptibility to illness and by taking control over areas of women's lives such as pregnancy and childbirth that were previously the domain of female lay practitioners and midwives. The dominant current in medical sociology failed to provide spaces for such criticisms. Most critiques advocate the 'empowerment' of patients, encouraging people to 'take back control' over their own health by engaging in preventive health activities. These were the trends of medical critique in the 1970s and into the 1980s. It remains the dominant approach in 1990s for feminist writers, for those who adhere to a Marxist perspective on health and illness and proponents of the consumerist approach to medicine. The problem with the orthodox critiques such as those of Ivan Illich is the rather black and white portrayal of scientific medicine, as largely detracting from, rather than improving people's health status, of doctors as intent on increasing their power over their patron rather than seeking to help them, and of patients as largely helpless, passive and disempowered, their agency crushed beneath the might of the medical profession [D. Lupton 1977]. 'The asymmetry of relationship is exaggerated to the point that the lay client becomes not the beneficiary but the victim of consultation' [Atkinson 1995]. In their efforts to denounce medicine as an oppressive force, orthodox critics undermine the positive contributions of medicine. They also fail to acknowledge the ambivalent nature of the feelings and opinions that many people have in relation to medicine or the ways by which patients willingly participate in medical dominance. This complicity inevitably incorporates latent conflict and resistance, 'a shifting balance between manifest collaboration and tacit opposition in relations between those who come for help and those who profess to provide it' [de Swaan 1997]. So, there is no struggle for power between the dominant party (doctors) and less powerful party (patients), but rather, there is collusion between the two to reproduce medical dominance. Foucault's writings emphasize the positive and productive rather than the repressive nature of power [Lupton 1997]. Further, Foucault argued that the very seductiveness of power in modern societies is that it is productive rather than simply confining:

> What makes power hold good, what makes it accepted, is simply the fact that it doesn't weigh on as a force that says no, but that it traverses and produces things, it produces pleasure, forms knowledge, produces discourse. It needs to be considered as a productive network, which runs through the whole social body, much more than as a negative instance whose function is repression [Foucault 1984a quoted by Lupton 1997: 98].

From this perspective, medical power may be viewed as the underlying resource by which diseases and illness are identified and dealt with. The power that doctors have in relation to the patient, therefore, might be thought of as a facilitating capacity or resource, a means of bringing into being the subjects 'doctor' and 'patient' and the phenomenon of patient's illness. From this perspective, doctors are not considered to be 'figures of domination', but rather 'links in a set of power relations', 'people through whom power passe(s) who are important in the field of power relation' [Foucault 1984b quoted by D. Lupton 1997: 99]. Unlike orthodox critiques, Foucauldian perspective argues, therefore, that it is impossible to remove power from members of the medical profession and hand it over to patients; power is not a possession of particular social groups, but is relational, a strategy that is invested in and transmitted through all social groups [Lupton 1997]. The orthodox critiques tend to view members of the medical profession as consciously seeking to gain power and status and limit other groups' power, largely by eliciting the state's support. In contrast, Foucauldian scholars tend to argue that the classical gaze is not intentional in terms of originating from a particular type of group seeking domination over others. There is not a single medicine but a series of loosely linked assemblages each with different rationalities [T. Osborne 1997: 100]. People are constantly urged to conduct their everyday lives in order to avoid potential disease or early death. As a result, 'sociologically speaking everyone lives under the medical regime, a light regime for those who are not yet patients, stricter according to how dependent on doctors one becomes' [de Swaan 1997].

Neither the orthodox critique nor the Foucauldian perspective has adequately taken account of the mutual dependencies and the emotional and psychodynamic dimensions of the medical encounter, preferring to rely upon a notion of the rational actor. Yet, as I argued, a recognition of the 'irrational' and contradictory aspects of the relationship that lay people have with members of the medical profession goes some way to explaining why it is that 'power, after investing itself in the body finds itself exposed to a counter attack in the same body' [Lupton 1997].

Psychology and Health

The day to day practice of psychological researchers in mainstream, bourgeois psychology is governed by 'variable model'. Under this model, the subject matter of psychology is conceived of as a universe of actually or a potentially measurable variables, the relation among which forms the basis for all of the discipline's scientific propositions and laws. The rise of capitalism was at the same time the rise of the middle class, the 'bourgeoisie'. The prevailing social scientific theories and their underlying philosophy will reflect these bourgeois values. Psychology in general, and health psychology in particular, is not an exception. Health psychology is the offshoot of this bourgeois, positivist psychology. It is claimed that psychology and medicine have a long history of collaboration and at least psychology's involvement in health and illness go back well over a century. The emergence of health psychology took place at a time when it became apparent that the leading causes of death were no longer acute infectious diseases, but had been replaced by chronic illness, said to be closely related to particular types of individual behaviour and lifestyles that developed with the growth of a consumerist bourgeois culture. This was the first set of events that deepened the involvement of psychologists in health care. The second set of events which helped to shape the new subdiscipline of health psychology and behavioural medicine came from within psychology and involved the development of behaviour modification, that is, changing behaviour by manipulating reinforcement in order to obtain a desired behaviour. The third event was the interest in bio-feedback, which is a process whereby information about such physiological conditions as heart rate or brain wave activity is made available to the person so that she/he can learn to gain control over those responses. Researchers such as Brown and Miller indicated that 'increased physical control could be learned for involuntary as well as voluntary responses' [Stone 1979].

These three are considered important causes in the development of the new subdiscipline of health psychology. In simple terminology, health psychology is an attempt to understand relationships between what people think, feel, and do about their health problems. As far as definitions are concerned, there have been several definitions proposed, perhaps the most frequently quoted one is by Joseph Matarazzo (1980), 'health psychology, is the aggregate of the specific educational, scientific and professional contributions of the discipline of psychology to the promotion and maintenance of health, the prevention and treatment of illness, and the identification of etiologic and diagnostic correlates of health, illness and related dysfunction'. This definition was modified to include psychology's contribution to the health care system and health policy formulation [Matarazzo 1982]. Psychology claims to be an interdisciplinary field of scientific enquiry. But it remains one, which investigates person-oriented health problems such as smoking, obesity, dental hygiene, etc., with a reductionist paradigm of individual psychology [Matarazzo 1980].

With the development of health psychology, a new popular health consciousness pervades the western countries and even among the elite of the developing countries. This new health consciousness is more inclusive and the more general heightened awareness and interest in health often includes environmental and occupational health concerns as well as a concern for personal health enhancement. A focus on personal health and individual lifestyle modifications may co-exist with and even act to stimulate attempts to change social conditions detrimental to everyone's health. As Katz and Levin (1980) and Gartner and Riessman (1977) point out with respect to self-care and self-help, there are numerous examples of politically activated groups that identify with these increments. As an ideology that promotes heightened health awareness, along with personal control and change, it may prove beneficial for those who adopt a more health promoting lifestyle [Belloc and Breslow 1972]. But it may, in the process, also serve the illusion that individuals control their own existence, and that taking personal action to improve health will somehow satisfy the longing for a much more varied complex of needs. This is important: lifestyles only explain a small proportion of the morbidity and mortality between social classes. Yet the focus on 'lifestyles' serves to obviate the larger differentials which are mediated by class. Such an ideology, contributes to the protection of the social order from the examination, critique and restructuring which would threaten those who benefit from the malaise, misery and deaths of others.

How health is popularly understood is in large part reflected in a society's therapeutics. In turn, those therapeutics further structure cultural understanding [Friedson 1972]. Popular notions about health, in other words, help produce and are partially reproduced by the therapeutic mode. The new health consciousness entails further medicalization of culture, and in particular, a medicalization of how the problem of health is understood. Medicalization refers to the extension of the range of social phenomena mediated by the concept of health and illness, often focusing on the importance of that process for understanding the social control of deviance. As Illich notes:

> By naming the spirit that underlies deviance, authority places the deviant under the control of language and custom and turns him from a threat into a support of the social system. Aetiology is socially self-fulfilling [Illich 1975].

The medical naming of that spirit increasingly circumscribes social existence. Deviant behaviour is defined in terms of sickness and normality in terms of health. Alcoholism, child abuse, opiate addiction, obesity, problems with sexual functioning, and violence have all become matters for medical diagnosis, and the label of illness has been attached to them [Conrad and Schneider 1988]. This is ironic since the problems of ill health and disease in the third world countries is entirely of a different order, located in hunger, poverty, and infection, all of which have social bases. Medicine as a therapeutic or clinical science locates the problem of disease in the individual body. The individual is both the locus of perception and intervention, more firmly so since the end of the 19th century when as, Foucault (1983) traces the transformation (the beginning of which he dates to the close of the 18th century), the very foundation of medical knowledge becomes lodged in the 'sovereignty of the gaze' fixed on individual signs and symptoms and then in deep anatomical structures. It is through the observation of individual signs and symptoms that it became 'possible to designate a pathological state... a morbid essence ... and an immediate cause' [Foucault 1983: 90]. And with the development of pathology, the medical understanding of disease turned even more fully toward 'the deep, invisible, solid, enclosed, but accessible space of the human body' [*Ibid:* 195]. Thus, what is known about disease is now a matter of positive knowledge of the individual. What is seen is what is known, and what is known becomes the space for intervention. Locked into a particular way of seeing, an imprisonment reinforced by institutional structures, medicine knows and acts upon disease bounded by an immediacy of perception which is physical (mechanical, biochemical, visual). In escaping from a nosology of morbid essences, it builds its science and chemical practice on the closed grounds of what becomes, in principle, an observed occurrence within the individual body. Notions of causation are compressed as well, limited to the boundaries of the individual in which disease takes its only meaningful existence. Anything, which cannot be shown to interact with the organism to produce a morbid state, is increasingly excluded. The local space of the disease is also, immediately, a causal space [*Ibid:* 189]. The solution to the problem of disease is directed towards breaking the most immediate cause link. Thus, medical perception pushes causal understanding toward the immediate and local, and solution toward the elimination of symptoms and the restoration of normal signs. As Foucault states, 'the space of the disease is, without reminder or shift, the very space of the organism' [*Ibid:* 191]. Medicine has become 'a science of the individual'. Foucault contrasts 'medical thought with an epidemiological tradition and perceptions' [1983: 22–36] which see the problem of disease as 'a nucleus of circumstances', a 'complex set of intersections', in which the only individuality is a 'historical individuality' [Dubos 1959: 113–143; Rosen 1979: 23–50].

In sum, medical practice is an individualized treatment mode, a mode which defines the client as deficient and which reconstructs the individual's understanding of the problem for which help is being sought. That reconstruction individualizes and compartmentalizes the problem, transforming it into its most immediate property: the answer to the problem is then logically held to be found in the same professionalized and individualized treatment, not in the reordering of the social, political, and environmental world. The response to individual disease experience, not denied here, thus becomes the field upon which selective explanations are authoritatively communicated and dominant social relations thereby reproduced. The spectre of a medicalized and medicated society, where already psycho-active drugs, sleeping aids and common pain relievers have become the standard response to almost every conceivable malaise, must at least raise questions about the wisdom of such heavy reliance upon medical problem solving. Despite the broadening, the use of psychology in the field of health awareness remains locked in a prison of reductionism and the modification of medical notions of causality is entirely unidimensional, towards psychologism, towards host resistance and adaptation. Jacoby has written much on contemporary psychology; the context is most often reduced to the immediate one of interpersonal relations and 'psychological atmospheres'. He notes:

> A social constellation is banalised to an immediate human network. It is forgotten that the relation between 'you and me' or 'you and the family' is not exhausted in the immediate: all of society seeps in [Jacoby 1975].

But, the study of the individual reduces the social context to the immediate context of interpersonal relations and psychological atmospheres. Ardell observes:

> The manner in which you organise your bedroom or work space, the kinds of friendship networks you create and sustain and the nature of the feedback about yourself which you invite by your actions, are all examples of the personal environment, or spaces you consciously or unknowingly set up for yourself [Ardell 1977].

In the reduction of 'social relations to immediate human ones', the society in which experience is lodged remain hidden; the part is isolated from the whole. Central to the self-care and awareness model is the concept of individual responsibility. This notion appears in virtually everything that has been written on these subjects. Ardell summarizes its importance:

> All dimensions of high level wellness are equally important, but self-responsibility seems more equal than all the rest. It is the philosopher's stone, the mariner's compass, and the ring of power to a high-level wellness lifestyle. Without an active sense of accountability for your own well being, you won't have the necessary motivation to lead a health enhancing lifestyle [Ardell 1977: 94]

Asserting a claim to individual responsibility partially delegitimizes existing authorities and throws open a new political terrain. To the extent that individual responsibility and related terms like self-help are experienced as symbols of empowerment, they may become one of the few ways that people conceive of themselves as actively political at all [Gartner and Reissman 1977].

However, like political language, individual responsibility is highly problematic. It risks all the myopia of classical individualism. It promotes a conception, which overlooks the social constraints against 'choosing'. Finally, as currently employed, the notion of individual responsibility promotes an assumption of individual blame as well. Self-care and changes in lifestyles are supposed to be the most important strategies to improve the life span of our individual citizens [Navarro 1976:126]. And behaviourists, psychologists, and 'mood' analysers are put to work to change the individual's behaviour [*Ibid*]. The basic cause of sickness or ill-health is located within the individual and not in the system. And the solution, therefore, is intervention, primarily behaviour modification, and not the structural change of the economic and social systems, which work to transform fundamental economic relationships. In this way, broad socio-economic dimensions are systematically excluded from the analysis and, instead, risk is considered largely in behavioural terms. Behaviourism, carried to an extreme, has to lead to unscientific and reactionary theories such as behaviour modification, which uses unethical and even brutal means to change behaviour. The predominant orientation of major research done in the health field as quoted in George C. Stone is related to behavioural aspect of health. Topics on mental health still dominate the studies. Other areas categorized in one survey include abortion, fertility, population control, accident, smoking, cancer, heart disease, psychosomatic illness, pain, death, etc. [G. Stone 1976: 60–61].

As far as theoretical developments in this field are concerned, there is no complete and comprehensive theory of the health system. However, Parson's sick role behaviour and rationality principle have found favour with this group. Sick role behaviour refers to what a person does to keep from getting sick, how she/he investigates the need for treatment and how he/she acts after being designed as sick [*Ibid*: 69]. The problem with this approach, which has already been discussed, is its personal and process orientation as opposed to situation and context orientation. The Health Belief Model (HBM) which developed in the 1950s provided theoretical support to the sick role approach. It focuses only on the rationality-irrationality of a person when she or he is sick. In essence, the theory says that the likelihood of taking a particular action is a function of perceived threat and perceived benefits while adding modifying factors which influence these actions [*Ibid*: 73].

Numerous studies follow the Health Belief Model. The basic thing this model talks about is why people seek health care. According to a review provided by Rosenstock and Krischt (1979), it becomes apparent that the effort is to explain preventive health behaviour in purely psychological terms. Most of these studies show racial differences and class differences in the utilization of health services. The explanation of the variance in utilisation is more astounding: among 'coloured' or among the poor, there is a low perceived susceptibility and low health motive. Other components in this model include readiness to use services, orientation to care, perceived severity, etc.

This abstract conceptual belief considered responsible for preventive health behaviour is open to question. Health Belief Model remains within the classical paradigm of medicine in which compliance, patient adherence, etc., are important concepts for understanding preventive health behaviour [Krischt and Rosenstock 1979:190]. Its weak explanatory power is reflected in the studies [Quah 1986]. As a consequence, its methodology is also its weakest component. Coburn and Pope mention that: 'Many of the studies, which we have examined, show responses of school, college students and, in some others, factory workers using mailed questionnaires to which response rates are terrible low' [Coburn and Pope 1974; K. Wurtele 1982].

This is the prevailing situation in western countries in general and is the epitome of bourgeois culture, in the United States of America. Psychology, even in the field of health, is used as exploitative tool for intervention or victim blaming.

People of other cultures often claim that western psychology is a subtle form of colonialism. Organized groups of ex mental patients claim that scientific appraisals and treatments have abused them. People of 'colour' find that scientific testing procedures are systematically biased against them. Black feminist activist, Bell Hooks claims that the white culture (including that of social science) has no right to speak for the black woman. And even studies from India, such as *KAP Studies* [K. G. Rao 1974], *Studies on Medical Students* [P. Ramalingaswamy, *et al.* 1972] and development of *Health Modernity Scales* [A. K. Singh 1984] show the biased nature of this empiricist and positivist social science. The KAP studies were conducted for introduction or imposition of various methods of contraception. The interventionist concept of motivation was used to change the attitude of the people towards such contraception. The concept of health modernity, which is located in 'rational' and 'irrational' principle which tends to neglect structural issues in the utilization of health services, is very much value loaded. These instances, therefore, indicate that psychology is indeed reductionist, mechanical, interventionist, and empiricist and thus a tool in the hands of capitalist material world. The question then arises, is whether there is a psychology which is not bourgeois in nature, or can be used for the purpose.

The question to be posited is, should there have been a subdiscipline called health psychology? Isolated perfunctory studies do not provide sufficient case for formulating such a subdiscipline. Behaviourism in psychology, such as the theories of J. B. Watson and B. F. Skinner, must be criticized as mechanical, as the reduction of the psychological process of human functioning to the psychological process of behaviour alone. On the other hand, there is the metaphysical theory of Freudianism, which focuses on an unconscious mind divorced from social and individual reality, and consciousness, which is seen as the basic source determining human attitude and behaviour. Thus, there is a need for a strong theoretical base, a critical social theory broadly similar to the attempt made by the Frankfurt school.

Erich Fromm, the only psychoanalytically trained member of this school extensively argued for using psychoanalytic typology, for an analytic social psychology. He said that analytic social psychology has its place within the framework of historical materialism. He investigates one of the natural factors that are operative in the relationship between the economic base and the formation of ideologies. Thus, analytic social psychology enables us to understand the ideological superstructure in terms of the process that goes on between society and nature [Eric Fromm 1970]. In other words, critical social psychology studies the social character, which is the practice of life, as it is constituted by the mode of production and the resulting social stratification. The social character is the structure of psychic energy that is moulded by any given society so as to be useful for its functioning. Empirically the important task for such an approach would be in revealing the nature of human need, the satisfaction of which makes human beings more alive and sensitive, and synthetic needs created by capitalism which tend to weaken them to make them more passive and enslave to their greed for things [Eric Fromm 1976]. Fromm had been critical of others who had used psychoanalytic concepts for a social theory on the ground that they had no clinical experience [*Ibid*: 210]. This criticism is against Herbert Marcuse who is alleged to have distorted psychoanalysis. Marcuse considers psychoanalysis as a set of 'meta psychological' speculation rather than a clinically oriented 'technical discipline', the main contention of Fromm for its distortion, is to limit the incompatibility of conjoining Marx and Freud [K. R. Nayar 1991].

The importance of Marcuse is for his dexterity in linking individual psyche with the social structure through needs and not for his psychoanalytic concepts. The concepts in psychoanalysis were taken to add a missing link in the Marxist approach [Marcuse 1968]. The need for such an integration is necessitated by a critical theory of society which would demonstrate that individuals would collectively regulate their lives in accordance with their needs and lay the foundation for a transformation of the economic order [*Ibid*: 141–42].

Following the Marxian concept of praxis, for Marcuse, 'knowledge of essence of an object or situation through reason would enable man to change the object in the light of his interest and needs and ensure his freedom' [*Ibid*: 75–87; Marcuse 1964]. Domination and freedom are contrary to each other. When the individual is provided with a goal and a purpose and means to strive for and attain, domination takes place. For Marcuse, domination can take many forms, to require an individual to do something by physical force, to coerce him by threats of disagreeable consequences, to condition the psyche. Systematic propaganda, to socialize or indoctrinate the individual so that she makes her choices within framework of a 'performed mentality', to plant certain desires in her by subliminal advertizing and such other measures, all constitute coercion.

It becomes apparent that psychoanalysis and its concepts have been given undue prominence for linking psyche with society. If one looks into Fromm's own analysis of Marx's contribution to the knowledge of man, it would be possible to point the incompatibility of Marxist and psychoanalytic thinking [Fromm 1970: 68–84]. Fromm's 'social character' is very relevant for social psychology and it can be used even in the health field. But Marcuse's attempt at understanding the concept of essence and the process of domination, again through need is more relevant and paves the way for critical social theory which integrates psychological correlates of social structure [K. R. Nayar 1991: 24]. In any case, the issue that has been brought to the limelight by these two viewpoints, not withstanding the weaknesses of relying on psychoanalysis for achieving it, is the integration of the missing individual in critical social theory despite the fact that both view points suffer from being too much pessimistic and as Wellmer puts it, 'as a protest impotent in practice'.[6] But Wexler notes differently:

> Despite the facile homologies, the mirroring of social processes at the microscopic level, despite the absence of description of social psychology of social interaction of the medicating process between the social matrix and the intro-individual dynamics, the Marxist Freudians, on the other hand, do provide a critical model of the relation between the social structure and the functioning of individual [Wexler 1983].

However, the Marxist Freudians remain at the periphery of American and English criticism of social psychology. This peripheral place, despite the accomplishment of Marxist-Freudians, is, in part, justified (though they have probably been ignored by liberal social psychologists for different reasons). A critical social psychology should include a description and analysis of precisely that intermediate level of social processes which the Marxist Freudians omit: how are the reproduction and transformation of social relations and the individual life processes which constitute them accomplished in social interaction? A critical psychology is an attempt to include that mediating process.

It is open to decide what kind of social sciences can be utilized to enrich the discipline of public health and enable it to have strong moorings in population based services. Existing deterministic models of social science have more or less perpetuated the status quo. A critical psychology can be the meeting point for health and epidemiology.

Acknowledgement: This paper originated as chapter II, of my M Phil dissertation 'Interdisciplinary Approach to Health: An Exploration into the Role of Social Psychology' at the Centre of Social Medicine and Community Health, School of Social Sciences, JNU, 1997. I would like to thank my supervisor, Mohan Rao for his guidance, encyclopedic knowledge and constructive comments on this paper. I am also indebted to Nilanjana for every kind of support.

Notes

1. Hippocrates as quoted in G. M. Howe, *National Atlas of Disease Mortality in the United Kingdom*, London, Nelson, 1963.
2. R. Descartes, *The Philosophical Works*, translated by E. S. Haldane and G. B. T. Ross, Cambridge University Press, 1967.
3. M. Taussing, as quoted in Robert Crawford, 'Healthism and Medicalisation of Everyday Life', *Int J. Hlth Serv.,* vol. 10, no. 3, 1980, pp. 365–388.
4. E. Chadwick, *Report on the Sanitary Condition of the Labouring Population of Great Britain*, 1842, as quoted in L. Doyal, The Political Economics of Health, Pluto Press, 1981, p. 144.
5. M. R. Lepsius, *Herausforderung and Forderung der Sozial Wissenschaft Lichen* as quoted in Manfred Pflanz, 'A Critique of Anglo American Medical Sociology', *Int J Hlth Serv*, 1974, vol. 4, no. 3.
6. Wellmer as quoted in T. Bottomore, *Sociology and Social Criticism*, George Allen and Unwin, 1975, p. 92.

References

Ackerknecht, E. (1953): *Rudolf Virchow: Doctor Statesman and Anthropologist*, University of Wisconsin Press, Madison.

Ardell, D. (1977): *High Level of Wellness: An Alternative to Doctors, Drugs and Disease*, Rodale Press, Emmaus.

Belloc, N. and L. Breslow (1972): 'Relationship of Physical Health Status and Health Practices', *Preventive Medicine*, vol. 1, no. 3, pp. 409–421.

Berry, J. W. (1972): 'Radical Cultural Relativism and the Concept of Intelligence' in L. J. Cronbacks and P. J. Drenth (eds.) *Mental Tests and Cultural Adaptation*, Humanities Press, New York.

Bloom, S. W. (1979): *From Learned Profession to Policy Science: A Trend Analysis of Sociology of Medical Education in United States* as quoted in George, C. Stone, C. Frances and Nancy E. Adler (eds.), *Health Psychology*, Jossey-Bass, San Francisco.

Cassel, C. K. (1983): 'Work, Peace and Professional Responsibility', *Soc Sci Med*, vol 17.

Coburn, D. and C. R. Pope (1974): 'Socio-economic Status and Preventive Health Behaviour', vol. 15, no. 2, pp. 67-78.

Conrad, P. and J. Schneider (1988): *Deviance and Medicalisation: From Badness to Sickness*, C V Moshy, St Louis.

Coulins, N. (1977): 'The Mysterious Placebo: How Mind Helps Medicine Work', *Saturday Review*, October 1, pp. 9-16.

de Swaan, A. (1997): *The Management of Normality: Critical Essay in Health and Welfare* in Alan Peterson and Robin Bunton (eds).

Doyal, L. (1981): *The Political Economics of Health*, Pluto Press.

Dubos, R. (1959): *Mirage of Health*, Harper Collins, New York, pp. 85-104

Eyer, J. and P. Sterling (1977): 'Stress Related Mortality and Social Organisation', *Review of Radical Political Economics*, vol. 9, nos. 1, 2, pp. 1-44.

Figlio, K. (1977): 'The Historiography of Scientific Medicine: An Invitation to Human Sciences', *Comparative Studies in Society and History*, vol. 19, p. 265.

Foucault, M. (1983): *The Birth of the Clinic: An Archaeology of Medicine Perception*, Pantheon, New York.

Freeman, H. E., S. Levine and L. G. Reeder (eds) (1979): *Handbook of Medical Sociology*, Prentice Hall Englewood Cliffs, NJ.

Friedson, E. (1972): *Profession of Medicine*, Dodd Mead and Co, New York.

Fromm, E. (1970): *The Crisis of Psychoanalysis: Essays on Freud, Marx and Social Psychology*.

——(1967): 'Human Psychoanalysis and Marxist Theory' in Erich Fromm (ed), *Socialist Man*, Allen Lane, Penguin Press, p. 216.

Gartner, A. and F. Reissman (1977): *Self Help in the Human Services*, Jossey-Bass, San Francisco.

Ginsburg, H. and S. Opper (1969): *Piaget's Theory of Intellectual Development: An Introduction*, Prentice Hall Englewood Cliffs, NJ.

Gouldner, A. W. (1971): *The Coming Crisis of Western Sociology*, Heinemann Education Books, London, p. 344.

Ilich, I. (1975): *Medical Nemesis: The Expropriate of Health*, Pantheon, New York.

——(1976): *Limits to Medicine*, London, Marion Boyers.

Israel, L. (1978): *Conquering Cancer*, Random House, New York.

Jacoby, R. (1975): *Social Amnesia: A Critique of Contemporary Psychology from Adler to Laig*, Beacon Press, Boston.

Jewson, N. (1974): 'Medical Knowledge and Patronage System in Eighteenth Century England', *Sociology*, vol. 8, no. 3, pp. 369-85.

——(1976): 'The Disappearance of the Sickman from Medical Cosmology, 1770-1870'; *Sociology*, vol. 10, no. 2, pp. 225-44.

Katz, A. and L. Levin (1980): 'Self-care is not A Solipsistic Trap: A Reply to Critics', *Int J Hlth Serv*, vol. 10, no. 2, pp. 329-36.

King, M. (ed.) (1966): *Medical Care in Developing Countries: A Symposium from Makerere*, Oxford University Press.

Knowles, J. H. (1977): *Introduction to Doing Better and Feeling Worse: Health in United States.*, Norton, New York, pp. 1-44.

Krischt, J. P. and I. M. Rosenstock (1979): 'Patient Problems in the Following Recommendations of Health Experts' in George, C Stone (1979), p. 190.

Kuhn, T. S. (1962): *The Structure of Scientific Revolution*, University of Chicago Press, Chicago.

Lilienfeld, A. M. and D. E. Lilienfeld (1980): *Foundation of Epidemiology*, Oxford University Press.

Lupton, D. (1997): 'Foucault and Medicalisation Critique' in Alan Peterson and Robin Bunton (eds), *Foucault, Health and Medicine*, Routledge.

Luria, A. (1971): 'Towards the Problem of Historical Nature of Psychological Processes', *Int J Psy*, vol. 6, no. 4, pp. 259-72.

Makrazzo, J. D. (1980): 'Behavioural Health and Behavioural Medicine: Frontiers for A New Health Psychology', *American Psychologist*, vol. 35, p. 815.

——(1982): 'Behavioural Health Challenge to Academic Scientific and Professional Psychology', *American Psychologist*, vol. 37, no. 1 pp. 1-14.

Marcuse, H. (1964): *One Dimensional Man*, Routledge and Kegan Paul.

——(1968): *Negations: Essays in Critical Theory, Cap on Hedonism*, Allen Lane, Penguin Press, pp. 159-200.

Navarro, V. (1976): *Medicine under Capitalism*, Prodist, New York.

——(1986): *Crisis, Health and Medicine: A Social Critique*, Tavistock Pub, p. 167.

Nayar, K. R. (1991): 'Interdisciplinary Approach in Social Science in Health: A Reexamination of the Linkages between Social Psychology and Health', Working Paper, Unpublished.

Neisser, U. (1976): *Cognition and Reality*, Freeman, San Francisco.

Olesen, V. L. (1975): 'Convergences and Divergences: Anthropology and Sociology in Health Care', *Soc Sci and Med*, vol. 9, pp. 421-25.

Osborne, T. (1997): 'On Anti Medicine and Clinical Reason' in Alan Peterson and Robin Bunton (eds), *Foucault Health and Medicine*, Routledge.

Patrick, D. L. and G. Scambler (eds.) (1982): *Sociology as Applied to Medicine*, Balliere Tindall, London.

Quah, S. R. (1986): 'Social Science and Illness Prevention: An Overview of Health Beliefs Models', *J Soc and Eco Studies* (ns), vol. 3, no. 4, pp. 345-57.

Ramalingaswamy, P. *et al.* (1972): 'Studies on Medical Students', NIHAE Research Report, no. 12.

Rao, K. G. (1974): *Studies in Family Planning in India*, Abhinav Pub.

Reich, W. (1970): *The Mass Psychology of Fascism*, Farrav Straus and Giroux, New York.

——(1972): *Character Analysis*, third edition, Simon and Schuster, New York.

Reiser, S. J. (1978): *Medicine and the Reign of Technology*, Cambridge University Press.

Rifkin, S. B. (1985): *Health Planning and Community Participation: Case Studies in South East Asia*, Croom Helm, London.

Rosen, G. (1979): 'The Evolution of Social Medicine', in Levine Freeman and Reeder (eds.), *Handbook of Medical Sociology*, Prentice Hall Englewood Cliffs, NJ, pp. 23-52.

Rosenstock and J. P. Krischt (1979): 'Why People Seek Health Care' in George, C Stone *et al.*

Rossdale, M. (1965): 'Health in a Sick Society', *New Left Review*, no. 34, pp. 82 - 90.

Rothman, K. J. (1981): 'The Rise and Fall of Epidemiology 1952–2000 AD, New Engl', *J Med*, 304, pp. 600-02.

Singh, A. K. (1984): 'Health Modernity: Concepts and Correlates', *Social Change*, vol. 14, no. 3, pp. 3-16.

Shylock, R. H. (1969): *The Development of Modern Medicine*, New York, Hasner.

Stark, E. (1977): 'Introduction to the Special Issue on Health', *Review of Radical Political Economics*, no 1, spring, p. V.

Stern, B. (1980): 'Society and Medical Progress', as quoted in Berliner and Salmon, 'The Holistic Alternative to Scientific Medicine: History and Analysis', *Int J Hlth Serv*, vol. 10, no. 1, pp. 133-47.

Strauss, R. (1981): 'The Nature and Status of Medical Sociology', in Peter Conrad and Rochelle Kern (eds.), *The Sociology of Health and Illness*, St Marlin's Press, New York, p. 6.

Waldron, I. (1977): 'Increased Prescribing of Valium Librium, and Other Drugs: An Example of the Influence of Economic and Social Factors as the Practice of Medicine', *Int J Hlth Serv*, vol. 7, no. 1, pp. 37-62.

Wartofsky, M. (1975): 'Organs, Organism and Disease: Human Ontology and Medical Practice', in H. T. Engel Hardt, Jr and S. Spicker (eds.), *Evaluation and Explanation in the Biomedical Sciences*, Reidel Publications, Boston.

Wexler, P. (1983): *Critical Social Psychology*, Routledge and Kegan Paul, p. 69.

Westfall, R. S. (1977): *The Construction of Modern Science: Mechanisms and Mechanics*, Cambridge University Press, Cambridge.

Wurtele, K. *et al.* (1982): 'Health Beliefs and Intentions: Predictors of Return Compliance in a Tuberculosis Detection Drive', *J Applied Soc Psy*, vol. 12, no. 2, pp. 128-36.

18

Ranchodlal Chotalal: Pioneer of Public Health in Ahmedabad

—Mridula Ramanna

Indian responses to western ideas of sanitation were not always negative, as has been generally assumed. The efforts of Ranchodlal Chotalal, the Chairman of the Ahmedabad Municipality and textile magnate, in the last two decades of the 19th century provides a glimpse of a different dimension in the interactions between the colonial power and Indians. He campaigned for a better water supply and sewage system, in the face of opposition from Ahmedabad's citizens, including leading educated reformers and the public. His initiative provides a contrast to the responses in other cities. The Sanitary Commissioner of Bombay considered the 'appalling' sanitary condition of Nasik an 'index of the little interest' that the municipality took in the sanitation 'of their picturesque city' [1] The Madras municipal council's scepticism of certain medical interventions in the early 1900s have been shown.[2]

Indian philanthropists had financed medical facilities in Bombay Presidency since the mid-nineteenth century.[3] Shethias Premabhai Hutteesing and Bechurdass Ambaidass, had established a hospital (1859), respectively. Ranchodlal Chotalal also funded dispensaries in Ahmedabad for the poor and for women and children. Ranchodlal's anxiety to start the Victoria Jubilee dispensary for women and children in the year of Queen Victoria's jubilee is apparent in his correspondence with the collector of Ahmedabad and the Bombay Government. He was made CIE in 1883 and given the title Rao Bahadur. Medical philanthropy has been seen as 'a part of a strategy of accommodation' with the ruling power.[4] Nevertheless, his concern for improving his city and his pursuit of this goal, almost singly, is significant.

Born in 1823, in a nagar brahmin family, Ranchodlal received elementary education in Gujarati and then studied Persian and English, with Rao Bahadur Bholanath Sarabhai. He continued his studies at the Subscription English School, a private institution. Like other English educated young men of his time, Ranchodlal entered government service as a clerk.[5] Subsequently, in ten years of government service, he rose to be *daftardar* and assistant political agent.[6] Ranchodlal left for the more lucrative field of cotton manufacture and set up the first cotton mill in Ahmedabad. He was so successful that he soon made a large fortune as a leading cotton manufacturer and entrepreneur, and, in the words of his biographer, became 'the father of the mill industry'.[7] He was nominated as a member of the Ahmedabad municipality, in 1869, made President in 1885, and was nominated an additional member of the Bombay Legislative Council, in 1892. Ranchodlal not only promoted sanitary reform, as will be shown in this paper, but also gave generously to education, to the Gujarat Vernacular Society, established a girls' school, named after him, and funded a scholarship at the Victoria Jubilee Technical Institute, Bombay. Like other liberal reformers of his time, he seems to have regularly attended the meetings of the Prarthana Samaj.

Sanitary Reform

The high mortality rates and the poor sanitary condition of Ahmedabad had been repeatedly pointed out by the Collector, Alfred Borradaile, since 1874. He had represented before each Governor of Bombay who visited the city, but to no avail.[8] The Sanitary Commissioner, Thomas Gilham Hewlett, erstwhile health officer of Bombay made an adverse report, which was widely circulated, on the preponderance of fevers, in Ahmedabad, in contrast to Bombay. He recommended the appointment of a health officer to tackle the problems. Piqued by the report, Borradaile countered that there was nothing to prove that his city was 'exceptionally unhealthy', and that any comparison with Bombay was fallacious. He pointed out that despite its sweet water, pure air, wide streets, qualified health officer and controlled cremation ghats and graveyards, hundreds were dying of cholera in Bombay. Besides it had a large floating population of men, in the prime of their life, who went to that city to seek their fortunes and returned home to die.[9] Notwithstanding these differences within the establishment, the officials were in agreement that the poor water supply and the deficient sanitation were responsible for the high mortality rates in Ahmedabad. The local press had also been writing about the neglect by the municipality. Thus, in 1868, the *Samsher Bahadur* (founded in 1854) compared the municipality to a *pinjrapole* (asylum for old animals).[10] The same paper reported a proposal made to the government by the Swami Narayan sect to have the Kankaria lake (in the neighbourhood of Ahmedabad) repaired and cleaned, on the condition that fishing in it would be prohibited. The lake had been fouled by washing and bathing, but the government declined the offer.[11]

It was as head of the municipality, that Ranchodlal prepared an elaborate memorandum, dated December 8, 1883, on the deteriorating public health in the city and made suggestions which were circulated among his colleagues in the municipality. He compared the city's high mortality rates with other cities; while Ahmedabad's death rate was 44 per 1000, in 1880–81, Calcutta's was 30 per 100, Bombay's was 27.87, and Poona's 25.1. The former also had the dubious distinction of having the highest number of deaths from fever in the same year: 35,365 per 1000, as against 33.96, in Kanpur, another industrial centre.[12] He contended that with a large river like the Sabarmati, a lake like the Kankaria (with a depth of 10 feet and an area of 72 acres), good potable spring water and wells, Ahmedabad had an abundant supply of water, though of poor quality. The sewage from houses was collected in cess pits, called *khalcooas*, which were dug close to the houses, to a depth of 15 to 20 feet. Since the sub-soil was porous, the *khalcooa* water found its way into the water supply, including springs and wells. The river water was used for bathing, washing and cleaning animals, making it unclean, too.[13] A pumping plant had been erected in 1847, from the City Walls Restoration Fund. Four years later, piped water supply was pumped up by the Persian wheel from the river. This had proved to be inadequate and many schemes to increase the supply were mooted, including two, in 1878, one by Borradaile, and the other by Pottinger, Executive Engineer of Irrigation, Gujarat, while Playford Reynolds, in 1883 and S. B. Doig, in 1884, also drew up plans. But none of these had been implemented.[14] 133,000 gallons of water was raised by steam pumps from the Sabarmati, but the spot selected was at the lowest point, where the water had already been fouled by washing. The water was raised at night, when the river had fewer impurities, by two small engines of five and six horse power, respectively. After being raised, the water passed through a filter tank and was distributed partly by earthen pipes and partly by iron pipes.[15] Since this supply did not meet the needs of the population many persons relied on cisterns, underground reservoirs, or *tankas*, in which rain water was stored, during monsoons.[16] To solve the problem of inadequate water supply, Ranchodlal suggested more efficient filtration of water, as had been done at Hooghly, and the cleaning out of the *tankas*, which, on chemical analysis, had been found to contain purer water than river water. Since there was a spring in the neighbourhood of the city, he recommended that a well, 63 or 78 feet in depth, could be dug.[17]

As for drainage, Ranchodlal maintained that there was no system at all. In 1872, the municipality had prohibited the construction of deep well privies and in 1879, closed existing ones. There were only the *khalcooas*, and he estimated that out of 41,000 houses in the city, 8,000 had *khalcooas*, and the remainder had no privies at all.[18] Those which had no provision for sewage threw it out, in front of their houses. Since the gullies were narrow, the sun's rays did not reach them. Consequently, dampness prevailed and malaria was rampant. The marks of decay were visible in the walls, bricks, and in the *chunam* and were proof of the unwholesome state of the sub-soil. Ranchodlal endorsed the opinion of the Army Sanitary Commission that the *khalcooa* system should be replaced and some arrangements made to carry away the sewage for those who had no facilities, whatsoever. He suggested the construction of public toilets, stricter sanitary inspection, use of disinfectants, re-location of night soil depots, and town sweepings from their current position at the Jamalpur and Shahpur gates to a distance of two miles to the south east of the city, and the construction of a light railway, to carry the sewage there, as had been done at Amritsar. His other recommendations included filling out the hollow walls where water stagnated, the removal of offensive trades, the widening of narrow streets and the regulation of cattle stables. He pointed out that while the principal roads were well drained and metalled, those in the *pols* (neighbourhoods of persons coming from the same village but restricted to Hindus and Jains) were unsatisfactory. They were devoid of even surfaces and storm water drains. Being constantly sodden they were 'a fertile source of cholera'.[19]

The other issue, which Ranchodlal dealt with, in his memorandum, was the density of the population in the city. He believed that the evils of overcrowding could be explained to the people through tract and lectures. The government and the municipality, on their parts, could adopt the following measures: (1) induce people to build houses outside the city, (2) not sell land in already crowded place, (3) open up new spaces and thoroughfares. He also suggested welfare schemes like the building of *chawls* (tenements) for the poor and the provision of medical facilities for the poor 'middle castes', who out of prejudice and honest pride could not afford to pay for competent medical attendance and were unwilling to go to hospitals used by the poor.[20]

Ranchodlal estimated that the cost of these improvements would be Rs. 15,00,000 and suggested that the municipality should take a loan for this amount, at five percent interest, repayable in fifty years. To meet this expenditure, he proposed a special tax amounting to twelve annas per head, which he contended would be less than what the public would have to pay for the upkeep of the *khalcooas* and *tankas*.[21] To prevent the tax from being a burden on the poorest, he contended that the municipality should make a valuation of all immovable property in the city and regulate the incidence of the tax on the basis of that valuation. He appealed to the government to advance a loan by conceding to the municipality the right to receive sale proceeds of the occupancy rights of all unoccupied lands within municipal limits, and by paying to that body compensation for the loss of octroi fees on country liquor, which had resulted from government acquiring the monopoly over liquor, in 1881.[22]

While appealing to his fellow commissioners in the municipality and the people of Ahmedabad to take seriously the subject that involved the lives of so many citizens, he recognized that the question of funds might come in the way. However, he felt that, 'when the importance of the subject is well understood, I hope the difficulty will soon be removed'.[23] It is noteworthy that Ranchodlal had done his homework before preparing his memorandum. He had consulted the lectures of a sanitary officer of Manchester, who had proposed that the old sewers should be used for surface water and new water tight sewers be constructed, for liquid refuse, which could then be conveyed to farm lands. Many English towns had adopted this system. He also referred to an essay, in Gujarati, on agricultural improvements, wherein the use of human manure had been suggested.[24] Ranchodlal visited an exhibition at Calcutta and secured estimates from firms, which had built the light railway in the Punjab.[25] He had corresponded with Florence Nightingale, who was in contact with Lord Reay, Governor of Bombay, about the Bombay Village Sanitation Act, which aimed at educating villagers in sanitary matters.[26]

Responses to the Schemes

Hewlett commended Ranchodlal's memorandum as 'a remarkable document for native gentleman', as it exhibited 'a breadth of view and a masterly appreciation of some of the main questions that affect public health in the city'.[27] The Army Sanitary Commission hailed it as a remarkable report, which threw additional light on the causes of fever in Indian towns.[28] Hewlett, in his report for 1885, pointed out most forcibly the need to improve the sanitary conditions of a city, whose mean death rate for the previous eleven years had been 53.15 per 1000.[29] It was more difficult convincing Ranchodlal's colleagues in the municipality and numerous meetings of the managing committee were held, in the first year of his office. He succeeded in obtaining sanctions for certain improvements like dealing with street sweepings and garbage, the construction of open gutters to carry away storm water, and the erection of reservoirs of water for use by cattle.[30]

At Ranchodlal's request, the Bombay Government used the services of Col. Walter M. Ducat, who was executive engineer at Poona. Ducat recommended improvements to the water supply and the introduction of a system of underground drainage.[31] Ducat's plans were received with great hostility both by Ranchodlal's colleagues and the public, who considered the schemes as impracticable and expensive. Daily protest meetings were held, presided over by Ranchodlal's opponents. The press reported the goings on. Despite rumours that there would be violence, if he went to the mass protest meeting to be held at Tanksal, Ranchodlal braved the hostility and attended. He was refused a hearing and, according to his biographer, was pelted with garbage and stones, and had to be escorted to his home by the police.[32] In June 1886, the municipality rejected Ducat's report. Gillian has attributed this opposition to various factors: religious prejudice, since piped water would be available to all, jealousy of Ranchodlal, and a fear that additional taxes would follow the introduction of these schemes. The opponents included reformers like Mahipatram Rupram, Padshahi Diwan Mirza Najaf Ali Khan, Valade Mirza Nawab, Ardeshir Kewasji Karanjwala, and Maganlal Sarup Chand.[33]

Ranchodlal had gathered the views of Dr. Thomas Blaney, coroner and a prominent doctor who had opposed underground drainage in Bombay. In a letter to the *Bombay Gazette*, Blaney had shown the unfavourable results of the system, when it was implemented in Kamatipura, Bombay. In his reply to Ranchodlal, Blaney referred to the deaths of four labourers from asphyxiation, when they had been sent down to clean out a sewer only nine days after its construction. Besides, the system most suitable to Ahmedabad had to be worked out with reference to that city's needs.[34]

In order to convince his colleagues in the civic body, Ranchodlal even improvised a scheme from the Sabarmati for his own mills, laid down small drainage works and a model farm in the compound of his house. But his opponents remained adamant and received unexpected support from Sir Theodore Hope, former collector of Ahmedabad and at one time a member of the Viceroy's executive council. Hope wrote a long minute from Simla in October, 1886 condemning Ducat's scheme. His views were circulated in Ahmedabad and published in the *Bombay Gazette*. Hope recommended the removal of sewage by hand and the surface removal of sullage. Ranchodlal realized that Hope had been misled by hasty generalizations, based on different conditions in Lahore, and defended his proposals in an elaborate memo, which was circulated among his colleagues and the public. He wrote letters to the press, countering the theories of his opponents and justifying Ducat's plans. Ducat himself wrote a caustic refutation of Hope's views.[35]

Regarding improvements in the water supply, Ducat had recommended a more efficient use of the Sabarmati, though Doig had been in favour of bringing water from the Kharee, a smaller river. Ranchodlal studied the relative cost and showed that if twenty gallons of water was the requirement per head, there would be a saving in the Sabarmati project which would cost Rs. 20,594; while the Kharee project would cost Rs. 45,880. Ducat had emphasized the need for ventilation in the water channels, based on his knowledge of Kolhapur, where four men, sent to clean out the channels containing pure drinking water, were killed as the air inside had become deadly. Hope, too, had favoured the Sabarmati as the source of water supply and had suggested that reservoirs of moderate size should be constituted in distinct sections, with iron rather than masonry pipes.[36] In the meanwhile, Ranchodlal reported in the annual report of the municipality, 1887–8, that the experiment to remove foul water from the *pols* and dyers' vats had been satisfactory. Nevertheless, Ducat's idea of a trial well 25 feet in diameter, in the river bed at Dudheshwar, was implemented and demonstrated that double the daily quantity of water could be raised by machinery, from a single well.[37]

After a long discussion, the municipal commissioners passed a resolution, 16 to 10, moved by professor Abaji Vishnu Kathavate and seconded by Hugh Fraser, that a modified version of Ducat's scheme be adopted.[38] A well was constructed in the bed of the river Dudheshwar at a cost of Rs 10,000. The object was to get naturally filtered water and save the expense of the construction of filtering and setting beds.[39] The cost of providing iron pipes was subsequently raised from Rs. 5,00,000 to 6,00,000. In April 1887, the municipality gave its approval to raise a loan for the latter amount. The Bombay Government sanctioned it promptly but the Government of India passed its orders only in May, 1888. The work commenced in March, 1889. Two years later, in June 1891, the Governor, Lord Harris opened the completed works which comprised of a pumping plant capable of supplying 13,00,000 gallons of water, working twelve hours, and piping for fifty one miles. The work was done under the supervision of Doig and his assistant, Fardunji Cooverji Taraporewala. On completion, the cost came to Rs 7,50,000. A second high level reservoir with a capacity of 3,18,000 gallon was built and a third, in 1898, which could deliver 1,800 gallons per minute to the high level reservoir.[40]

The question of drainage proved more contentious. The system of removal of night soil, by hand, to the depots at Jamalpur and Shahpur was replaced by its removal by train to a place outside city limits, called Bagh Firdaus. Ranchodlal reported that the number of deaths had consequently reduced from 6,729 in 1885 to 4,773 in 1886, the decrease was particularly noted in the areas, where the night soil depots had been located. More importantly, the labour of the *bhangis* had been reduced to keeping the privies clean.[41] A municipal subcommittee appointed in November, 1886 to discuss the issue recommended the removal of sullage water by pipes as a temporary measure. The municipality declined to sanction this proposal and declared its support for Hope's suggestion of removal of sullage by hand. However, the Collector, the Commissioner of the Northern Division, the Sanitary Commissioner and the Bombay Government rejected the proposal as expensive and inefficient. Another subcommittee recommended in its report of 1887, a system of main drains or sewers to carry off sullage water from the city. This too was rejected by the municipality, who reverted to the original proposal of removing sullage water by hand. Now the government emphatically vetoed this move and issued a firm resolution requiring the municipality to implement the underground drainage scheme.[42]

Since a number of members voted in favour of this proposal, the local press alleged that the commissioners had been pressurized to do so. The *Ahmedabad Times* held that several commissioners absented themselves from the general meeting of the municipality as they had been invited by a 'government servant' to his residence and told that government would carry out the scheme, even though they opposed it.[43] Among the other papers were the *Gujarati, Gujarat Gazette, Hitechchu, Bombay Samachar, Gujarat Darpan,* and *Yajdan Parast.* The *Nyaydarshak*, saw it as want of encouragement to local self government, and *Praja Mat* even welcomed rumours that Ranchodlal had resigned from the presidency of the municipality.[44] The citizens held a public meeting, at the invitation of Pitambardas Tribhuvandas Mehta, to adopt a memorial against drainage. Two of the speakers, Chaganlal Umedchand and Kalidas Sankalchad dwelt on the harm done to Bombay by drainage, and advised care in the future selection of municipal commissioners. A petition was submitted to the Viceroy claiming that their rights to self government had been infringed. The petitioners maintained that underground drainage was yet a matter of experiment even in England and experts had disagreed as to its efficacy. In Calcutta, the sewerage works had not proved an 'unmixed good'. They averred that unless the trapping in every house connection and street opening was completed, and underground drainage system was sure to become a nuisance and an active source of diseases. The petitioners wanted the removal of sullage by the pail system, which had long worked in Manchester and Glasgow. The petition was supported by Hope, Blaney, and signed by seven thousand persons and adopted at a public meeting.[45] The paper *Rast Goftar*, in a newsletter from Ahmedabad, remarked that except for a few agitators, few cared whether the drainage works were constructed or not. It held that those who wished to push forward their names to public notice pretended that they had consented, owing to the threats held out by the new Collector, H. E. M. James and by the City Magistrate, Dastur Firuz.[46] The petitioners decided next to send a deputation to Calcutta, to meet the Viceroy and explain to him, how difficult and impractical the new scheme was. Ahmedabad's lanes were three feet in breadth and people living on these lanes did not get fresh air. However, it seems that the inability of the delegation to procure a map led to the plan being dropped. In the meanwhile, the Viceroy, in his reply to the petition, declined to interfere with the Bombay Government's orders.[47]

Since many adverse opinions had been expressed against underground drainage, it was decided that the system be tried in a part of the town, before making further extensions.[48] Designs were made by the sanitary expert, Baldwin Latham, and the work was carried out by the public works department officers, Doig, Major H. D. Olivier, and Fardunji Taraporewala.[49] Even while the pipes were being laid, the public remained hostile and would refer to the pits as graves. Abuses were particularly heaped on Ranchodlal, women outvying men in doing so.[50] It was the success of the water works which gradually changed the opinion of Ahmedabad's citizenry. By 1897, there was a demand for the extension of the drainage to other parts of the city and under the direction of Ranchodlal plans were made, involving an expenditure of Rs 8,00,000. The approval of the government and the sanction of the loan, came only after Ranchodlal's death in 1898.[51] Ranchodlal had described these changes in the sanitation of Ahmedabad in a paper he submitted to the International Congress of Hygiene and Demography, held in London, in 1892.[52]

Promotion of Medical Facilities

Ranchodlal's interest in public health predated his assumption in the municipality. In 1879, he submitted a proposal to government endowing a building for the establishment of a charitable dispensary in the railway suburb just outside the city. This location was specially chosen, so that patients from Kathiawar could avail of the services offered at the dispensary.[53] A *dharamshala* for relatives attending on patients was also proposed. However, the government turned down Ranchodlal's request to pay the salary of the assistant surgeon, who would run the dispensary. On earlier occasions, too, the Bombay Government had been reluctant to subsidize medical salaries, when Jagannath Shankar Sheet had offered to extend the facilities of the charitable dispensary at Girgaum, Bombay in 1860, and when Bechurdass Ambaidass had offered to endow a dispensary in Ahmedabad, in 1862.[54] Ranchodlal was not deterred and, by 1881, had secured the services of a doctor for his dispensary, and was sanctioned grant-in-aid.[55] It was transferred to the municipality and he donated Rs. 20,000 towards its maintenance. Subsequently, he provided more funds for the extension of its buildings, so that inpatients could be admitted, and hospital staff could be increased.[56] He frequently visited the dispensary which was in the charge of assistant surgeon, Nilkant Dayabhai, LMS.[57] Surgical operations were performed and the number of patients, rose to 11,849, including 7,247 males, 1,613 females and 2,989 children, in 1898. The surgeon general, who inspected the dispensary, reported that it was kept in 'good condition'.[58]

In 1885, Ranchodlal again offered a sum of Rs. 20,000 for the establishment of a small hospital for women and children, provided the government took charge of it and appointed a qualified lady doctor, half of whose salary he would bear for a period of four years.[59] That he wished to support this scheme in view of the Queens Victoria's interest in medical aid for women in India is evident. He wanted the founding of the institution to coincide with her jubilee and in this connection met Lady Reay, who was vice-patroness of the Countess of Dufferin Fund. Surgeon General W. J. Moore interpreted this gesture as a desire to gain the credit for establishing a female hospital, without providing adequate infrastructure.[60] The government, as usual, dragged its feet on the question of subsidy. Moore had estimated the cost of its maintenance to be Rs. 5,626 per annum. On the Collector's intervention, the government finally agreed to grant Rs. 2,000 per annum.[61] The municipality, was willing to contribute Rs. 600 per annum for four years, and then raised it to Rs. 1,200.[62] The Local Fund Board provided Rs. 300 per annum, while the remainder was financed by the interest on the public fund of Rs. 15,469, collected for the support of the institution.[63] Ranchodlal agreed to fund the construction of the building and agreed to provide the land. The management committee included the collector, James, the civil surgeon, Ranchodlal, as president of the municipality, K. B. Shapurji Ratanji, vice-president of the local board, and Sheth Jehangir Pestonji, member of the Victoria Jubilee Fund.[64]

After considerable search for a lady doctor, Madame C. Blim, as she is referred to in the records, was appointed. A Parisian by birth, C. Blim was a widow, who had come to India as a governess to the two young daughters of General Sir Michael Biddulph. After the premature death of her charges, Blim gained experience at the Obstetrics Institution, attached to Jamsetji Jejeebhoy Hospital, and trained as a midwife at Grant Medical College, Bombay. Then, she moved to Madras, where she studied the curriculum of the L. M. and S degree of that university, but was not awarded the degree, because she was not a matriculate, which was the prescribed requisite qualification. Her training was therefore regarded on par with an apothecary, lower than a full fledged doctor. Blim knew Hindustani and assured the authorities that she would soon learn Gujarati.[65] The Victoria Jubilee Dispensary, with provision for eight beds, opened on April 1, 1889.[66] Blim served for a short period and was succeeded by Motibai Kapadia, a certified practitioner from Grant Medical College.[67] Motibai was very popular and the attendance at the dispensary rose to 11,437 patients, including 7,415 women and 4,022 children, in 1898.[68] The annual inspection reports of the dispensary for the 1890s record that it was in 'excellent order'. The most common cases treated at both the dispensaries, were malaria fevers, respiratory complaints, and diseases of the skin, eye, and ear. Patients were categorized community wise, Hindus, constituting the largest number of patients, others being Muslims, Parsis, Indian Christians, Europeans and Eurasians.

Yet another medical facility financed by Ranchodlal, was the Medical Home Relief Scheme, 1894, for poor patients who were unable to go to a dispensary. The scheme particularly benefited bed ridden patients. A retired hospital assistant named Laxman Singh was hired for the first year, and the total cost of the scheme was shared by Ranchodlal and the municipality. Thereafter, the former made an endowment of Rs. 25,000 and handed over charge to the latter. The number of men, women and children, who used this facility in 1898 was 608.[69] The Lord Harris Travelling Dispensary was also established by Ranchodlal in the taluka of Daskroi. The services of a doctor and a compounder were provided, to distribute medicines among the villagers of the taluka. In 1898, it is recorded that 5,099 patients including 4,983 Hindus, 111 Muslims and 5 Indian Christians availed of this facility.[70]

Concluding Remarks

Ranchodlal's involvement with public health was so complete that, as Gillian has shown, there was a deterioration in the public health of the city, after his death in 1898.[71] In fact, there were a series of editorials in the second decade of the next century castigating the same municipality, which he had led in the promotion of sanitary improvements, for their negligence.[72] Whatever he achieved was in the face of hostility from Ahmedabad's citizenry, led by western educated champions of social reforms, like Mahipatram Rupram. In Bombay, Vishwanath Narayan Mandlik, the chairman of the municipality and Dr. Blaney, had opposed underground drainage, for financial and socio-religious reasons.[73] Mandlik had asserted that there was not enough water, and had favoured open sewers. He had felt that the whole question had been handled by the administration of Sir Richard Temple in a high handed manner and that municipal administration ought to be 'untramelled by the fetters of officialism'.[74] While Ranchodlal's opponents saw the new schemes and the government's decision to implement them as an infringement on their rights, he believed that civic progress had been made, with the introduction of local self government. These differences in the perceptions of western sanitation among Indians are significant. Ranchodlal was doubtless accommodating to the British and named the women's dispensary after the Queen, but the fact remains that the municipal improvements that he initiated led to a decline in mortality rates. Focus at the micro level on efforts such as Ranchodlal's is necessary for an overall analysis of Indian attitudes towards western medicine and colonial conceptions of public health.

Acknowledgement: An earlier version of this paper was published in *Radical Journal of Health*, n.s., vol. II, April–Sep., 1996.

References

1. *Report of the Sanitary Commissioner*, Bombay: Government Central Press, 1888, p. 60.
2. V. R. Muraleedharan and D. Veeraghavan, 'Disease, Death and Local Administration: Madras City in the Early 1900s', *Radical Journal of Health* n.s., i, January, 1995, p. 23.
3. See Mridula Ramanna, *Western Medicine and Pubic Health in Colonial Bombay, 1845–1895*, Hyderabad: Orient Longman, 2002.
4. David Arnold, *Colonizing the Body: State Medicine and Epidemic Disease in Nineteenth Century India*, Berkeley: University of California Press, 1993, p. 271. A nagar shet, Premabhai Hutteesing was a generous benefactor, donating towards the establishment of Gujarat College, the Gujarat Society for promoting vernaculars, and the Grant Medical College, Bombay. A greater expression of his generosity was evident in his religious benefactions, endowing Jain temples, *dharamshalas* and

pinjrapoles. Representative Men of Bombay Presidency, Philadelphia: Historical Publishing Co., 1900, p. 197.

5. Bhagwanlal Badshah, *Rao Bahadur Ranchorelal Chhotala, C.I.E.*, Ahmedabad: Times of India Press, 1899, pp. 5-8.
6. *Representaive Men*, p. 204.
7. Badshah, *Ranchorelal*, p. 37.
8. GD, 97, 1876, pp. 107–8.
9. *Ibid.*, pp. 117-148, 125. The population of Ahmedabad comprised of 58,477 males and 58,396 females. *Ibid*, p. 129.
10. *Report on Native Newspapers of the Bombay Presidency*, (hereafter *RN*), Samsher Bahadur, 17 Oct., 1868.
11. *Ibid.*, 20 May, 1874.
12. General Department volumes, Maharashtra State Archives, Mumbai (hereafter GD), 104, 184, p. 89.
13. GD, 104, 1884, p. 90.
14. S. M. Edwardes, *A Memoir of Rao Bahadur Ranchodlal Chhotalal, C.I.E.*, Exeter: William Pollard and Co., 1920, p. 32.
15. GD, 148, 1885, p. 254.
16. *Annual Report of the Municipality of Ahmedabad* (hereafter *ARMA*), 1882–3, pp. 61-2, in GD, 3, 1884.
17. GD, 104, 1884, p. 90.
18. *ARMA*, 1883–4, p. 26, in GD, 26, 1884.
19. GD, 104, 1884, p. 90-1.
20. *Ibid.*
21. *ARMA*, 1883–4, p. 26, in GD, 26, 1884.
22. Edwardes, *Memoir*, p. 31.
23. GD, 104, 1884, p. 91.
24. Badshah, *Ranchorelal*, pp. 84-6.
25. GD, 26, 1884, p. 27.
26. Kenneth Gillian, *Ahmedabad. A Study in Indian Urban History*, Canberra: Australian National University, 1969, p. 133. Cecil Woodham Smith, *Florence Nightingale*, London: 1950, p. 565.
27. GD, 104, 1884, p. 83.
28. GD, 148, 1885, p. 256-7.
29. *RSC*, 1885, in GD, 101, 1886, p. 281.
30. Edwardes, *Memoir*, p. 30.
31. GD, 148, 1885, p. 185.
32. Edwardes, *Memoir*, p. 33.
33. Gillian, *Ahmedabad*, p. 137.
34. Badshah, *Ranchorelal*, pp. 44-45.
35. Edwardes, *Memoir*, pp. 35-7.
36. Badshah, *Ranchorelal*, pp. 47-63.
37. *ARMA*, 1887–8, p. 2, in GD, 13, 1889; Edwardes, *Memoir*, p. 35.

38. *Ibid.*, p. 36.
39. *ARMA*, 1887–8, p. 2, in GD, 13, 1889.
40. Edwardes, *Memoir*, pp. 36-7.
41. *ARMA*, 1886–7, p. 27, in GD, 8, 1888.
Ranchodlal showed the relative fall in deaths, in his covering letter forwarding the *ARMA*, 1887–8.
Average of deaths

Years	**Number of deaths**	**Rates per 1,000**
1877–8 to 1886–7	6,040	49.49
1882–3 to 1886–7	5,310	41.74
1887–8	4,719	37.09

42. GD, 103, 1889, pp. 130-1.
43. RN, *Ahmedabad Times*, 15 May, 1858.
44. RN, May 1888.
45. GD, 103, 1889, pp. 93-103.
46. RN, *Rast Goftar*, 3 June, 1888.
47. GD, 103, 1889, pp. 103 & 141.
48. *ARMA*, 1887–8, p. 3, in GD, 13, 1889.
49. GD, 45, 1893, p. 108.
50. Badshah, *Ranchorelal*, p. 89.
51. Edwardes, *Memoir*, p. 40.
52. *Transactions of the VII International Congress of Hygiene and Demography*, London: Eyre and Spotiswode, 1892, pp. 166-9 in GD 29, 1892.
53. Badshah, *Ranchorelal*, p. 50.
54. GD, 7, 1860, p. 237; GD, 8A, 1864, p. 113.
55. Confidential vol., 16, 1885, p. 390.
56. Edwardes, *Memoir*, p. 53.
57. *Report of Civil Hospitals and Dispensaries*, Bombay, App. 1., p. 39.
58. *Administration and Progress Report on the Mofussil Civil Hospitals and Dispensaries*, Bombay, 1893–1898, (gereafter *ARCHD*)
59. GD, 45, 1886, pp. 30-31.
60. GD, 40, 1887, p. 67.
61. GD, 47, 1888, pp. 95-99.
62. GD, 45, 1886, p. 47.
63. GD, 40, 1887, p. 208.
64. GD, 54, 1889, p. 206
65. GD, 54, 1889, pp.119-121.
66. GD, 40, 1887, pp. 56-57.
67. GD, 54, 1889, p. 207.
68. *ARCHD*, 1896, p. 32; *ARCHD*, 1898, pp. 128-129.
69. *Ibid.*, 1898, p. 70; Edwardes, *Memoir*, p. 54.

70. *ARCHD*, 1898, pp. 128-129.
71. Gillian, *Ahmedabad*, p. 142.
72. *Praja Bandhu, 1918*. Started in 1898, this Anglo-Gujarati paper took A keen interest in public health and even started a relief fund for influenza victims in 1918.
73. Thomas Blaney and Viswanath Narayen Mandlik, *The Drainage of Bombay, its History and Prospects*, Bombay: Union Press, 1883, p. 22.
74. *Writings and Speeches of Late Honourable Rao Saheb Visavanath Narayan Mandlik*, ed. N. V. Mandlik, Bombay: Native Opinion Press, 1896, p. 416.

19

Voluntary Associations and Public Health in Bengal 1900–1947

—*Kabita Ray*

Public health in Bengal was in a deplorable condition during British rule. The colonial government concerned itself mainly with the maintenance of law and order and collection of revenue and was indifferent and callous to the problems of public health. To compensate for this neglect, the voluntary associations of Bengal played a notable part and in some cases had a better record than that of the government.

Central Co-operative Anti-malaria Society

The most important popular effort in Bengal for fighting against malaria and other diseases was made by the Central Co-operative Anti-malaria Society,[1] a purely non-official organization, founded in 1919 by Dr. Gopal Chandra Chatterji.

The main function of the Society was to help in the organization of a network of autonomous, co-operative, anti-malaria public health societies throughout the villages of Bengal, for the prevention through such societies of malaria and other epidemic diseases. It acted as an advisory and guiding agency of the numerous rural societies. By 1943, the number of branch societies gradually increased to 3000 of which about 1200 were registered.[2]

The Central Society also carried out propaganda by holding or taking part in meetings, demonstrations, and conferences of the branch anti-malaria societies. The Society also issued bulletins, posters, and leaflets on public health subjects to the branch societies. Reprints of publications of scientific bodies of the United States received by the Central Society were translated into Bengali and distributed to the branch societies for their guidance. The Society also published a monthly billingual journal, *Sonar Bangla* containing information of the activities of the different branch societies and discussions on public health problems; these were also circulated among the branch societies. The anti-malaria week was first inaugurated by the Society in 1945.

For preventing cholera and other water-borne diseases, the Central Society carried out extensive propaganda and was able to popularize, against terrible opposition, the utility of deep tubewells as cheap and safe source of pure drinking water for rural areas of Bengal. Through the cooperation of the local medical volunteers and the local anti-malaria societies, the Central Society carried out anti-cholera preventive inoculation in Swarupnagar thana (24 parganas). The method was popularized in the province with definite beneficial results. The Governor-in-Council appreciated the admirable work of the cholera brigade of the Society. Anti-*kala-azar* work was also carried out in different districts by the Society. With the help of the local medical practitioners, the Society carried out systematic treatment of *kala-azar* patients by a course of intravenous injections of *sodium antimony tartrate* for which numerous free treatment centres were organized by the Society in different districts.

The branch societies prevented indiscriminate breeding of mosquitoes, by filling up many useless, shallow, insanitary ditches and *dobas* (ponds); many stagnant drains were regularly kerosinized. Acquatic vegetations causing obstructions to drainage of many natural channels were removed by the voluntary efforts of the local anti-malaria societies.

Most of the important branch societies established *kala-azar* centres, employed doctors, made arrangements for free treatment of the poor, and sold medicine at a cheap rate. They also formed volunteer corps and tried to eradicate malaria by cutting jungles, destruction of mosquitoes, and clearing drains. On the outbreak of cholera, small-pox, and other diseases in the villages or in the neighbouring areas, the societies with the help of the volunteers and doctors tried to put down the epidemics. The societies also tried to make provisions for pure water.[3] Some of the societies also carried out anti-malaria propaganda through posters. Posters with quotations, such as, 'clear the jungles, kill the mosquitoes', 'why should you die, kill the mosquitoes',[3A] etc. were stuck on the walls. Anti-malaria propaganda was also carried out through '*Swasthya Sankirtan*' (health songs).

Among the branch societies, special mention should be made of the Ghola Anti-malaria Co-operative Society in 24 Parganas. The village Ghola was divided into sections and a group of volunteers was formed for each section under a leader. The duty of the volunteers consisted in mopping out, every Sunday, every stagnant pool within their areas with crude kerosine oil; not a single puddle was left untreated. The result was marvellous. Many other societies (Harinavi, Bistoopur, Nobogram) took up this plan of work and were successful in carrying out their objectives.

The Ghola Society also carried out extensive anti-malaria propaganda work. Placards were posted in prominent places in the villages. When occasions arose, the members of the Society went to villages to sing popular songs composed by the volunteers as part of anti-malaria propaganda work.[4] The volunteers thus attempted to make the people aware of malaria and anti-malaria works. Taranath Chattopadhyay composed a Bengali song through which he called upon the people of Bengal and especially the youths of the country to wake up fight against malaria, which hampered their education and fight for *Swaraj*.[5]

The volunteers of the Society also staged a drama *Banglar Satru* in 1923 at the Calcutta University Institute and subsequently in other exhibitions.[6] The services of the Society was appreciated by many including the then Director of Public Health, Dr. C. A. Bentley, to whom the system of stamping out malaria and *kala-azar* appeared excellent.[7]

The Co-operative Anti-Malaria Societies, described by the *Indian Medical Gazette* as 'modern St. Georges'[8] were unique organizations not only in Bengal but in the whole of India. No such society existed in the world till 1921. Though ridiculed by many, the voluntary workers of the Society worked enthusiastically and waged an aggressive war against malaria.

In the report of 1936–1937, the London School of Hygiene and Tropical Medicine praised the work of the Society thus: 'The result of fostering interest in the prevention of malaria in villages by the societies has been the general uplift of the village community and it has led to the development of small holdings to such an extent that compared with a few years ago, the whole outlook to some villages has changed'.[8A] The great poet Rabindranath Tagore while presiding over the fourth annual meeting of the Society on 29th August, 1923 appreciated Gopal Chandra Chatterjee for his service to the people by setting up an anti-malaria society.[9]

The paper *Lancet* congratulated the efforts of the organizers of the system in their attempts to awaken the sanitary conscience of the village population of Bengal and to promote the idea of self-help in local sanitation.[10] The Society created an urge to act in groups for the benefit of the people.

However, the policy of the government not to dole out any anti-malaria grant to the rural societies in the districts brought about a definite setback to their activities. Although the demand for services of the organizers from the Central Society daily increased, want of funds compelled the Society to diminish the organizing staff.

British Empire Leprosy Relief Association (BELRA)

In Bengal leprosy constituted a major public health problem. The Bengal Branch of the British Empire Leprosy Relief Association[11] founded in 1926, carried out anti-leprosy work for controlling this dreadful malady.[11A] The Association conducted leprosy surveys for ascertaining the incidence of leprosy. Their activities also included treatment of leper cases, inspection of leprosy clinics of district boards and municipalities, training of medical officers, giving lecture-demonstrations to students of medical institutions, examination of school children, group discussions, and public meetings. The Association also carried out anti-leprosy propaganda work and distributed pamphlets such as 'Leprosy, How it is Measured', 'Leprosy, the Sign of the Disease', 'Leprosy, How to Conduct a Campaign', etc. These were also inserted in the journal of the Anti-Malaria Co-operative Society.

While conducting leprosy surveys, the workers met with opposition from many people which was overcome by PTS method (propaganda, treatment, survey) adopted in 1930. The work of the Association drew the attention of the local authorities to the problem of leprosy; by 1935, 200 leprosy clinics were established in the districts.

In 1936, the Association established the Leprosy Investigation Centre at Bankura, taken over by the Indian Council of the Association in 1938. The Centre was established in order to make a study of the epidemiology of leprosy in the rural areas. The main activities of the Centre included detection and recording of all new cases, and periodical re-examination of all persons with suspicious signs of leprosy. No real attempt was made at leprosy control since the main object of the centre was the epidemiological study of leprosy.

As an offshoot of the work of the Association private dispensaries were started in highly endemic areas, the most successful of these was the one established in the neighbourhood of Raniganj where in a week, there was an average attendance of 230 leprous patients.

Mission to Lepers

Another organization which devoted itself to the care and treatment of lepers was the Mission to Lepers founded in 1874 by Mr. Wellesley C. Bailey with its head-office at London. In Bengal, the asylums at Raniganj, Bankura, Kalimpong, and Chandrakona of the Mission, deserve mention.[12] 'For one and fifty years', noted *The Statesman* in 1925 'the Mission to

Lepers has been providing hospitality for thousands of men, women and children, who, but for the Mission's asylums would look in vain for sympathetic care'.[13]

Tuberculosis Association of Bengal

Tuberculosis was also a veritable scourge of Bengal. The work for the prevention of tuberculosis was first organized on a voluntary basis by the Tuberculosis Association of Bengal in 1929 at the initiative of Florence Backer of Washington.

The Association maintained dispensaries both in Calcutta and mofussil. The number of patients treated in these dispensaries increased from 2,079 in 1929 to 75,355 in 1947.[14] Anti-tuberculosis campaigns were also carried out from these dispensaries. A team of home visitors, trained and maintained by the Association visited the patients in their homes to educate them in the prevention of infection.[15] Instructions for prevention of tuberculosis were also sent to the poor villagers by post. A nourishment fund was started by the Association in 1932 and twelve tuberculosis patients were supplied extra food for three months.[16] The Association also organized training courses on tuberculosis for health officers and Diploma of Public Health Students.[17]

The publicity staff of the Association organized lectures in educational institutions, clubs, parks, *bustees* (slums), both in Calcutta and mofussil and participated in health exhibitions, and also made arrangements to broadcast a talk on tuberculosis every month from All India Radio (Calcutta Station).[18] Anti-tuberculosis day was observed by the Association on 8th February, 1936.[19] For educating the people in preventive methods of tuberculosis, the Association published a journal, the *Journal of the Tuberculosis Association of Bengal* and also published a Bengali edition of a book *Rogta Jakhan TB* by Amiya Jiban Mukherjee.

The Association was able to make appreciable headway with its noble mission, wrote the *Amrita Bazar Patrika* in 1936[19A] but the work of the Association was hampered by insufficiency of resources.

In 1939, the Tuberculosis Association of Bengal was renamed Bengal Tuberculosis Association, affiliated to the Tuberculosis Association of India.[19B] District branches of the Association in Bengal began to be established from 1940. In 1946, the Association started domiciliary treatment of those who were unable to attend clinics.[20]

Bengal Health Association

Inaugurated under the auspices of the All Bengal Young Men's Association in 1923, the Bengal Health Association was principally engaged in anti-*kala-azar* work and also carried out anti-cholera work.

The principle on which the Association's activities was based appeared to be a careful searching out of those who were suffering from *kala-azar* and to administer immediate treatment through its *kala-azar* centres. While speaking to a representative of *The Statesman*, a prominent member of the Association remarked that 'one of our policy is to win confidence of the common people by instructing them of the baneful effects of the disease and demonstrating that medical treatment is not unnecessary and terrible thing which many of them imagine to be'.[21]

The voluntary workers of the *kala-azar* centre of the Association at Dogachia (24 Parganas) carried out blood examination and aldehyde test and provided free treatment to hundreds of sufferers. There being no hospital or sanitorium, the accommodation of patients was confined to a mango tope.[22] The Minister for Public Health, S.N. Banerjee praised the work of the Association and noted thus: 'I visited the Dogachia centre of the Bengal Health Association and was greatly impressed with the splendid work which they were doing...'.[23] In his opening speech at the Second All Bengal *Kala-azar* Conference (1925) the Governor of Bengal spoke highly of the Bengal Health Association's work regarding *kala-azar*.[24]

The Association also carried out anti-cholera work. A 'Kodali brigade' of the Association formed by the students from Calcutta in 1924, visited Birbhum where cholera had broken out due to acute scarcity of water in consequence of short rainfall. The brigade visited the cholera affected areas, and by digging *kutcha* (mud-built) wells in beds of dried up tanks, succeeded in doing much to relieve the situation.[25]

Bengal Public Health Association

The Bengal Public Health Association,[26] a voluntary association with branches in all the districts throughout the province was composed mainly of public health workers, under government and local bodies and eminent sanitarians of the province. The Association tried to advance the cause of public health by cooperating with the public health organization of the province in the most intimate and useful way. It rendered useful services to the cause of public health by means of important suggestions. The resolution passed by the Association was found to be useful and at the instance of the Association, the government approved some of the suggestions such as restoration of the help of the *chowkidars* (village watchmen) in public health work, arrangements for coordination of activities of various departments for training of medical and health officers and health workers in anti-tuberculosis work and introduction of the scheme for establishment of maternity and child welfare centres.

The Association served also as a Public Health Information Bureau and one of the ambitious and very useful projects taken up by it was the establishment of the Public Health Library. The Association also published a journal of its own viz., the *Bengal Public Health Journal*. Besides original articles by experts, it contained extracts from important public health articles published in other countries, public health notes and news of the province, and important public health law cases. Apart from its value as a medium for health propaganda, it helped the public health workers to keep themselves abreast of the latest public health activities.

The Association further advanced the cause of public health by organizing public health conferences with sections dealing with different public health problems. In these conferences experts took part in deliberations and these helped focus the attention of the public and the administration towards the various intricacies of public health problems. The Association was perhaps the only body of its kind throughout India.

Birnagar Palli Mandali

Anti-malaria work at Birnagar (Nadia) started by a Society called Birnagar Palli Mandali in October 1923, roused the deepest interest in view of its notorious association with the history of malaria epidemic in Bengal.[27] The Society maintained an anti-mosquito department and a quinine department and paid house to house visits to find out cases of malaria and administer quinine. The Malaria Commission of the League of Nations praised the work of the Society.[28]

The Society's anti-malaria operation of 1926 reveals the method of work of the Society. During the rainy season, the work of kerosinization was carried out by two work-sarkars (staff of the anti-mosquito department) along with the coolies on the northern and the southern areas of Birnagar and they spent their spare time in clearing aquatic vegetation form *dobas* (ponds) and tanks, filling up tree holes with rubbish and cutting down jungles and draining off stagnant water. Individual health cards of the entire population were filled in periodically by the work-sarkars. In their daily round they also administered quinine and kept a record of the quantity of quinine issued on separate cards. The medical officer personally examined these cards and helped people with suggestions where necessary. The medical officer himself administered quinine to the school boys during school hours and kept a record of their spleen index. He also personally attended to all complicated cases brought to his notice by the work-sarkars.[28A]

Public health propaganda was carried out by house to house visit and by placards. The meetings of the Palli Mandali also served to disseminate knowledge of hygiene and malaria. The Chief Medical Adviser delivered lectures in special meetings, occasionally convened by the Society. The publicity officer of the Public Health Department delivered lantern lectures during the Ulai Chandi Mela days.[28B]

Saroj Nalini Dutt Memorial Association

The Saroj Nalini Dutt Memorial Association was founded in 1925 by Gurusaday Dutt, a Bengali civil servant, with the object of carrying out welfare work among women. With the object of familiarizing the village women with ideas on hygiene and sanitation, the *mahila samitis* (women's associations) under this association carried on a systematic campaign; the *samitis* also took prominent part in maternal and child welfare work, training of midwives, and in health exhibitions. The Association published a monthly magazine titled *Banga Lakshmi*.[29]

Bengal Social Service League

The Bengal Social Service League was founded in 1915. The First Health and Social Welfare Exhibition was opened in the Calcutta University Institute by the League in 1918, which also inaugurated a Travelling Exhibition and Lecture Movement in the districts and a permanent Health Exhibition in Calcutta.[30] The Society also provided medical relief during epidemics.[31]

The Minister for Local Self-Government recorded his appreciation of the valuable work done by Dr. D. N. Maitra, Secretary of the Bengal Social Service League.[32]

The Ramkrishna Mission

The Ramkrishna Mission[33] maintained free dispensaries and organized inoculation of pilgrims at important centres. The Mission was selected as one of the government agencies for free distribution of quinine.[34]

Indian Red Cross Society

A great part of the income of the Indian Red Cross Society[35] was spent upon its peacetime programme, specially on child welfare. In Calcutta, four baby clinics and milk kitchens run entirely by voluntary lady workers were maintained by the Bengal Provincial Branch of the Indian Red Cross Society.[36] As part of an all India movement, the Bengal Health Welfare Committee of the Provincial Branch inaugurated the Baby Week Movement (which grew into the Health Welfare Week) in 1924, and this became an annual function. Nearly all the districts arranged baby weeks with exhibitions and lectures.[37] A training school for health visitors was established in Calcutta under the auspices of the Red Cross Society, largely supported by the government.[38]

National Association for Supplying Female Medical Aid to the Women of India

Maternal and infantile mortality attracted the attention of voluntary workers which resulted in the establishment of the National Association for Supplying Female Medical Aid to the Women of India (more commonly known as the Dufferin Fund) in 1885.[39] Its object was to impart medical education and to provide medical relief to women. Branch associations were formed in most parts of the country. The main activity of the Bengal Branch of the Association was the foundation of the Dufferin Hospital at Calcutta.[40]

Youth Association and Palli Unnayan Samitis

Local youth associations also did valuable work. The Yubak Sangha of Adamdighi, Bogura came forward to help the villagers in times of outbreak of epidemics.[41] The Baruipur Yubak Samiti arranged anti-malaria film show at the Baruipur Show House in September 1945. About eight hundred people of the locality highly appreciated the film.[42]

Lastly, reference should be made to the 'Palli Unnayan Samitis' (village welfare societies) which established dispensaries, cleared tanks of water hyacinth and made provisions of pure water, and performed maternity and child welfare work.[43] They were also selected as government agencies for free distribution of quinine.[44]

Thus a great deal of the burden of public health was shared by the voluntary associations. However beneficial the effects of British rule, in many other respects, as regards any serious improvement in health of the inhabitants, the results of British administration was to a great extent a failure. This was admitted by G. B. Williams, the then Chief Engineer, Public Health Department, Bengal.[45] Amelioration of public health was a stupenduous task, but in Bengal, the health of the people was in the hands of a few unqualified sanitary inspectors, incapable of doing anything substantial for the improvement of public health. The district health officers also were too distant and detached from the people.

The administration was top-heavy; there was lack of coordination among the various interdependent branches of public health administration. There was poverty of ideas among the administrators themselves. The result was that only some fragmentary and wasteful public health measures were undertaken in the urban areas; the rural population was hopelessly neglected. With a hopelessly inadequate amount earmarked for public health, the Public Health Department of Bengal made some sporadic, meagre, and belated attempts to control epidemics. Further the government unwisely enforced complicated legislation upon the illiterate, helpless, and poor people.

It must be admitted that an official public health agency like a Health Department, whether at the national, or state or district or even at the village level, has certain limitations in carrying out public health work. This was specially the case with the Public Health Department of Bengal during British rule when people were suspicious of anything in the nature of publicity carried out by the government. The people often avoided the lectures and demonstrations and ascribed political motives behind public health propaganda work carried out by the government.

However, the voluntary agencies close to the people with their well thought out programme took important steps towards combating diseases and educating the people about the rules of sanitation. They succeeded in mobilizing voluntary labour for carrying out quite a number of activities and tried to complete for the neglect of the government. Scores of voluntary workers worked for the organization of measures against epidemic diseases and to ameliorate public health conditions. They succeeded in rousing the dormant energies of the population and organizing them for taking effective measures against diseases. The establishment of the anti-malaria and the welfare societies led to what appears as a reform movement in the villages of Bengal.

The Report on the Administration of Bengal (1923–1924) described the progress made in the treatment and prevention of various diseases by the voluntary organizations as 'very active and encouraging'. *The Report of the Royal Commission on Agriculture* (1928) noted that 'in course of our tour we have been much impressed by the great awakening of non-official interest in the health and welfare of the countryside'.

It must be remembered, as pointed out by Dr. B. C. Roy in the Second All Bengal *Kala-azar* Conference (1925), that voluntary agencies could not enforce regulations regarding prevention of epidemic diseases with the same measure of authority as the government. Further they had not the authority to collect huge sums of money needed for any public health scheme.[46] In spite of the difficulties, the work of the government was supplemented by the splendid efforts of the voluntary associations with very small funds at their disposal. It was the total dedication and commitment on the part of these organizations that produced the desired results.

References

1. Facts regarding the objects and functions of the Central Co-operative Anti-Malaria Society have been collected from the Annual Reports of the Society unless otherwise mentioned.
2. For development of Branch Anti-Malaria Societies year by year and district by district vide Appendices I and II.
3. Gopal Chandra Chattopadhyaya, 'Vange Malaria Nibaran', *Banglar Katha* (Cal.) 16 June 1928; *Palliswaraj*, 2nd year, no. 12, Bhadra 1342 BS, pp. 407–408; 3rd year no. 1, Aswin 1342 BS; no. 10, Asar 1342, BS, p. 239.

3A. These posters were written in Bengali.

4. 'Co-operative Campaign Against Malaria' (Read in a public meeting, held on the 29th August 1923, under the auspices of the Visva Bharati Sammilani and presided over by Rabindra Nath Tagore, vide *The Bengal, Bihar and Orissa Co-operative Journal* (Cal.), vol. 9, 1923–24, p, 129.
5. Quoted in *Swasthya* (Cal.), First year, Aswin no. 8, 1330, p. 252. The song was sung by the volunteers of the Ghola Society at an annual conference at Panihaty. It was highly praised by P. C. Roy who presided over the conference.
6. Letter from Haridhan Banerjee, dt. Ghola, 24 Parganas, Jan. 17, 1924, to the Secretary, Local Self Govt. Dept. Bengal, Proceedings of the Govt. of Bengal, Local Self Govt. Dept., Public Health Branch, File no. PH 1B–18. Progs. B 2–4, Oct. 1925.
7. *The Bengal, Bihar and Orissa Co-operative Journal*, (Cal.) 1923–24, vol. 9, p. 131.
8. *Indian Medical Gazette* (Cal.) Sept. 1925, p. 451.

8A. Quoted in the *Annual Report of the Central Co-operative Anti-Malaria Society* (Cal.) 1940, p. 112.

9. 'Gopalbabu has devoted himself to a great cause. Good sense devoid of any excitement from greed, anger or hatred has inspired him to perform this work. This example of greatness in no less valuable than killing of mosquitoes'. *Rabindra Rachanabali*, Viswabharati, vol. 27, p. 572.
10. *Lancet* (London) 25 April 1925, p. 891. Quoted in *Malaria in India* by Patrick Hehir, OUP, 1927, p. 376.
11. British Empire Leprosy Relief Association (BELRA) was founded in 1924 in London under the patronage of the Prince of Wales. The Association decided to make its campaign empire-wide. In 1925, the Indian Council of the Association was inaugurated by the then Viceroy of India, Marquis of Reading, for according to census figures India contained by far the largest number of lepers in the empire and perhaps in the world.

11A. Facts regarding the activities of the British Empire Leprosy Relief Association (BELRA) have been collected from the *Annual Reports of BELRA* (Indian Council) Cal. and *Bengal Public Health Reports*, Public Health Dept. Govt. of Bengal (cited hereafter as *BPHR*).

12. K. V. Mathew (ed.), *All India Medical Directory and WHO's WHO*, Travancore, 1951, p. 58; *Report on Leprosy and its Control in India* by the committee appointed by the Central Advisory Board of Health, Govt. of India, New Delhi, 1942; *Leprosy in India* (Cal.), vol. 27, no. 4, Oct. 1945.
13. *The Statesman* (Cal.), 10 Dec, 1925, quoted in *The Indian Medical Gazette* (Cal.), March, 1926, p. 14.
14. *BPHR*, relevant years.
15. *Annual Report of the Tuberculosis Association of Bengal*, Bengal Govt. Press, Cal.; K. V. Mathew, *op.cit.*, p. 35.
16. Letter by the Publicity Officer, Bengal Tuberculosis Association, to the *Bangabani* (Cal.), 13 Jan., 1931, p. 8.
17. *BPHR*, 1938, 1940.
18. *BPHR*, 1940; *Annual Report of the Tuberculosis Association of Bengal*, Bengal Govt. Press (Cal.), 1932.
19. A. C. Ukil, 'The Tuberculosis Problem, Our Responsibility', *Amrita Bazar Patrika* (Cal.), 8 Feb, 1936, p. 14.

19A. *Amrita Bazar Patrika* (Cal.), 8 Feb, 1936, p. 8.

19B. The Tuberculosis Association of India was formed incorporating the King George Thanksgiving Anti-Tuberculosis Fund (1930) and King Emperor's Anti-Tuberculosis Fund (1937). For details vide *An Indian Medical Review* by E.W.C. Bradfield, Govt. of India, 1938, p. 276-277.

20. *BPHR*, 1938, 1940, 1946.
21. 'Fighting Kala-azar in Bengal', *The Statesman* (Cal.), June 14, 1923.
22. Leader, 'Kala-azar in India, the Present Position', *The Indian Medical Gazette* (Cal.), July 1923, p. 318.
23. Letter dt. 9th June, 1925, from the Secretary, Bengal Health Association to the Secretary to the Govt. of Bengal, Public Health Dept., Proceedings of the Govt. of Bengal, Local Self-govt. Dept., Public Health Branch, File no. P H G-1, progs. A. 112–133, Dec. 1925.
24. *Amrita Bazar Patrika* (Cal.), Nov. 22, 1925, p. 6.
25. *Report on the Administration of Bengal*, 1923–1924, Bengal Secretariat Press, Cal., p. XXXVII.
26. Facts regarding the Bengal Public Health Association have been collected from *BPHR*, 1941, and *Health of India: Indian Public Health Association Souvenir, Inaugural session*, by S. C. Seal, Cal., 1956, p. 193.
27. Krishna Sekhar Bose, 'Malaria Control at Birnagar', *Calcutta Medical Journal*, vol. 21, no. 7, Jan. 1927, p. 350; C. F. Strickland, *Review of Rural Welfare Activities in India*, London, 1932, p. 47.
28. *Indian Medical Journal* (Cal.), vol. 25, March 1931, p. 112; C. F. Strickland, *op. cit.*

28A. Krishna Sekhar Bose, *op. cit.*, pp. 352-353.

28B. *Ibid*, p. 354.

29. *Annual Report of the Public Health Commissioner with the Govt. of India*, 1933, Delhi, p. 276; C. F. Strickland, *op. cit.*, p. 52.
30. D. N. Maitra's radio talk on 'Calcutta, Health Welfare Week, What is Health?' *Amrita Bazar Patrika* (Cal.), 1st Feb., 1933, p. 6.
31. Edward Blunt, *Social Service in India*, London 1938, p. 383.
32. Resolution No. 401 P. H., Govt. of Bengal, L. S. G. Dept., Public Health, Cal., 1st March 1924, on the Report of the Director of Public Health, 1922, Proceeding of the Govt. of Bengal, Local Self-Govt. Dept., Public Health Branch, File no. P H IR–40, Progs. A. 43–44, April 1924.
33. The activities of the Ramkrishna Mission, founded in 1897, included the organization of social services and emergency relief works.
34. Letter dt. Feb. 9, 1940, from Addl. Dy. Secy., Govt. of Bengal, Local Self-Govt. Dept., Public Health Branch, File no. P H 10–12 of 1939, progs, A. 60–61, April 1940; C. F. Strickland, *op. cit.*, p. 51.
35. The Indian Red Cross Society Act (Act XV of 1920) set up an independent Indian Red Cross Society. For further details vide *The Indian Year Book*, 1922, edited by Sir Stanley Reed, Cal., p. 484.
36. Reply by Minister S. N. Banerji to a question by Mahendra Mitra Bahadur at a meeting of the Legislative Council, Proceedings of the Govt. of Bengal, Local Self-Govt. Dept., Public Health Branch, File no. P H 20–37, Progs. A. 57–58, March 1923.
37. *BPHR*, 1923, 1924; *Amrita Bazar Patrika* (Cal.), 11th Dec. 1939, p. 5 and 25th April 1939, p. 15.
38. Presidential Address by Lt. Col. A. C. Chatterji, Director of Public Health Bengal, at the fifth session of the All Bengal Public Health Conference, 7th April 1939, Bengal Govt. Press, p. 12.
39. The National Association for Supplying Medical Aid by Women to the Women of India is known more commonly as the Dufferin Fund, after its first president Countess of Dufferin.
40. E. W. C. Bradfield, *op. cit.*, pp. 264-266.
41. '*Pallibarta*', *Bangabani* (Cal.), Feb. 2, 1931.
42. *Amrita Bazar Patrika* (Cal.), 1st Oct. 1945, p. 3.
43. *Bangabani* (Cal.), 10th March 1931, p. 8; *Palliswaraj*, 3rd year, no. 10, 1343 B S, p. 239.
44. Letter dt. Feb. 9, 1940, from Addl. Dy. Secy., Govt. of Bengal, to All Commissioners of Divisions, Proceedings of the Govt. of Bengal, Local Self-Govt. Dept., Public Health Branch, File no. P H IQ–12, Progs. A. 60–61, April 1940.
45. *Amrita Bazar Patrika* (Cal.), 27th June 1929, p. 10.
46. *Amrita Bazar Patrika* (Cal.), 25th Nov. 1925, p. 5.

Appendix-I

Department of Anti-Malaria Society in Bengal, 1919–1940

Year	*No. of Societies*	*Total No. of Societies Registered*
1919	4	2
1920	19	4
1921	21	8
1922	31	9
1923	85	19
1924	384	29
1925	500	43
1926	869	263
1927	1090	444
1928	1236	566
1929	1367	668
1930	1434	769
1931	1640	868
1932	1730	907
1933	1855	927
1934	2000	940
1935	2064	931
1936	2117	985
1937	2198	1024
1938	2281	1045
1939	2362	1091
1940	2389	1112

Source : Annual Report of the Central Co-operative Anti-Malaria Society, 1943.

Appendix-II

District	*Total No. of Societies*	*Total No. of Societies Registered*
Burdwan	208	131
Birbhum	75	32
Bankura	45	30
Midnapur	123	64
Hooghly	247	154
Howrah	47	41
Rajshahi	78	56
Malda	22	21
Dinajpur	14	7
Jalpaiguri	4	0
Rangpur	17	6
Bogra	16	6
Pabna	77	30
Darjeeling	2	2
24 Parganas	305	100
Khulna	283	166
Jessore	216	84
Nadia	189	54
Murshidabad	32	9
Dacca	32	9
Mymensingh	24	4
Faridpur	140	41
Bakarganj	50	5
Chittagong	31	8
Noakhli	68	45
Tipperah	33	7

Source : Annual Report of the Central Co-operative Anti-Malaria Society, 1943.

Index

C

D

L

M

N

Q

R

S

T

U

V

W

Y

Z